Becoming a Helper

Sixth Edition

Marianne Schneider Corey
Consultant

Gerald Corey
California State University, Fullerton
Diplomate in Counseling Psychology
American Board of Professional Psychology

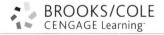

BROOKS/COLE
CENGAGE Learning™

Australia • Brazil • Japan • Korea • Mexico • Singapore • Spain • United Kingdom • United States

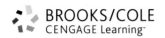
BROOKS/COLE
CENGAGE Learning

Becoming a Helper, Sixth Edition
Marianne Schneider Corey
Gerald Corey

Counseling Editor: Seth Dobrin
Developmental Editor: Julie Martinez
Assistant Editor: Arwen Petty
Editorial Assistant: Rachel McDonald
Media Editor: Dennis Fitzgerald
Marketing Manager: Trent Whatcott
Marketing Assistant: Darlene Macanan
Marketing Communications Manager: Tami Strang
Content Project Manager: Rita Jaramillo
Creative Director: Rob Hugel
Art Director: Caryl Gorska
Print Buyer: Paula Vang
Rights Acquisitions Account Manager, Text:
Roberta Broyer
Production Service: Ben Kolstad, Glyph International
Text and Cover Designer: Denise Davidson
Copy Editor: Kay Mikel
Cover Image: Heceta Head Lighthouse at Sunset,
© Craig Tuttle/CORBIS
Compositor: Glyph International

For product information and technology assistance, contact us at **Cengage Learning Customer & Sales Support,
1-800-354-9706.**

For permission to use material from this text or product, submit all requests online at **www.cengage.com/permissions.**
Further permissions questions can be e-mailed to **permissionrequest@cengage.com.**

Printed in the United States of America
1 2 3 4 5 6 7 13 12 11 10 09
Library of Congress Control Number: 2009928381
ISBN-13: 978-0-495-81226-5
ISBN-10: 0-495-81226-9

Brooks/Cole
20 Davis Drive
Belmont, CA 94002-3098
USA

Cengage Learning is a leading provider of customized learning solutions with office locations around the globe, including Singapore, the United Kingdom, Australia, Mexico, Brazil, and Japan. Locate your local office at: **www.cengage.com/global.**

Cengage Learning products are represented in Canada by Nelson Education, Ltd.

To learn more about Brooks/Cole,
visit **www.cengage.com/brookscole.**

Purchase any of our products at your local college store or at our preferred online store **www.ichapters.com.**

To you, our readers.

We hope that this book will help you

make a significant difference

in the lives of others.

About the Authors

MARIANNE SCHNEIDER COREY is a licensed marriage and family therapist in California and is a National Certified Counselor. She received her master's degree in marriage, family, and child counseling from Chapman College. She is a Fellow of the Association for Specialists in Group Work and was the recipient of this organization's Eminent Career Award in 2001. She also holds memberships in the American Counseling Association; the Association for Specialists in Group Work; the American Group Psychotherapy Association; the Association for Spiritual, Ethical, and Religious Values in Counseling; the Association for Counselor Education and Supervision; and the Western Association for Counselor Education and Supervision.

Marianne has been involved in leading groups for different populations, providing training and supervision workshops in group process, facilitating self-exploration groups for graduate students in counseling, and co-facilitating training groups for group counselors and weeklong residential workshops in personal growth. With her husband, Jerry, Marianne has conducted training workshops, continuing-education seminars, and personal-growth groups in the United States, Germany, Ireland, Belgium, Mexico, China, and Korea. She sees groups as the most effective format in which to work with clients and finds it the most rewarding for her personally.

In addition to *Becoming a Helper*, Sixth Edition (2011, with Gerald Corey), which has been translated into Korean and Japanese, Marianne has co-authored the following books, all with Brooks/Cole, Cengage Learning:

- *Issues and Ethics in the Helping Professions*, Eighth Edition (2011, with Gerald Corey and Patrick Callanan), which has been translated into Korean, Japanese, and Chinese
- *Groups: Process and Practice*, Eighth Edition (2010, with Gerald Corey and Cindy Corey), which has been translated into Korean, Chinese, and Polish
- *I Never Knew I Had a Choice*, Ninth Edition (2010, with Gerald Corey), which has been translated into Chinese

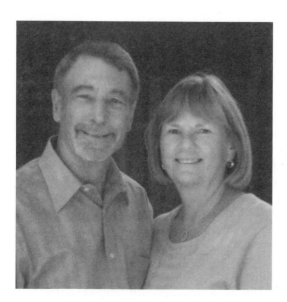

- *Group Techniques*, Third Edition (2004, with Gerald Corey, Patrick Callanan, and J. Michael Russell), which has been translated into Portuguese, Korean, Japanese, and Czech

Marianne has made two educational video programs (with accompanying student workbooks) for Brooks/Cole, Cengage Learning: *Groups in Action: Evolution and Challenges—DVD and Workbook* (2006, with Gerald Corey and Robert Haynes); and *Ethics in Action* CD-ROM (2003, with Gerald Corey and Robert Haynes).

Marianne and Jerry have been married since 1964. They have two adult daughters and three grandchildren. Marianne grew up in Germany and has kept in close contact with her family and friends there. In her free time, she enjoys traveling, reading, visiting with friends, bike riding, and hiking.

GERALD COREY is Professor Emeritus of Human Services at California State University at Fullerton. He received his doctorate in counseling from the University of Southern California. He is a Diplomate in Counseling Psychology, American Board of Professional Psychology; a licensed psychologist; a National Certified Counselor; a Fellow of the American Psychological Association (Counseling Psychology); a Fellow of the American Counseling Association; and a Fellow of the Association for Specialists in Group Work. Jerry received the Eminent Career Award from ASGW in 2001 and the Outstanding Professor of the Year Award from California State University at Fullerton in 1991. He regularly teaches both undergraduate and graduate courses in group counseling and ethics in counseling. He is the author or co-author of 15 textbooks in counseling currently in print, along with numerous journal articles. Many of his books have been translated and are popular throughout the world.

Along with his wife, Marianne Schneider Corey, Jerry often presents workshops in group counseling. In the past 30 years the Coreys have conducted group counseling training workshops for mental health professionals at many universities in the

United States as well as in Canada, Mexico, China, Hong Kong, Korea, Germany, Belgium, Scotland, England, and Ireland. In his leisure time, Jerry likes to travel, hike and bicycle in the mountains, and drive his 1931 Model A Ford.

Recent publications by Jerry Corey, all with Brooks/Cole, Cengage Learning, include the following:

- *Issues and Ethics in the Helping Professions*, Eighth Edition (2011, with Marianne Schneider Corey and Patrick Callanan), which has been translated into Korean, Japanese, and Chinese
- *Groups: Process and Practice*, Eighth Edition (2010, with Marianne Schneider Corey and Cindy Corey), which has been translated into Korean, Chinese, and Polish
- *I Never Knew I Had a Choice*, Ninth Edition (2010, with Marianne Schneider Corey), which has been translated into Chinese
- *Theory and Practice of Counseling and Psychotherapy*, Eighth Edition (and *Manual*) (2009), which has been translated into Arabic, Indonesian, Portuguese, Turkish, Korean, and Chinese
- *Case Approach to Counseling and Psychotherapy*, Seventh Edition (2009)
- *The Art of Integrative Counseling*, Second Edition (2009)
- *Theory and Practice of Group Counseling*, Seventh Edition, (and Manual) (2008), which has been translated into Korean, Chinese, Spanish, and Russian
- *Group Techniques*, Third Edition (2004, with Marianne Schneider Corey, Patrick Callanan, and J. Michael Russell), which has been translated into Portuguese, Korean, Japanese, and Czech

Jerry is co-author (with Barbara Herlihy) of *Boundary Issues in Counseling: Multiple Roles and Responsibilities*, Second Edition (2006) and *ACA Ethical Standards Casebook*, Sixth Edition (2006); he is also co-author (with Robert Haynes, Patrice Moulton, and Michelle Muratori) of *Clinical Supervision in the Helping Professions: A Practical Guide*, Second Edition (2010); and is the author of *Creating Your Professional Path* (2010), all four of which are published by the American Counseling Association. He is co-author, with his daughters Cindy Corey and Heidi Jo Corey, of an orientation-to-college book entitled *Living and Learning* (1997), published by Wadsworth, Cengage Learning.

Jerry has also made several educational video programs on various aspects of counseling practice: (1) *Theory in Practice: The Case of Stan—DVD and Online Program* (2009); (2) *Groups in Action: Evolution and Challenges—DVD and Workbook* (2006, with Marianne Schneider Corey and Robert Haynes); (3) *CD-ROM for Integrative Counseling* (2005, with Robert Haynes); and (4) *Ethics in Action CD-ROM* (2003, with Marianne Schneider Corey and Robert Haynes). All of these programs are available through Brooks/Cole, Cengage Learning.

Contents

CHAPTER 7

Understanding Diversity 184

CHAPTER 8

Ethical and Legal Issues Facing Helpers 217

CHAPTER 9

Managing Boundary Issues 254

CHAPTER 10
Getting the Most From Your Fieldwork and Supervision   *281*

CHAPTER 11
Stress, Burnout, and Self-Care   *304*

CHAPTER 12
Working With Groups   *331*

CHAPTER 13

Working in the Community   351

Preface

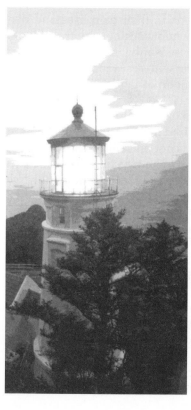

Many books deal with the skills, theories, and techniques of helping. Yet few books concentrate on the problems involved in becoming an effective helper or focus on the personal difficulties in working with others. In writing this book, we had in mind both students who are planning a career in human services, counseling, social work, psychology, couples and family therapy, sociology, or related professions and helpers who have just begun their careers. This book provides a general overview and introduction, and you will eventually take a separate course on each chapter topic we present here. It is our hope that we are able to introduce you to these topics in such a way that you will look forward to learning more about the issues we raise. We intend this book to be used as a supplement to textbooks dealing with helping skills and with counseling theory and practice. *Becoming a Helper* has proved useful for introductory classes in human services, introduction to helping, introduction to counseling, and social work as well as for classes such as pre-practicum, practicum, fieldwork, and internship.

In this book we focus considerable attention on the struggles, anxieties, and uncertainties of helpers. In addition, we explore in depth the demands and strains of the helping professions and their effects on the practitioner. Readers are challenged to become aware of and examine their motivations for seeking a career in the helping professions. We assist readers in assessing what they will get from their work.

Values are an integral part of the client–helper relationship, and we devote considerable attention to an analysis of how values influence the helping process. We develop the thesis that the job of helpers is not to impose values but to help clients define their own value system. We explore the belief systems of helpers and discuss the positive and negative effects that a variety of beliefs and assumptions can have on one's practice.

We discuss the importance of helpers knowing themselves and encourage readers to explore their family-of-origin experiences, focusing on how earlier relationships continue to influence the quality of later ones. We look at how helpers understand the developmental transitions in their own lives and discuss the implications of this self-understanding when working with transitional phases in the lives of clients. Beginning and seasoned helpers encounter common problems in their work related to dealing with resistance, transference and countertransference, and clients who are sometimes perceived as "difficult," and we address these critical topics in depth.

This book provides an overview of the stages of the helping process, with a brief discussion of the skills and knowledge required to be a successful helper at each of these stages. The focus of this discussion is not on skill development but on the personal characteristics that enable helpers to be effective. Because helpers ask clients to examine their behavior to understand themselves more fully, we ask helpers to be equally committed to an awareness of their own lives. Without a high level of self-awareness, a helper may obstruct clients' progress, especially when these clients are struggling with issues the helper has avoided facing. We also provide an overview chapter of various theories with the emphasis on key concepts and practical applications. There is a discussion of an integrative approach to counseling practice, which offers guidelines on how to select a theoretical orientation.

Special consideration is given to understanding and working with diverse client populations whenever this topic is relevant. In addition, Chapter 7 addresses a range of diversity issues. Forming a sense of ethical awareness and learning to resolve professional dilemmas is a task facing all helpers. We raise a number of challenges surrounding current ethical issues as a way to sensitize readers to the intricacies of ethical decision making and managing boundaries.

We challenge students to take a proactive stance in their educational program. Being proactive applies to selecting field placements and internships as well as to getting the most from supervision. Therefore, we offer some practical strategies for ensuring quality experiences in fieldwork and profiting from supervision.

Other topics covered in the book are stress, burnout, and the importance of self-care. Throughout the book we have kept the focus on how helpers may be affected by the problems they face and the choices they make in service to their clients. We discuss the group process and the value of working with groups in human services work, and we also deal with understanding one's role as a helper in the community.

Although this book should be useful to any student planning to enter the helping professions, our backgrounds are in the field of counseling, and this orientation comes through in this book. Therefore, those who want to work in the counseling aspects of the human services are likely to find this book especially meaningful. We have tried to write a personal book that will stimulate both thought and action. At the end of each chapter we encourage readers to commit to some specific action that will move them closer to their goals. In addition, exercises from the *Ethics in Action* CD-ROM (Corey, Corey, & Haynes, 2003) have been incorporated in the chapter activities for Chapters 2, 7, 8, and 9.

New to This Edition

Chapter 1 has new information on rehabilitation and substance abuse counseling organizations. Specific areas of value conflicts are highlighted in Chapter 2 along with an expanded discussion of how to work ethically in the therapeutic process. Chapter 3 has been condensed and focuses on self-awareness and the value of self-exploration for the helper. The discussion of transference and countertransference has been expanded, and Chapter 4 also has a new section on recognizing competence and learning when to refer. New resources for gaining skills and specific competencies have been added in Chapter 5.

Chapter 6 contains a new section on narrative therapy, and Chapter 7 has been extensively updated, including a new section on social justice competencies. Chapter 8 (ethical and legal issues) and Chapter 9 (managing boundaries) benefit from new research on these controversial topics discussed in a contemporary framework. Chapter 10 has been largely rewritten to focus on student helpers getting the most from fieldwork and supervision, and Chapter 11 has new material on staying alive as a person and a professional. Chapter 12, which describes group counseling, encourages helpers to consider participating in a group themselves. An increased focus on the roles of advocacy and social activism in community work in Chapter 13 expands the role of helper to a wider client base. New emphasis is also given to crisis intervention work in this final chapter. Whenever possible, new references have been added to bring discussions up to date and to provide a springboard for further investigation of topics of interest.

Supplements

Instructor's Resource Manual

An *Instructor's Resource Manual* is available for this edition. It contains suggestions for teaching the course, course objectives, key terms, class activities to stimulate interest, PowerPoint slides, and a bank of test items, discussion questions, and online test items. The instructor can choose from the many multiple-choice, true-false, matching, and short essay questions provided.

Codes of Ethics for the Helping Professions

Each of the major mental health professional organizations has its own code of ethics. Many of these codes are contained in a booklet titled *Codes of Ethics for the Helping Professions* (4th., 2011), which is available at a nominal cost when bundled with this textbook. We recommend that students become familiar with the basic standards for ethical practice of the various mental health professions. Codes of ethics for specific organizations also can be accessed through the Internet or by contacting the professional organizations directly.

Ethics in Action *CD-ROM*

An integrated learning package designed to enhance the sixth edition of *Becoming a Helper*, entitled *Ethics in Action* CD-ROM (Corey, Corey, & Haynes, 2003), brings to life, through video role-play segments, the ethical issues and dilemmas that helpers often encounter. The program provides ample opportunity for discussion, self-exploration, and problem solving through self-inventories and exercises designed for interactive learning geared directly to the vignettes shown.

The *Ethics in Action* CD-ROM is divided into three parts: Ethical Decision Making, Values and the Helping Relationship, and Boundary Issues and Multiple Relationships. This interactive self-study program challenges students to deal with the complexity of ethical issues and encourages reflection on their perspectives on each of the issues presented. By viewing the video program and completing the exercises, students will be in a better position to get involved in class discussions. The more students become involved in this learning package, the more their understanding of ethical practice will be enhanced.

Ethics in Action CD-ROM is available from Brooks/Cole, Cengage Learning, and can be purchased at a discount when packaged with *Becoming a Helper*.

Acknowledgments

In preparation for this revision, a Web survey was conducted with responses from 45 instructors. The comments of these instructors were helpful in guiding our revision process, especially by focusing our attention on the diversity of courses for which this book is selected, including counseling, human services, psychology, and social work.

We also want to express our appreciation for those individuals who reviewed the revised manuscript of this Sixth Edition of *Becoming a Helper*. Although we could not incorporate all of their suggestions, we relied on their input in developing the final version of this edition. We appreciate the insights, comments, and perspectives of the following people:

- Randy Alle-Corliss, California State University at Fullerton
- Leslie Joan Allen, Mt. Hood Community College
- Emily B. Anderson, Borough of Manhattan Community College CUNY
- Malachy Bishop, University of Kentucky
- Richard L. Brewer, Southwest Baptist University
- Patrick Callanan, California State University at Fullerton
- Robert Haynes, Borderline Productions
- Kathy Keefe-Cooperman, Long Island University
- Patrice Moulton, Northwestern State University
- Mark A. Stebnicki, East Carolina University
- Vanessa van Orden, Hudson Community College
- Gary Villereal, Western Kentucky University
- Daniel Weigel, Southeastern Oklahoma State University

We acknowledge the valuable contribution of the following people for reviewing and providing feedback on Chapter 13 (Working in the Community): Hugh C. Crethar, Oklahoma State University; Allison Donahoe Beggs, Riverside County Children's Services; and Kristie Kanel, California State University at Fullerton. We thank James Bitter, East Tennessee State University, for his review and editing of Chapter 3 (Helper, Know Thyself).

We appreciate the members of the Brooks/Cole, Cengage Learning team who continue to offer support for our projects: Seth Dobrin, acquisitions editor for counseling, social work, and human services; Julie Martinez, developmental editor, who monitored the review process; Caryl Gorska, for her work on the interior design and cover of this book; Arwen Petty, assistant editor, for work on the supplements; Trent Whatcott, senior marketing manager; and Rita Jaramillo, project manager. We thank Ben Kolstad of Glyph International, who coordinated the production of this book; and Kay Mikel, the manuscript editor of this edition, whose exceptional editorial talents continue to keep this book reader friendly. We appreciate the careful work of Susan Cunningham in preparing the index. The efforts of these dedicated professionals have contributed greatly to the quality of this sixth edition.

Marianne Schneider Corey
Gerald Corey

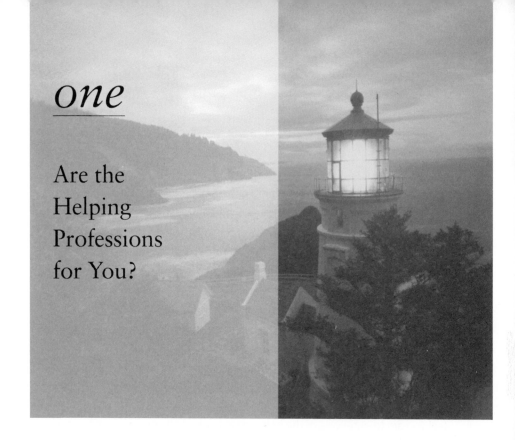

one

Are the Helping Professions for You?

Focus Questions

1. What has attracted you to the helping professions? Who in your life has influenced your decision to consider this role for yourself?

2. What is your main motivation for wanting to be a helper? What personal needs of yours are likely to be met through your work as a helper?

3. Think of a time when you needed help from a significant person in your life or from a counselor. What did you most want from this person? What did he or she do that either helped or hindered you?

4. Think about the attributes of an effective helper. What traits or characteristics would you identify as being the most important?

5. What can you do to make your educational program more meaningful? How can you derive the maximum benefit from your academic courses?

6. At this time in your life, how prepared (from a personal standpoint) do you feel you are to enter one of the helping professions? If you were applying to a graduate program or for a job in the field, you might be asked these questions: "What qualities, traits, attitudes, values, and convictions are central to being an effective helper?" "How might these personal characteristics be either assets or liabilities for you as a helper?"

7. If you were to pursue a career in one of the helping professions, what would your ideal vision be? What kind of work appeals to you? With what clients would you most like to work? What kind of human service work would bring you the greatest meaning and satisfaction?

Aim of the Chapter

As you consider a career in one of the helping professions, you are probably asking yourself these questions:

- Are the helping professions for me?
- Do I know enough to help others?
- Will I be able to secure a job?
- Will my career provide me with financial security?
- Will I be able to apply what I am learning to my job?
- Will this career be satisfying for me?
- For which specific profession am I best suited?
- How do I select the best school?

This book is intended to help you with these and other questions about your career. The focus of the book is on *you* and on what you need personally and professionally to be the best helper possible. We also emphasize the realities you are certain to face when you enter the professional world. You will be best able to cope with the demands of the helping professions if you get an idea now of what lies ahead. In addition to presenting the obstacles that you may encounter, we also want to point out the joys and rewards of making a commitment to helping others as a way of life. Perhaps one of the most meaningful rewards for helping professionals is the opportunity to assist people in creating their own paths.

We begin this chapter by inviting you to examine your reasons for wanting to become a helper. To help you clarify your personal and professional motivations, we share our own experiences as beginning helpers and demonstrate that learning to become a helper is a process that has both joys and challenges. This chapter also introduces you to the attributes of an effective helper. There is no one pattern of characteristics that identifies "ideal helpers," but we encourage you to think about the characteristics you possess that could either help or hinder you in your work with others.

Most students have questions about which professional program will best help them attain their career objectives, and we explore the differences among various educational routes. Although you may think you know the career path you want to pursue, we encourage you to keep your options open while you are reading this book and taking this course. You will probably work in several different positions within a career that you eventually choose, and many human service professionals change careers at different points in their lives. For example, you may begin by providing direct services to clients in a community agency but later on shift to administering programs.

Finally, keep in mind as you read this book that we use the terms **helper** and **human services professional** interchangeably to refer to a wide range of practitioners, some of which include social workers, counselors, clinical and counseling psychologists, couples and family therapists, pastoral counselors, mental health nurses, rehabilitation counselors, and community mental health workers.

Examining Your Motives for Becoming a Helper

In choosing a career in the helping professions, it is imperative that you reflect on the reasons you are considering entering this field. For many of us, becoming a helper satisfies some of our personal needs, such as the need to make a difference in the lives of others. It is gratifying to know that we can make a significant difference, especially when people do not have a great deal of hope that they can change or faith in themselves to create a better life. You can be a change agent for such people and facilitate their belief in themselves. As you reflect on the needs and motives we discuss in this section, ask yourself this question, "How do my personal needs influence my ability to be an effective helper?"

Typical Needs and Motivations of Helpers

Our students and trainees have had a variety of motivations for pursuing careers in the helping professions. We want you to recognize your motivations and needs, and to become aware of how they influence the quality of your interactions with others. Let's examine some of the reasons you may have for becoming a helper.

The need to make an impact. Perhaps you hope to exert a significant influence on the lives of those you serve. You may have a need to know that you are making a positive difference in someone's daily existence. Although you recognize that you will not be able to change everyone, you are likely to derive satisfaction from empowering individuals. When clients are not interested in changing or do not want your help, however, you may become frustrated. If your worth as a person is too dependent on your need to make a difference, you are likely to become disillusioned and disappointed. Your professional work is one source for finding meaning in your life, but we hope it is not your only source of satisfaction.

The need to reciprocate. The desire to emulate a role model sometimes plays a part in the decision to be a helper. Someone special, perhaps a teacher or a therapist, may have influenced your life in a very special way, or the influential person may be a grandmother, an uncle, or a parent. Practicing therapists often acknowledge that they were greatly influenced by their experience in their own personal therapy to seek the education needed to become competent professionals.

The need to care for others. You may have been a helper from an early age. Were you the one in your family who attended to the problems and concerns of other family members? Do your peers and friends find it easy to talk to you? If you are a "natural helper," you may have sought training to improve and enhance your talent. One professional we contacted reported that half of the 33 people in the training program at his institute identified themselves as "rescuers" in alcoholic families. In his view, they were recruited at birth and trained daily to stabilize the family. Many of our own students are adult children of alcoholics who adopted the role of peacemaker in their families.

Although this pattern is not necessarily problematic, it is important that such helpers become aware of their dynamics and learn how they function in both their personal and professional lives.

One of the pitfalls of being a caregiver to significant people in your life is that very often no one attends to your needs. As a result, you may not have learned to ask for what *you* need. You can easily become personally and professionally burned out, or emotionally exhausted, if you do not learn to ask for help for yourself. Skovholt (2001) writes about the importance of sustaining the personal self: "Individuals in the caring professions are experts at one-way caring. Others are attracted to them because of their expertise and caring attitude" (p. 147). He cautions helping professionals to become aware of the dangers of one-way caring in their professional lives. If you hope to function effectively in a professional role, it is essential that you learn and practice the art of self-care. If you burden yourself with the responsibility of always being available for everyone who might need your help, you are likely to find that soon you will have little left to offer. It is crucial to have a healthy balance between taking care of others and taking care of yourself.

The need for self-help. An interest in helping others may stem from an interest in dealing with the impact of your own struggles. The wounded healer can be authentically present for others searching to find themselves. If you have struggled successfully with a problem, you are able to identify and empathize with clients who come to you with similar concerns. For example, you may have experienced the difficulties of growing up in an abusive family, and you are sensitive to this early wounding. In your professional work you are likely to encounter a number of individuals with similar struggles. Some women who were involved in abusive relationships may become counselors who specialize in working with battered women. Some men who were abused as children develop particular professional interests in counseling abused children and youth.

Stebnicki (2009a) believes that professionals who have experienced a wounded spirit need to be open to questioning their own spiritual health so they can be of assistance to their clients as they struggle with existential concerns of loss, grief, trauma, and stressful life events. He reminds us that "remembering emotions related to such painful events and re-creating an internal emotional scrapbook can be extremely painful and difficult for both clients and counselors, especially for counselors new to the helping profession" (p. 54).

Sometimes individuals who are psychologically impaired study to become helpers. If you are not on the road to your own healing, it is unlikely that you will be effective in helping others. Furthermore, engaging in intense work with others can stimulate and intensify your own pain. Before you attempt to deal with the lives of others, examine your own life situation. For example, a female counselor who works with women who are victims of partner abuse may try to work out her own unfinished business and conflicts by giving advice and pushing these women to make decisions they are not yet ready to make. Because of her unresolved personal problems, she may show hostility to a controlling husband. She might make the assumption that what "worked" for her will work for everyone.

The need to be needed. Very few helpers are immune to the need to be needed. It can be psychologically rewarding to have clients say that they are getting better because of your influence. These clients are likely to express their appreciation for the hope that you have given them. You may value and get a great deal of satisfaction from being able to take care of other people's wants. Satisfying this need is perhaps one of the greatest rewards of being a helper. It is not necessary to deny that you like being wanted, approved of, and appreciated. However, if this dynamic is consistently in the forefront, it can overshadow the needs of your clients. Helpers can foster client dependence due to the helpers' need to be needed.

If you depend exclusively on your clients to validate your self-worth, you are on shaky ground. In reality, many clients will not express appreciation for your efforts, nor will some of them make changes in their lives. Furthermore, agencies often provide feedback only when your performance does not meet the expected standards. No matter what you accomplish, the institution may expect more of you. Eventually, you may realize that whatever you do it is not enough. Wanting to feel appreciated for what you are doing for others is certainly understandable, but you are likely to be disappointed if you tell yourself that you *must* receive appreciation and recognition to feel worthwhile.

The need for prestige, status, and power. You may have hopes of acquiring a certain level of prestige, if not a certain income level. If you work in an agency, however, many of the consumers of the services you offer will be economically disadvantaged. You may be working with people on probation, those with various addictions, and people who are mandated to see you. This work may not bring you the financial rewards, prestige, and status you seek. However, the field offers many opportunities for those who continually work to enhance their education and training.

Conversely, you may work in a setting where you can enjoy the status that goes along with being respected by clients and colleagues. If you have worked hard and are good at what you do, accept the recognition you have earned. You can be proud yet still be humble. If you become arrogant as a result of your status, you may be perceived as unapproachable, and clients may be put off by your attitude. You also may come to accept far more credit for your clients' changes than you deserve. Some clients will put you on a pedestal, and you may come to like this position too much. If you want your self-esteem to rest on a solid foundation, it is essential that you look within yourself to meet your status needs rather than looking to others to provide you with affirmations that you are indeed a worthwhile person, whether by verbal acclaim or by financial gain.

The need to provide answers. Some students seem to have a need to give others advice and to provide "right answers." They may say that they feel inadequate if friends come to them with a problem and they are not able to give them concrete advice. Yet their friends may really need to be listened to and cared for rather than to be told "what they should do." Although you may find satisfaction in influencing others, it is important to realize that your answers may not be best for them. Many times there is not a "correct" answer at all. Your purpose is to provide direction and to assist clients in discovering their own course of action. If your need for providing advice and answers sometimes gets in the way of effectively relating to others, we suggest that you explore this in personal counseling.

The need for control. Related to the need to provide others with advice and answers is the need to control others. All of us have some need for self-control and may also have the need to control others at times. Some have a great need to control what others are thinking, feeling, and doing. You might ask yourself these questions: Are you convinced that some people should think more liberally (or more conservatively)? When people are angry, depressed, or anxious, do you sometimes tell them that they should not feel that way and do your best to change their state of mind? Do you at times have a strong need to change the way people who are close to you behave, even if what they are doing does not directly affect you? Although some helpers have a need to control under the guise of being helpful, it can be a productive exercise to reflect on what the outcomes might be if you gave more control to those you encountered. Is your role to control the lives of others, or is it to teach others how to regain effective control of their own lives?

How Your Needs and Motivations Operate

We often say that in the ideal situation your own needs are met at the same time that you are meeting your clients' needs. Most of the needs and motives we have discussed can work either for or against a client's welfare. If you are unaware of your needs, however, there is a much greater likelihood that your own needs will determine the nature of your interventions. If you are attempting to work through conscious or unconscious personal conflicts by focusing on the problems of others, for example, there is a greater chance that you will unconsciously use your clients to meet your own needs. In addition, you may be in trouble if some of these needs assume such a high priority that you become obsessed with them. For instance, if your need for control is so high that you consistently attempt to determine the path that others take, you could easily interfere with your clients' development of independence and self-determination.

In one counseling program we are familiar with, instructors expect their students to examine their own vulnerabilities, struggles, and faulty beliefs as part of the process of becoming effective helpers. This program is based on the premise that it is as much the "wounded" parts of us as the "healthy" parts that drive us to become helpers. Students are asked to examine the ways in which their personal issues and psychological histories will be an asset or a liability in their future professional work.

Helpers who meet their own needs at the expense of their clients are depriving their clients of the quality of care to which they are entitled. If you feel a strong need to provide solutions to every problem a client presents, for example, you are meeting your own needs rather than working in the best interest of your client. One guiding principle we find useful is to remain invested in the client's *process* rather than the *outcome*. If a client is considering divorce, for example, and if our values are strongly against divorce, we can help the client explore the pros and cons of either choice. We should remain neutral with respect to the client's final decision. As helpers, it is important to remember that it is our clients—not us—who have to live with the consequences of the decisions made.

As you reflect on the needs we have discussed, think about how they might either enhance or interfere with your ability to help others. If you have not yet worked with clients, recall your actions in situations with friends or family members who were struggling with some problem. How did you respond to them when they were looking for the best course of action? Do your best to identify how any of these needs can become problematic if you deny them, become obsessed with them, or meet them at the expense of others.

It is unlikely that any single motive drives you; rather, needs and motivations are intertwined and can change over time. Even though your original motives and needs change, your desire to be a helper may remain unchanged. Because personal development is an ongoing process, we suggest that you periodically reexamine your motives for being a helper. It can be a valuable tool toward self-awareness and client welfare.

Our Own Beginnings as Helpers

This is a personal book in two ways. It is personal in that we encourage you to find ways to apply the book to yourself. In addition, we have written the book in a personal manner, sharing our own views and experiences whenever we think it is appropriate and useful. As a concrete illustration of how personal motives and experiences can affect career choice, we discuss some of our own motivations for becoming helping professionals and remaining in the field.

Beginning a helping career is not always easy and can involve anxiety and uncertainty. Although at this point we feel more confident than when we were beginning our careers, we have not forgotten our own struggles. We, too, had to cope with many of the fears and self-doubts that are addressed in this book. By sharing our own difficulties with you, we hope to encourage you not to give up too soon.

At this point in our professional lives, we continue to take time to reflect on both what we are giving and what we are getting through our varied work projects.

Marianne Corey's Early Experience

I was a helper long before I studied counseling in school. From childhood on I responded to the needs of my brothers and sisters. At age 8, I was made almost totally responsible for my newborn brother. I not only took care of him but also attended to other members of an extended family.

My family owned a restaurant in a German village. The restaurant, which was in our home, was the meeting place for many of the local men. These men came mostly to socialize rather than to eat and drink. For hours they would sit and talk, and I was taught that I had better listen attentively. Furthermore, I learned that I should not repeat the personal conversations and gossip to other townspeople. At this early age I learned three very important skills: attentive listening, empathic understanding, and confidentiality. It became apparent to me that a variety of people found it easy to talk to me and tell me about their personal problems.

In my growing-up years I felt liked and respected by most people. Even as a small child, I remember feeling compassion, especially for those who had a difficult or unusual life situation. For example, I recall seeing a woman who had a psychotic episode standing naked by an upstairs window. She threw her clothes and furniture out of the window as onlookers baited her. I felt sad and thought that she must be very unhappy. I also had special feelings for two persons in my village who were considered alcoholics. I was curious about why they drank so much.

I have always been interested in looking beyond the facade that people present to others. I became convinced that people could be more than they appeared if they were willing to make an effort to change. My belief was not typical. In my immediate cultural environment the normative message was that "this is fate, and there is nothing you can do about it."

In my own life I overcame many obstacles and exceeded my dreams. As a result, I am often successful in challenging and encouraging my clients not to give up too soon when limits are imposed on them. Through my work I derive a great sense of satisfaction when I have been instrumental in the lives of individuals who are willing to take risks, to tolerate uncertainty, to dare to be different, and to live a fuller life because of their choices. When clients show appreciation for what I have done for them, I enjoy hearing it. However, I always let them know that their progress stems only partially from my efforts; the rest comes from their hard work.

In my life now I find it easy to give to my friends, family, and community as well as to clients. It seems natural to me to give both personally and professionally. It continues to be a struggle for me to find a good balance between giving to others and taking care of myself. Although I am considered a good giver, I realize that I am not as good when it comes to making my needs known and asking for what I want.

It is interesting for me to compare my cultural conditioning and early role in my family with my development as a professional caregiver. Although I seemed to assume the role of caring for my brothers and sisters "naturally," I did not feel quite as natural when I began formal helping. In my first practical experiences as part of my undergraduate program in behavioral sciences, I had my share of self-doubt.

In one of my earlier internships I was placed in a college counseling center. I remember how petrified I was one day when a student came in and asked for an appointment and my supervisor asked me to counsel this client. The feedback that I received later from my supervisor on how confident I had appeared was very incongruent with what I had felt. Here are some of the thoughts that ran through my head as I was walking to my office with this client: "I'm not ready for this. What am I going to do? What if he doesn't talk? What if I don't know how to help him? I wish I could get out of this!" In my self-absorption I never once considered any of my client's feelings. For instance, how might he be approaching this session? What fears might he be having?

I was much more aware of myself than of my clients. I took far too much responsibility, put much pressure on myself to "do it right," and worried a lot about what harm I might do. I did not allow my clients to assume their rightful share of the responsibility for making changes. I often worked much harder than they did, and sometimes it seemed that I wanted more for my clients than they wanted for themselves. I think I had a tendency to exaggerate my capacity for causing harm because of my fears and insecurities as a helper. When I shared with my supervisor my concern about feeling overwhelmingly responsible for the outcomes of our sessions and about hurting my clients, she responded, "You are assuming more power than you have over your clients."

Another time I told my supervisor that I had doubts about being in my profession, that I was overwhelmed by all the pain I saw around me, and that I was concerned that I was not helping anybody. I remember being very emotional and feeling extremely discouraged. My supervisor's smile surprised me. "I would be very concerned about you as a helper," he said, "if you never asked yourself these kinds of questions and were not willing to confront yourself with these feelings." In retrospect, I think he was telling me that he was encouraged for me because I was acknowledging my struggles and was not pretending to be the all-competent counselor who was without fears.

As a beginning counselor I was acutely aware of my own anxieties. Now I am much better able to be present with my clients and to enter their world. Although I am not anxiety-free, I am not watching myself practicing therapy. Furthermore, although I take responsibility for the counseling process, I do not see myself as totally responsible for what goes on in a session, and I am usually not working harder than my clients.

At one time I wanted to abandon the idea of becoming a counselor and instead considered teaching German. I was very aware of comparing myself with professionals who had years of experience, and I thought I should be as effective as they were. I eventually realized that my expectations were extremely unrealistic: I was demanding that I immediately be as skilled as these very experienced people. I had been giving myself no room for learning and for tolerating my rudimentary beginnings.

One of my professional activities now is working with beginning helpers. I find that they are often in the same predicament I was in when I began working with others. These students seem focused on how much I know and how easy interventions seem to come to me. By contrast, they feel discouraged with their lack of knowledge and with how much they have to struggle to find "the right thing to say." They usually sigh with relief when I tell them about some of my beginnings and admit that I do not see myself as an expert but as someone who has a certain amount of expertise in counseling. I want most to convey to them that learning never stops, that beginnings are difficult and, at times, discouraging.

Jerry Corey's Early Experience

When I was in college studying to become a teacher, I hoped to create a different learning climate for students than I was experiencing as a learner. I wanted to help others, and it was important for me to make a difference. I recognize now that the need to make a significant difference has been a theme for the more than 45 years I have been in the helping professions. As a child and as an adolescent, I did not feel that my presence made that much difference. In many ways, during my early years, I felt that I did not fit anywhere and that I was invisible. I was surrounded by a large, extended immigrant Italian family who often spoke in their native language, which I did not understand. There was a good deal of pain attached to feeling ignored, and one of my early decisions was not to let myself be ignored. This took the form of me becoming a nuisance, which of course resulted in negative attention. But I thought this type of recognition was better than being ignored! In college I experienced some success and found some positive routes to being recognized. Later, when I began my teaching career, I began to see that I could make a difference, at least within the confines of my classroom. In addition to helping students enjoy learning, I also got personal satisfaction from knowing that I was a useful person, which was quite different from my perception of myself during my youth. In fact, I think that I depended (and still do) to a large extent on my professional accomplishments for my sense of identity.

At the beginning of my career as a counseling psychologist, I did not feel confident, and I often wondered whether I was suited for the field. I recall the times that I co-led a group with my supervisor as being particularly difficult. I felt incompetent and inexperienced next to my co-leader, who was an experienced helper. Much of the time I didn't know what to say or do. It seemed that there was little place for me to intervene because my co-leader was so effective. I had many doubts about my ability to say anything meaningful to the members. It just seemed that my supervisor was so insightful and so skillful that I would never attain such a level of professionalism. The effect of working with an experienced group leader was to heighten my own sense of insecurity and inadequacy. In retrospect, however, I realize that this was an invaluable learning experience.

Another thing that I found difficult was practicing individual counseling in a university center. When I began as a practicing counselor, I frequently asked myself what I could do for my clients. I remember progress being very slow, and it seemed that I needed an inordinate amount of immediate and positive feedback. If a client was still talking about feeling anxious or depressed after several weeks of sessions, I immediately felt my own incompetence as a helper. I frequently found myself thinking: "How would my supervisor say this? What would he do?" I even caught myself copying his gestures, phrases, and mannerisms. Many times I felt that I did not have what it took to be an effective counselor, and I wondered if I had pursued the wrong path.

I often had no idea of what, if anything, my clients were getting from our sessions. Indications of whether clients were getting better, staying the same, or getting worse were typically very subtle. What I did not know at the time was that clients need to struggle as a part of finding their own answers. My expectation was that they should feel better quickly, for then I would know that I was surely helping them. I also did not appreciate that clients often begin to feel worse as they give up their defenses and open themselves to their pain. When I saw clients expressing their fear and uncertainty about their future, it brought out my own lack of certainty that I could help them. Because I was concerned about saying "the wrong thing," I often listened but did not give too many of my own reactions in return.

Even though it is uncomfortable for me to admit this, I was more inclined to accept clients who were bright, verbal, attractive, and willing to talk about their problems than clients who seemed depressed or unmotivated to change. I encouraged those whom I considered "good and cooperative clients" to come back. As long as they were talking and working, and preferably letting me know that they were getting somewhere with our sessions, I was quick to schedule other appointments. Those clients who seemed to make very few changes were the ones who increased my own anxiety. Rather than seeing their own part in their progress or lack of it, I typically blamed myself for not knowing enough and not being able to solve their problems. I took full responsibility for what they did during the session. It never occurred to me that the fact that they did not return for another session might have said something about them and their unwillingness to change. I had limited tolerance for uncertainty and for their struggle in finding their own direction. My self-doubts grew when they did not show up for following appointments. I was sure that this was a sign that they were dissatisfied with what they were getting from me.

I particularly remember encouraging depressed clients to make an appointment with one of the other counselors on the staff. I learned in my own supervision that working with depressed clients was difficult for me because of my reluctance to deal with my own fears of depression. If I allowed myself to really enter the world of these depressed clients, I might get in touch with some of my anxiety. This experience taught me the important lesson that I could not take clients in any direction that I had not been willing to explore in my own life. Had I not challenged my fears and self-doubts, I am quite certain I would have missed out on many of the meaningful and enjoyable facets of my work.

Is a Helping Career for You?

As is clear from our accounts, both of us had self-doubts. If you keep the question of whether you want to pursue a helping career open, you are bound to have periods of self-doubt. At times you may feel excited about the prospects of your career choice, and at other times you may feel hopeless and discouraged. Be tolerant of these ambivalent feelings. Don't make the decision to pursue a helping career or not based on your initial experiences. Remain open to the pattern of consistent feedback you receive from faculty members, supervisors, and your peers. In some situations you may hear that you are not suited for a particular field. Such feedback is certainly hard to accept. But if someone has concerns about your entering a helping profession, be willing to listen and to consider what that person has to say. Your first inclination may be to decide that the person does not like you, yet the advice may be in your best interest. If you hear such a recommendation, ask for specific reasons for this evaluation and find out what alternatives the person can suggest to you.

Realize that you can always work toward becoming more effective, both in your personal and professional life. You can develop your interpersonal skills if you are committed to self-reflection and taking action to change. Give yourself credit for being willing to change. If you are willing to remain open and apply the effort needed to change, you may find that your limitations can become your assets.

The inclination to give up too soon is often greatest when you first have to apply what you have learned in your courses to a situation in the real world. Chances are that you will find that what worked in the lab does not work so well in real-life helping situations. In the lab you may have worked with fellow students who role-played clients who were cooperative. Now you are facing some clients who, no matter how hard you try, are not responding to you. It takes time and experience to learn how to apply your knowledge of theories and techniques to actual situations. At first your attempts at helping may seem artificial and rehearsed. You will probably be more aware of this artificiality than your clients. Again, allow yourself time to gain a greater sense of ease in applying what you have learned and in functioning in your role as a helper.

Portrait of the "Ideal Helper"

Imagining the characteristics of the "ideal helper" can be a useful exercise, but even the most effective helpers cannot meet all of these criteria. If you try to match the ideal picture we are about to paint, you could be needlessly setting yourself up for failure and frustration. But it is surely possible to become a more effective helper if you are aware of areas that you need to strengthen. You can improve your existing skills and acquire new ones. You can integrate knowledge that will enhance your abilities. You can make personal changes that will enable you to be more present and effective as you intervene in the lives of your clients. With these possibilities in mind, consider this picture of a helper who is making a significant difference:

- You are committed to an honest assessment of your own strengths and weaknesses. You recognize that who you are as a person is one of the most important instruments you possess as a helper.
- You have a basic curiosity and are open to learning. You realize what you do not know, and you are willing to take steps to fill the gaps in your knowledge.
- You have the interpersonal skills needed to establish good contact with other people, and you can apply these skills in the helping relationship.
- You genuinely care for the people you help, and this caring is expressed by doing what is in their best interest. You are able to deal with a wide range of clients' thoughts, feelings, and behaviors.

- You realize that change is typically hard work, and you are willing to stay with clients as they go through this difficult process. You are able to enter the world of your clients and see the world through their eyes rather than imposing your own vision of reality on them.
- You realize that clients often limit themselves through a restricted imagination of possibilities for their future. You are able to invite clients to dream and to take the steps necessary to fulfill their dreams. You know that you cannot inspire clients to do in their lives what you are unable or unwilling to do in your own life.
- You are willing to draw on a number of resources to enable clients to fulfill their goals. You are flexible in applying strategies for change, and you are willing to adapt your techniques to the unique situation of each client.
- In working with clients whose ethnic or cultural background is different from your own, you show your respect for them by not fitting them into a preconceived mold.
- You take care of yourself physically, mentally, psychologically, socially, and spiritually. You do in your own life what you ask of your clients. If you are confronted with problems, you deal with them.
- You question life and engage in critical self-examination of your beliefs and values. You are aware of your needs and motivations, and you make choices that are congruent with your life goals. Your philosophy of life is your own creation, not one that has been imposed on you.
- You have established meaningful relationships with at least a few significant people.
- Although you have a healthy sense of self-love and pride, you are not self-absorbed.

Our intent in presenting this list is not to overwhelm you but to provide you with some characteristics that are worthy of reflection. You might be telling yourself that you lack many of these characteristics. An unskilled helper can become a skilled one, and all of us can become more effective in touching the lives of the clients we encounter. In addressing the question "Are the helping professions for me?" you are encouraged to use this book as a catalyst for honest self-reflection. We also strongly encourage you to question and interview people in the helping professions from a variety of settings to assist you in exploring the possibilities of a future as a helper. Ask about their journey into their chosen profession and the struggles they encountered along the way.

Many training programs offer some self-exploration experiences in which students can become more aware of how their personal attributes manifest themselves in relationships. Practicum and internship seminars typically provide opportunities for you to focus on ways in which your personal style influences your ability to establish helping relationships with clients. If your program does not offer formal personal-growth experiences, seek these resources in the community. Much of the rest of this book deals with the interplay between you as a person and your work as a professional helper. Our underlying assumption is that the best way to prepare for a dynamic career is to appreciate the richness of your own being and to be able to use your own life experiences in your evolution in the helping professions.

Creating Meaning in Your Education

Regardless of the structure of the course in which you are using this book, you can find ways to become personally involved. *You* can decide to be either actively engaged or marginally involved. *You* can make this class different. Once you become aware of those aspects of your education that you don't like, *you* can decide to change your style of learning to make it more meaningful for you.

Investing in Your Educational Program

At the beginning of your educational program, you may feel that you will have to remain in school forever to do what you want professionally. However, if you are enjoying and gaining from the experience, you will likely be surprised at how soon you complete your program. The key is to be personally involved in your educational program and to see a connection between your formal studies and your personal and professional goals. Think about how much time and energy you are prepared to devote to making your education meaningful. It may help to consider your education as an investment, and then decide what you can do to get the most from this investment. Most of all, find ways to enjoy the process.

Investments are often evaluated by their cost-benefit ratio. The cost of your educational investment includes not just money but your time and energy as well. Look at the potential benefits of this investment, including what you hope to gain. Ask yourself if what you are putting in (costs) is worth what you hope to get out of it in return (benefits). What are the benefits of putting a great deal of yourself into your formal studies? What will taking responsibility for your education cost you in terms of time taken away from other facets of your life?

Learning to Cope With the System

You will encounter external and internal barriers to achieving your goals and maximizing your potential as learners and professional helpers. We have found that students, as well as professionals, often underestimate the ways in which they do have power. For example, we know of a student who was responsible for changing several unfair practices within her academic institution merely by raising her concerns and bringing them to the attention of the faculty and administrators. Many systems impose limitations, and you will be challenged to learn how to work creatively within them without sacrificing your integrity. People often are so busy that they fail to question the practices and procedures within the systems in which they work. It can be empowering to question and strive to change these institutions and systems.

You will undoubtedly face a number of challenges in your educational program, a few of which involve grades, requirements, courses, and evaluation. You may feel anxious about being evaluated and think that grades are not an accurate measure of your learning. It is a mistake to assume that grading stops when you graduate from a university. There are reviews and evaluation practices on all levels in the professional world. In a business, for example, your supervisors rate you and determine whether you get a promotion or a raise. If you are a professional, both your clients and your place of work will evaluate your performance.

Students sometimes assume that there are worlds of difference between the roles they play in college and the roles they will assume as professionals. Many of the traits that you have as a student will most likely carry over into your behavior as a worker. If you have great difficulty in showing up for classes regularly, for example, you are likely to carry this habit into your work appointments. Getting a position in a community agency is a highly competitive effort. If you hope to gain entry into the professional world, it is essential that you be prepared to cope with the realities of the marketplace.

We ask our students to think about their time in school as a long job interview. The connections you make in school and the reputation you build for yourself are critical in gaining access to future jobs and professional opportunities. How you performed as a learner will undoubtedly influence how strongly your professors state their degree of support or their recommendation for opportunities you may pursue in your professional life.

Selecting a Professional Program and Career Path

In this section we introduce you to a range of considerations in selecting your educational program and your career in the helping professions. We encourage you to think about how the following topics apply to you: the rewards of being a helper, creating realistic expectations and testing them, and deciding which educational and professional route to pursue.

The Joys and Rewards of Being a Helping Professional

Your involvement in working intimately in the lives of others can yield many benefits and gifts to you personally. In very few other kinds of work do you have as many opportunities to reflect on the quality of your own life. Helping others can provide you with the satisfaction of knowing that you are making a significant difference to others, which in itself enhances the meaning of life.

In their research study, Radeke and Mahoney (2000) found that mental health practitioners recognize that the impact of their work makes them better and wiser and increases their self-awareness. The work that helpers do tends to accelerate their psychological development, amplify their emotional life, and results in them feeling both stressed and satisfied. As a result of their professional commitment, helpers report a deeper appreciation for human relationships, an increased tolerance for ambiguity, a greater capacity to enjoy life, a sense of doing spiritual work, and an opportunity to examine and change, when necessary, their personal values. These are but a few of the psychological benefits often reported by helping professionals.

Create Realistic Expectations

Students planning to enter one of the helping professions sometimes fall into the trap of idealizing the profession. In their minds, they may be overly focused on the appreciation they expect to receive from their clients. They may envision themselves as being able to help anyone who comes to them, and even reaching those who do not seek their counsel. Although having ideals and goals to strive for is part of being a helper, it is easy to paint an unrealistic picture of what your career as a helper will be like. You need to engage in ongoing reality testing to maintain a balanced outlook. You can test your vision by talking to various practitioners in many different settings. Ask them to tell you what they do in a typical week. Inquire about their motivations for choosing and remaining in the helping professions. Ask especially about the rewards, challenges, demands, and frustrations of their work.

When you begin fieldwork, you will be able to test many of your ideas and expectations against the real world of work. This is a good time to reflect on your motives and needs for considering helping as a career. Observations in various field settings and practical experience working with different client populations will provide a more accurate picture of how your career is likely to satisfy your needs for becoming a helper in the first place. We have met students who remained in a course of study even though they had discovered that they were not enthusiastic about the field. If you find yourself in a program that you really do not like, consider whether it is worth it for you to stay in the program. Be sure you evaluate the overall direction of the program rather than a specific course or requirement that you do not like.

Deciding Which Educational and Professional Route to Take

At this point, you may not even be certain you want to pursue a career in the helping professions. If you are enrolled in a 2-year community college program in human services, you may be wondering whether it would be best for you to get a job when you complete your program. A wide range of human services jobs are available, including social service assistants, outreach workers in the community, work with parolees or in prison settings, work with the physically challenged, addictions counseling, and a host of positions in community agency settings. It is generally true that the higher your educational level the more career options are open to you. However, you may want to get a job for a time to gain experience once you complete a community college program. Later you may see the need to return to school for further study.

Human services programs at the bachelor's degree level train students for entry into a wide range of jobs, some of which include family and children's services, youth corrections, crisis shelters, career counseling, youth programs, residential treatment centers, mental health units, senior citizens centers, nursing homes, and agencies for people with disabilities.

Whether you are an undergraduate or a graduate student, you have probably experienced some anxiety in selecting the right program. We encourage students to be open to new ideas, especially when participating in fieldwork placements. There are no absolute guidelines or perfect choices, and you don't need to have a specific career goal in mind when you enter a program. Gather program material from several universities and talk with professors and students. Talking with professionals about their work experience can also broaden your perspective. Ask about the specific educational and practical background that they most value. In selecting a program, ask yourself these questions: "Will the program give me what I need to do the work I want to do? Does the orientation of the program fit with my values? Am I compatible with the program?"

You can take many routes as a helper in the human services: social worker, psychiatric technician, couples and family therapist, mental health counselor, psychologist, or school counselor. Each of these professional specialties has a different focus, yet all have in common working with people. Much depends on what you want to do, how much time you are willing to invest in a program, where you want to live, and what your other interests are. There is no "perfect profession," and each profession has advantages and drawbacks.

At the undergraduate level, human services programs train practitioners for community agency work. Human service workers generally carry out specific roles and functions under the supervision of clinical social workers, psychologists, and licensed counselors. At the master's degree level, students can choose among various types of programs, some of which include school counseling, mental health counseling, addiction counseling, rehabilitation counseling, counseling psychology, clinical psychology, couples and family therapy, and clinical social work. At the doctoral level, there are generally four approved programs for those wanting to become practitioners: social work, counselor education, counseling psychology, and clinical psychology. Each specialization has its own perspective and emphasizes different roles and functions for practitioners.

Regardless of which of the helping professions interests you the most, you are likely to discover many different positions within an area of specialization. Do not become overly anxious about making the "right decision" or delay making any choice because you cannot decide which career or program to pursue. View your professional life as a developmental process, and explore new possibilities as you gain additional work experience.

Overview of Some of the Helping Professions

As you read about the various specialty areas of practice described in this section, think about the characteristics that most meet with your own expectations. Each specialty has much to recommend it, but you probably will find yourself drawn more to one than to the others. The professional organization for each specialty is described, and we have provided contact information for these organizations to facilitate further inquiries about membership, conferences, and the code of ethics of the organization.

Social Work

This specialization attends not only to the individual dynamics of a person but also to an understanding of the person in the environment. A master's program in **social work** (MSW) prepares students broadly for casework, counseling, community intervention, social policy and planning, research and development, and administration and management. The course work tends to be broader than that in counseling and focuses on developing skills to intervene and bring about social change on levels beyond the individual. Although clinical social workers are engaged in assessment and treatment of individuals, couples, families, and groups, they tend to view environmental factors as contributing strongly to an individual's or a family's problems. In addition to academic courses, a supervised internship is part of the social worker's preparation for either direct or indirect social services.

National Association of Social Workers (NASW). NASW membership is open to all professional social workers, and there is a student membership category. The NASW Press, which produces *Social Work* and the *NASW* News as membership benefits, is a major service in professional development. NASW also provides a number of pamphlets on relevant topics. For further information about NASW, contact:

National Association of Social Workers
750 First Street, NE, Suite 700
Washington, DC 20002-4241
Telephone: (202) 408-8600 or (800) 638-8799
Fax: (202) 336-8311
Website: www.socialworkers.org

Couples and Family Counseling

The specialization of **couples and family therapy** is primarily concerned with relationship counseling. It deals with assessing and treating clients from a family-systems perspective. Students in a master's or a doctoral program in couples and family therapy take a variety of courses in assessment and treatment, as well as theory courses. They also do extensive supervised fieldwork with children and adults, couples, and families.

American Association for Marriage and Family Therapy (AAMFT). The AAMFT has a student membership category. The organization sponsors a conference each October. For membership applications or for further information, contact:

American Association for Marriage and Family Therapy
112 South Alfred Street
Alexandria, VA 22314-3061
Telephone: (703) 838-9808
Fax: (703) 838-9805
Website: www.aamft.org

International Association of Marriage and Family Counselors (IAMFC). IAMFC members have the opportunity to have online discussions and to network with others who have similar research interests. Topics of interest include blended families; counseling offenders; separation and divorce counseling; substance abuse; mediation; MFT training; gay, lesbian, and bisexual issues; military families; sexual offenders; systemic interventions in mental illness; survivors of sexual abuse; family interventions in schools; multicultural counseling; and families and violence. For further information, contact:

International Association of Marriage and Family Counselors
American Counseling Association
5999 Stevenson Avenue
Alexandria, VA 22304-3300
Telephone: (800) 347-6647 extension 222
Fax: (800) 473-2329
Website: www.iamfc.com

Clinical and Counseling Psychology

Although clinical and counseling psychology are different specializations, there are no rigid boundaries separating their professional functions so we will discuss them together. Although you can be licensed as a social worker, counselor, and couples and family therapist with a master's degree, this is not the case if you wish to refer to yourself as a psychologist. Both counseling and clinical psychology require a doctorate for licensure. **Clinical psychologists** focus on assessment, diagnosis, and treatment procedures of mildly to severely disturbed persons. They interview clients and write case studies. **Counseling psychologists** assist relatively healthy people in solving developmental problems and functioning more effectively. They help clients find and use information to make better personal, educational, and occupational choices. Professional psychologists in both specialties often offer psychotherapy to individuals, couples, families, and groups; they may teach or conduct research. Both specializations focus on evaluation of treatments and programs and help clients develop action plans. Clinical and counseling psychologists often work in the same settings.

American Psychological Association (APA). The APA has a Student Affiliates category rather than student membership. Each year in August the APA holds a national convention. For further information, contact:

American Psychological Association
750 First Street, NE
Washington, DC 20002-4242
Telephone: (202) 336-5500 or (800) 374-2721
Fax: (202) 336-5568
Website: www.apa.org

American Counseling Association (ACA). Student memberships are available to both undergraduate and graduate students enrolled at least half-time or more at the college level. The organization sponsors a national convention each year in March or April. The ACA puts out a resource catalog that provides information on the various aspects of the counseling profession, as well as giving detailed information about membership, journals, books, home-study programs, video and DVD programs, and liability insurance. For further information, contact:

American Counseling Association
5999 Stevenson Avenue
Alexandria, VA 22304-3300
Telephone: (703) 823-9800 or (800) 347-6647
Fax: (703) 823-0252
Website: www.counseling.org

School Counseling

Neukrug (2007) traces the historical development of school counseling from its beginning as a response to the needs of vocational guidance to its growing viability as a profession today. Accreditation guidelines for school counseling have been implemented over the past 20 years, which has moved school counseling forward in terms of accountability as a helping profession. All states now require a master's degree in school counseling, and professional organizations advocate and lobby for legislative initiatives and the establishment of credentialing.

School counselors perform a wide variety of roles and functions in elementary, middle, and secondary schools, including individual counseling, group guidance, group counseling, consultation, and coordination. In addition to working with students, many school counselors consult with teachers, administrators, and, at times, with parents. School counselors work with students on a variety of educational issues, but many of them provide some personal and social counseling as well. From a multicultural perspective, school counselors have the challenge of striving to lessen language barriers, advocating for minority students, sensitizing the school community to cultural diversity issues, ensuring that educational materials are relevant for students' culture, and establishing a comprehensive developmental counseling and guidance program (Neukrug, 2007).

American School Counselors Association (ASCA). The ASCA is the major professional organization devoted to school counseling. ASCA has a student membership category. For additional information, contact:

American School Counselors Association
1101 King Street, Suite 625
Alexandria, VA 22314
Telephone: (703) 683-2722 or (800) 306-4722
Fax: (703) 683-1619
Website: www.schoolcounselor.org

Rehabilitation Counseling

Rehabilitation counseling focuses on person-centered programs and services for persons with medical, physical, mental, developmental, cognitive, and psychiatric disabilities to help them achieve their personal, career, and independent living goals in the most integrated setting possible. The profession itself is founded on humanistic values and the belief that each person has unique cultural attributes. Rehabilitation counseling is a holistic and integrated program of medical, physical, psychosocial, and vocational interventions (Commission on Rehabilitation Counselor Certification [CRCC], 2003). Rehabilitation counselors use career, vocational, mental health, case management, and counseling strategies to empower persons with chronic illnesses or disabilities to achieve their maximum level of independence and psychosocial adjustment through personally fulfilling, socially meaningful, and functionally effective interaction with their environment.

Historically, rehabilitation counselors have worked within the state-federal program of vocational rehabilitation under the primary occupational title of "rehabilitation counselor." However, for more than 27 years, the majority of rehabilitation counselors have specialized and practiced under a variety of other occupational titles such as substance abuse counselor, case manager, vocational or career counselor, job placement specialist, and, more recently, licensed professional counselor (Dew & Peters, 2002; Goodwin, 2006).

Commission on Rehabilitation Counselor Certification (CRCC). Current day rehabilitation counseling practices began to develop in 1972 when the Council on Rehabilitation Education (CORE, 2009) established the core content and competencies required to practice as a master's level rehabilitation counselor. In 1974, the Commission on Rehabilitation Counselor Certification (2009) became the first credentialing body in the counseling profession. This organization developed professional standards of practice and a code of ethics establishing the master's level certified rehabilitation counselor (CRC) credential (Stebnicki, 2009a).

A recent survey of all CORE-accredited programs reports that 60% of all rehabilitation counselor training programs offer a specialty concentration or emphasis. The most frequently identified areas include substance abuse counseling, clinical mental health counseling, and deafness and hearing impairment

(Goodwin, 2006). For additional information on the rehabilitation counseling profession, contact:

Commission on Rehabilitation Counselor Certification
1699 East Woodfield Road, Suite 300
Schumburg, IL 60173
Telephone: (847) 944-1325
Website: www.crccertification.com

Drug and Alcohol Counseling

Addiction is one of the main public health issues in the United States today. Substance abuse counselors are actively involved in education, prevention, intervention, and treatment for a variety of addictions. Practitioners in the field provide treatment in a variety of settings: private and public treatment centers, residential treatment facilities, hospitals, private practice, and community agencies.

The Association for Addiction Professionals (NAADAC). NAADAC is the major national professional organization devoted to ethical standards for addiction professionals. NAADAC's mission is to lead, unify, and empower addiction-focused professionals to achieve excellence through education, advocacy, knowledge, standards of practice, ethics, professional development, and research. For additional information, contact:

The Association for Addiction Professionals
1001 N. Fairfax Street, Suite 201
Alexandria, VA 22314
Telephone: (800) 548-0497
Website: www.naadac.org

Paraprofessional and Nonlicensed Human Service Workers

It is clear that there are not enough professionally licensed practitioners willing to meet the demand for psychological assistance to a diverse range of client populations within a community. Moreover, mental health services have not always been available to those unable to pay. Faced with these realities, many in the mental health field have concluded that nonlicensed workers could be given the training and supervision they need to provide some psychological services.

Nonlicensed human service workers, sometimes referred to as **paraprofessionals,** may have a graduate degree, an undergraduate degree, an associate of arts degree, a certificate of competence in some aspect of human services, or some formal training from experts in the field. **Paraprofessional helpers** perform some of the helping services licensed mental health professionals traditionally provide, but they also engage in broader roles, such as advocacy and community mobilization. The term *paraprofessional* denotes "persons with some of the skills and natural helping talents of the professional. They usually work directly with helpees under the professional's supervision for training and accountability"(Brammer & MacDonald, 2003, p. 17).

Paraprofessionals are often **generalist human service workers** who have education and training at the undergraduate level. These generalists have a variety of job titles, a few of which include community support worker, human services worker, social work assistant, alcohol or drug abuse counselor, mental health technician, child care worker, community outreach worker, residential counselor, client advocate, crisis intervention counselor, community organizer, psychiatric technician, church worker, and case manager (Woodside & McClam, 2009).

The question of how best to deliver services to the people who are most in need of them is a controversial one. Not all mental health professionals are enthusiastic about the increased use of nonlicensed workers and paraprofessional helpers. Some point to the danger that inadequately trained people might do more harm than good. Others contend that the poor will receive inferior service. Still others fear that more and more helpers will be allowed to practice without supervision and necessary training. Some fear that their own jobs or income may be jeopardized if nonlicensed helpers are allowed to provide services similar to those rendered by professionals.

Although there is some controversy regarding the relative effectiveness of professional and paraprofessional helpers, current evidence suggests that paraprofessional helpers are effective additions to helping services (Brammer & MacDonald, 2003), filling a vital role in the mental health field today (Trull, 2005). Paraprofessional helpers have demonstrated a positive influence in the human service field, effectively carrying out roles and assuming responsibilities that were not anticipated by the field (Woodside & McClam, 2009). Service agencies have discovered that paraprofessional workers can indeed provide some services as effectively as trained professionals—for much less cost. Tan (1997) asserts that paraprofessional helpers are able to provide support through fostering a sense of community and decreasing the isolation that many clients experience. Tan believes they can make unique and significant contributions in treatment planning and implementation.

The trend toward the increased use of nonlicensed workers and paraprofessional helpers means that licensed mental health professionals will have to assume new and expanding roles. Tan (1997) observes that mental health professionals can be expected to spend less time providing direct services to clients and more time teaching, supervising, and consulting with community workers. In-service workshops for entry-level human service workers and volunteer workers, educating the public about the nature of mental health, consulting, working as agents for change in the community, designing new programs, conducting research, and evaluating existing programs may all become part of the job for mental health professionals.

National Organization for Human Services (NOHS). The National Organization for Human Services (NOHS) is made up of members from diverse educational and professional backgrounds with the mission of fostering excellence in human service delivery through education, scholarship, and practice. Regular membership is open to educators and practitioners, and student memberships are available. NOHS schedules a conference each October. For further information, contact:

National Organization for Human Services
5341 Old Highway 5, Ste. 206, #214
Woodstock, GA 30188
Telephone: (770) 924-8899
Fax: (678) 494-5076
Website: www.nationalhumanservices.org

Becoming a Licensed Professional

Obtaining a master's degree or a doctoral degree in counseling, counselor education, social work, psychology, or couples and family counseling may be the beginning of your educational journey as a mental health professional, not the final destination. If you hope to establish even a part-time private practice, or to work in some positions in mental health agencies, you need to secure a license to practice. The main licenses available in most states include licensed professional counselor, licensed mental health counselor, licensed clinical social worker, licensed psychologist, and licensed marital and family therapist. To qualify for a license, an applicant generally must first secure a degree (or level determined by the licensing board) in the professional area of specialization. Beyond the degree a minimum number of hours of supervised clinical work is required, and the applicant must pass both a written and sometimes an oral examination. Licensure statutes determine and govern professional practice, specifying what the holder of the license can do. A person with a professional license is assumed to have minimal competence in the general practice of clinical work.

Licensure assures the public that practitioners have completed minimum educational programs, have had a certain number of hours of supervised training, and have gone through some type of evaluation and screening. Licenses do not, and probably cannot, ensure that practitioners will competently do what their licenses permit them to do. The main advantages of licensure are protection of the public from grossly unqualified and untrained practitioners and formal representation to the public that practitioners are part of an established profession.

Licenses and credentials usually do not specify the clients or types of problems practitioners are competent to work with, nor do they specify the techniques that counselors are competent to use. Most licensing regulations do specify that licensees are to engage only in those therapeutic tasks for which they have professional competence, but it is up to the licensee to put this rule into practice. If you are interested in securing more information about the licensure process, research the specific licenses available in your state and the requirements for making application for these licenses.

Values to Consider in Choosing Your Career Path

As we have previously stated, making career choices is an ongoing process rather than an isolated event. People generally go through a series of stages when choosing a career path. Information from practitioners and professors can help you define a professional direction. But you cannot rely solely on the advice of others when making your career decisions. In today's world, it is increasingly important to become a generalist. Your chances of gaining employment in a managed care system are greater if you are able to work with a range of client populations in a variety of problem areas. Although you may develop expertise in an area of specialization, flexibility is often necessary to meet the changing demands in the marketplace.

Ultimately you must decide for yourself which path is likely to best tap your talents and bring you the most fulfillment. In your career decision-making process, consider your self-concept, motivation and achievement, interests, abilities, values, occupational attitudes, socioeconomic level, parental influence, ethnic identity, gender, and any physical, mental, emotional, or social disabilities. Your values will affect your choice of a career path, and it is important to assess, identify, and clarify your values to match them with your career aspirations.

Your **work values** pertain to what you hope to accomplish in an occupation. Work values are an important aspect of your total value system. Recognizing those things that bring meaning to your life is crucial in finding a career that has personal value for you. A few examples of work values include helping others, influencing people, finding meaning, prestige, status, competition, friendships, creativity, stability, recognition, adventure, physical challenge, change and variety, opportunity for travel, moral fulfillment, and independence. Because certain work values are related to certain occupations, they can be the basis of a good match between you and a position. Take time to complete the following self-inventory as a way of clarifying some of your values pertaining to work.

Decide how important each of the following values is to you in your work. Write the appropriate number next to each:

4 = most important to me
3 = important, but not a top priority
2 = slightly important
1 = of little or no importance

____ 1. *High income:* opportunity for high pay or other financial gain.
____ 2. *Power:* opportunity to influence, lead, and direct others.
____ 3. *Prestige:* opportunity for respect and admiration from others.
____ 4. *Job security:* security from unemployment and economic changes.
____ 5. *Variety:* chances to do many different things in a job.
____ 6. *Achievement:* opportunities to accomplish goals.

_____ 7. *Responsibility:* chance to be in charge of others; being able to show trustworthiness.

_____ 8. *Independence:* freedom from rigid hours or controls.

_____ 9. *Family relationships:* time to be with family in addition to the job.

_____ 10. *Interests:* work that matches my field of interest.

_____ 11. *Opportunity to serve people:* being able to make a difference in the lives of others; helping others help themselves.

_____ 12. *Adventure:* a high level of excitement on the job.

_____ 13. *Creativity:* opportunities to come up with new ideas and do things in creative ways.

_____ 14. *Inner harmony:* peace and contentment through work.

_____ 15. *Teamwork:* opportunities to cooperate with others toward common goals.

_____ 16. *Intellectual challenge:* opportunity for a high level of problem solving and creative thinking.

_____ 17. *Competition:* the need to compete against others.

_____ 18. *Advancement:* opportunities for promotion.

_____ 19. *Continued learning:* chances to update learning and knowledge.

_____ 20. *Structure and routine:* a predictable routine on the job that requires a certain pattern of responses.

Go over the list again and identify your top three values—the ones you deem to be essential in a job you would accept. What does your list tell you? What other values do you consider to be extremely important in work? To clarify some of these values, ask yourself these questions: "Do I like working with a wide range of people? Am I able to ask for help from others when I am faced with problematic situations? Do I value doing in my own life what I encourage others to do in theirs? How do I feel about offering help to others with their problems? Am I interested in organizing, coordinating, and leading others in work projects? Do I value working on projects I have designed, or do I tend to look to others to come up with ideas for projects with which I can become involved?" Your values and interests are intertwined; knowing them can help you identify areas of work where you will find the most personal satisfaction.

Suggestions for Creating Your Professional Journey

In Conyne and Bemak's (2005) book, *Journeys to Professional Excellence: Lessons From Leading Counselor Educators and Practitioners,* 15 leaders in the counseling field share their personal and professional journeys. They talk about how they chose their career paths, what challenges they have faced, what factors contributed to their successes and failures, how they balance their personal and professional lives, and what advice they have for those entering the helping professions.

We have summarized some of the common themes of these contributors' stories and offer these suggestions to students and people new to the profession:

- Look for opportunities to stretch yourself. Focus on what you can do rather than the limitations you have.
- Seek help when you need it, both personally and professionally.
- Find a group of people who are supportive and can offer you encouragement.
- Seek out at least one mentor and become closely networked with others in the helping professions.
- Get supervision and be open to feedback and learning.
- Remain connected to those people who mean the most to you in your life. Take time for your family and your spiritual core.
- Strive to integrate your personal and professional journeys. Be committed to taking care of yourself in all ways.
- Learn about people from cultures different from yours and become culturally competent.
- Stay humble and open. Be your genuine self. Learn from others and integrate that into who you are.
- Listen to your intuitive voice and create your own path.
- Don't think of mistakes as failures but rather as opportunities for growth and change.
- Establish both long-term and short-term goals.
- Realize that much of your education will soon be out of date.
- Recognize that obstacles, disappointments, and failures are all teachable moments.
- Maintain a sense of humor.
- You're a part of the future. You can make a significant difference. Become an agent of individual and social change.
- Work hard and set high standards for yourself.
- Don't become easily discouraged.
- Think globally, act locally.
- Give back to the profession. Join a professional organization and attend conferences.
- Read, discuss, reflect, and keep a journal.
- Don't focus on the financial aspects of a job.
- Develop interests outside of the counseling field.
- Identify your strengths and limitations. Seek out self-exploration and therapeutic experiences.
- Keep life simple and passionate.
- Dare to dream and have the courage to pursue your passions.
- Identify your sphere of influence, and act when you have the power to do so.

At times you may feel discouraged, and it may be difficult to focus on what is really important. Review this list, and use it as a way to regain your momentum. Reflect on the points that most speak to you. What kind of future do you want for yourself both personally and professionally? Begin taking action now to get what you most want.

Self-Assessment: An Inventory of Your Attitudes and Beliefs About Helping

Self-assessment is an ongoing process for all helping professionals. Completing this inventory will help you clarify your beliefs and values. The inventory is designed to introduce you to issues and topics presented in this book and to stimulate your thoughts and interest. You may want to complete the inventory in more than one sitting, giving each question your full concentration.

This is not a traditional multiple-choice test in which you must select the "one right answer." Rather, it is a survey of your basic beliefs, attitudes, and values on specific topics related to the helping process. For each question, write in the letter of the response that most clearly reflects your viewpoint at this time. In many cases the answers are not mutually exclusive, and you may choose more than one response if you wish. In addition, a blank line is included for each item so you can provide a response more suited to your thinking or qualify a chosen response.

Notice that there are two spaces before each item. Use the space on the left for your answer at the beginning of the course. At the end of the course, take this inventory again, placing your answer in the space on the right. Cover your initial answers so you won't be influenced by how you originally responded. Then you can see how your attitudes have changed as a result of your experience in this course.

____ ____ 1. **Effective helpers.** The personal characteristics of helpers are
   a. not really that relevant to the helping process.
   b. the most important variable in determining the quality of the helping process.
   c. shaped and molded by those who teach mental health workers.
   d. not as important as the skills and knowledge helpers possess.
   e. _____

____ ____ 2. **Personal traits.** Which of the following do you consider to be the most important personal characteristic of a good helper?
   a. Willingness to serve as a model for clients
   b. Courage
   c. Openness and honesty
   d. A sense of being "centered" as a person
   e. _____

____ ____ 3. **Self-disclosure.** I believe helpers' self-disclosure to their clients
   a. is essential for establishing a relationship.
   b. is inappropriate and merely burdens the client.

    c. should be done rarely and only when helpers feel it would be of benefit to clients.

    d. is useful to reveal how helpers feel toward their clients in the context of the professional relationship.

    e. _____

4. **Fees.** If I were working with a client who could no longer continue because of his or her inability to pay my fees, I would most likely

    a. be willing to see this person at no fee, but in return expect him or her to do some type of volunteer work in the community.

    b. give my client the names of several referrals.

    c. suggest some form of bartering of goods or services for therapy services.

    d. adjust my fee to whatever the client could afford.

    e. _____

5. **Change.** Which of the following factors is most important in determining whether the helping process will result in change?

    a. The kind of person the helper is

    b. The skills and techniques the helper uses

    c. The motivation of the client to change

    d. The theoretical orientation of the helper

    e. _____

6. **Key attribute.** Which of the following do you consider to be the most important attribute of an effective mental health practitioner?

    a. Knowledge of the theory of counseling and behavior

    b. Skill in using techniques appropriately

    c. Genuineness and openness

    d. Ability to specify a treatment plan and evaluate the results

    e. _____

7. **Fieldwork.** With respect to a fieldwork placement,

    a. I do not feel at all ready to participate in fieldwork.

    b. I would treat it like a job.

    c. I expect to limit myself to working with the kind of clients that I think I want to eventually work with in a job position.

    d. I want to work with clients that I think would be a challenge for me.

    e. _____

8. **Effectiveness.** To be an effective helper, I believe I

    a. must have an in-depth knowledge of my client's cultural background.

    b. must be free of any personal conflicts in the area in which the client is working.

    c. need to have experienced the same problem as the client.

    d. must be aware of my own needs and motivations for wanting to enter the helping field.

    e. _____

____ ____ 9. **Helping relationship.** With regard to the client–helper relationship, I think

    a. the helper should remain objective and anonymous.

    b. the helper should be a friend to the client.

    c. a personal relationship, but not friendship, is essential.

    d. a personal and warm relationship is not essential.

    e. _____

____ ____ 10. **Being open.** I should be open and honest with my clients

    a. when I like and value them.

    b. when I have negative feelings toward them.

    c. rarely, if ever, so that I will avoid negatively influencing the client–helper relationship.

    d. only when it intuitively feels like the right thing to do.

    e. _____

____ ____ 11. **Ethical decision making.** If I were faced with an ethical dilemma, the first step I would take would be to

    a. talk to my supervisor or seek consultation.

    b. attempt to solve the problem myself.

    c. identify the nature of the problem or problems.

    d. talk to my client and strive to involve him or her in working through this dilemma.

    e. _____

____ ____ 12. **Inadequate supervision.** If I were not getting the kind of supervision I thought I needed and want, my inclination would be to

    a. make the best of the situation and not cause any trouble.

    b. demand that my supervisor provide adequate supervision.

    c. learn assertiveness skills and consistently ask for what I need by way of supervision.

    d. suggest that my peers and I form our own peer-supervision group to talk about the concerns we are facing.

    e. _____

____ ____ 13. **Competence.** If I were an intern and was convinced that my supervisor was encouraging trainees to take on clients with problems beyond their level of education and competence, I would

    a. first discuss the matter with the supervisor.

    b. ask my supervisor to give me extra help and perhaps work with me directly.

    c. ignore the situation for fear of negative consequences.

    d. refuse to engage in delivering any services that I thought were beyond my level of competence.

    e. _____

_____ _____ 14. **Cultural competence.** Practitioners who work with culturally diverse groups without having multicultural knowledge and skills
   a. are certainly not going to be able to provide effective services.
   b. are probably guilty of unethical behavior.
   c. will need to acquire the knowledge and skills by taking a course, reading, or engaging in continuing education.
   d. are making themselves vulnerable to a malpractice suit.
   e. _____

_____ _____ 15. **Difficult client.** If I were working with a difficult and resistant client, my approach would likely be to
   a. discuss my reactions to my client's behavior with him or her.
   b. keep my reactions to myself and figure ways that I might get the upper hand with my client.
   c. discuss strategies for reaching difficult clients with a supervisor or colleague.
   d. strive to honor and respect the resistances my client displays and encourage my client to explore his or her attitudes and behaviors.
   e. _____

_____ _____ 16. **Being ready.** I won't feel ready to offer professional help to others until
   a. I have completed the program I am now in.
   b. I have developed a specialization that will make me an expert in a particular area.
   c. I feel very confident and know that I will be effective.
   d. I have become a self-aware person and developed the ability to continually reexamine my own life and relationships.
   e. _____

_____ _____ 17. **Managing attractions.** If a client evidenced strong feelings of attraction or dislike for me, I think I would
   a. immediately want to discuss this matter in my supervision.
   b. not have a clue as to how to respond.
   c. quickly refer my client to another professional.
   d. engage in self-disclosure, letting my client know how I was affected by what he or she said to me.
   e. _____

_____ _____ 18. **Diversity.** Practitioners who counsel clients whose sex, race, age, social class, or sexual orientation is different from their own
   a. will constantly be tested by these clients, which will make trust almost impossible.
   b. need to understand the meaning of the differences between their clients and themselves.
   c. are likely to be very effective if they are willing to acquire a range of knowledge and skills that will enable them to become culturally competent helpers.

    d. are probably not going to be effective with such clients because of these differences.

    e. _____

19. **Value priorities.** When I consider being involved in the helping professions, I value most the
    a. money I expect to earn.
    b. status and recognition that will be associated with the job.
    c. knowledge that I will be intimately involved with people who are searching for a better life.
    d. personal growth I expect to experience through my work.
    e. _____

20. **Value judgments.** With respect to making value judgments in the helping relationship, I believe helpers should
    a. feel free to make value judgments about their clients' behavior.
    b. actively teach their own values when they think clients need a different set of values.
    c. remain neutral and keep their values out of the helping process.
    d. encourage clients to question their own values and decide on the quality of their own behavior.
    e. _____

21. **Helper tasks.** Helpers should
    a. teach desirable behavior and values by modeling them for clients.
    b. encourage clients to look within themselves to discover values that are meaningful to them.
    c. reinforce the dominant values of society.
    d. very delicately, if at all, challenge clients' value systems.
    e. _____

22. **Making referrals.** I would refer a client to another professional if
    a. I were convinced that I was no longer able to be effective with this client for any reason.
    b. I didn't have much experience working with the kind of problem the client presented.
    c. any sort of conflict of values existed between my client and me.
    d. the client seemed resistant and was not willing to be open to my suggestions.
    e. _____

23. **Confidentiality.** Regarding confidentiality, I believe
    a. there is little hope that trust will be established unless clients can be guaranteed absolute confidentiality.
    b. it is ethical to break confidence when there is reason to believe that a client will do harm to someone else or will harm him- or herself.

    c. it is essential for me to discuss in detail the purpose and limits of confidentiality at the first session with a client.

    d. it is ethical to inform the authorities when a client is breaking the law.

    e. _____

_____ _____ 24. **Sex with former client.** A sexual relationship between a former client and a therapist is

    a. ethical if the therapist can prove that the relationship will not harm the former client.

    b. considered ethical 5 years after the termination of the professional relationship.

    c. ethical only when client and therapist discuss the issue and agree to the relationship.

    d. never ethical, regardless of the time that has elapsed.

    e. _____

_____ _____ 25. **Accepting gifts.** If a client were to offer me a gift, I would

    a. possibly accept it, but only after fully discussing the matter with my client.

    b. never accept it under any circumstances.

    c. accept the gift only if this was the termination of our professional relationship.

    d. accept the gift if gift-giving were a part of the client's culture and if refusing the gift would be insulting to my client.

    e. _____

_____ _____ 26. **Spiritual and religious values.** With respect to the role of spiritual and religious values in the helping process, I would be inclined to

    a. do my best to keep my own values out of the professional relationship for fear that I would unduly influence my client.

    b. recommend to my client that he or she think about how spirituality or religion could bring new meaning to his or her life.

    c. avoid introducing such topics in a session unless my client initiated this discussion.

    d. routinely conduct an assessment of my client's spiritual and religious beliefs during the intake session.

    e. _____

_____ _____ 27. **Goals of helping.** Regarding the issue of who should select goals in the helping process, I believe

    a. it is the helper's responsibility to select goals.

    b. it is the client's responsibility to select goals.

    c. the responsibility for selecting goals should be a collaborative venture by both client and helper.

    d. the question of who selects the goals depends on what kind of client is being seen.

    e. _____

____ ____ 28. **Community.** Concerning the helper's responsibility to the community, I believe
    a. the helper should educate the community concerning the nature of psychological services.
    b. the central role of a helper is that of a change agent.
    c. it is appropriate to function as an advocate for underrepresented groups in the community.
    d. helpers should become involved in helping clients use the resources available in the community.
    e. _____

____ ____ 29. **Systems.** When it comes to working in institutions or a system, I believe
    a. I must learn how to survive with dignity within a system.
    b. I must learn how to subvert the system so that I can do what I deeply believe in.
    c. the institution will stifle most of my enthusiasm and block any real change.
    d. I cannot blame the institution if I am unable to succeed in my programs.
    e. _____

____ ____ 30. **Philosophical conflicts.** If my philosophy were in conflict with that of the institution I worked for, I would
    a. seriously consider whether I could ethically remain in that position.
    b. attempt to change the policies of the institution by any means possible.
    c. agree to whatever was expected of me in that system so that I would not lose my job.
    d. quietly do what I wanted to do, even if I had to be devious about it.
    e. _____

By Way of Review

Near the end of each chapter we list some of the chapter's highlights. These key points serve as a review of the messages we have attempted to get across. After you finish each chapter, we encourage you to spend a few minutes writing down the central issues and points that have the most meaning for you.

• Become active in getting the most from your education. No program is perfect, but you can do a lot to bring more meaning to your course of study.

• Just as you are evaluated and graded in your educational program, you will be evaluated in the professional world. Evaluation can create stress, but it is part of your educational program and your future career.

• Remain open to the question of whether a career in one of the helping professions is right for you. In deciding whether to pursue one of the helping professions, do not give up too soon. Be prepared for doubts and setbacks.

• Although the "ideal helper" does not exist in reality, a number of behaviors and attitudes characterize effective helpers. Even though you might not reach the ideal, you can progress, especially with the willingness to question what you are doing.

• It is essential that helpers examine their motivations for going into the field. Helpers meet their own needs through their work, and they must recognize these needs. It is possible for both client and helper to benefit from the helping relationship.

• Some of the needs for going into the helping professions include the need to be needed, the need for prestige and status, and the need to make a difference. These needs can work both for you and against you in becoming an effective helper.

• In selecting an educational program, follow your interests. Be willing to experiment by taking classes and by getting experience as a volunteer worker.

• Be willing to seek information about careers in mental health from others, such as professionals in the field and faculty members, but realize that ultimately you will decide which career path is best for you.

• Do not consider the selection of a career as a one-time event. Instead, allow yourself to entertain many job possibilities over your lifetime.

• Realize that you must have a beginning to your career. Be patient, and allow yourself time to feel comfortable in the role of helper. You don't have to be the perfect person or the perfect helper.

• Your career as a professional helper can be highly beneficial to you personally. In very few other kinds of work do you have as many opportunities to reflect on the quality of your own life and have opportunities to make a significant difference in the lives of others.

What Will You Do Now?

After each chapter review, we provide concrete suggestions you can put into action. These suggested activities grow out of the major points developed in the chapter. Once you have read the chapter, we hope you will find some way to develop an action program. If you commit yourself to doing even one of these activities for each chapter, you will become more actively involved in your own learning.

1. If you are an undergraduate and think you would like to pursue a graduate program, select at least one graduate school to visit and talk with faculty members and students. If you are in a graduate program, contact several community agencies or attend a professional conference to determine what kinds of positions will be available to you. If you have an interest in obtaining a professional license, contact the appropriate board early in your program to obtain information on the requirements.

2. Ask a helper whom you know about his or her motivations for becoming a helper and for remaining in the profession. What does this person get out of helping clients?

3. Conduct an interview with a mental health professional who works in a position similar to the one you hope to obtain. Before the interview, develop a list of questions that you are interested in exploring. Write up the salient points of your interview, and share the results in your class.

4. The career-guidance center in your college or university probably offers several computer-based programs to help you decide on a career. If you are interested in a more comprehensive self-assessment that describes the relationship between your personality type and possible occupations or fields of study, we strongly recommend that you take the *Self-Directed Search* (SDS), which is available online at Psychological Assessment Resources (www.self-directed-search.com). The SDS takes 20 to 30 minutes to complete and costs $9.95. Your personalized report will appear on your screen.

5. Create your own activity or project (for this chapter or any of the chapters to follow). Find some ways to get involved by taking action. Think of ways you can apply what you read to yourself. Decide on something specific, a step you can take now, that will help you get actively engaged in a positive endeavor. After reading this chapter, for example, you could decide to reflect on your own needs and motives for considering a career in the helping professions. Review some significant turning points in your life that might have contributed to your desire to become a helper.

6. If you are in a training program, now is an ideal time to get involved in professional organizations. Become an active student member in at least one of the organizations described in this chapter. By joining an organization, you can take advantage of its workshops and conferences. Membership also puts you in touch with other professionals with similar interests, gives you ideas for updating your skills, and helps you make excellent contacts.

7. We cannot stress enough the value of keeping a journal as an adjunct to reading this book and taking this course. Write in your journal in a free-flowing and unedited style. Be honest, and use journal writing as an opportunity to get to know yourself better, to clarify your thinking on issues raised in each chapter, and to explore your thoughts and feelings about working in

the helping professions. At the end of each chapter, we will provide a few suggestions of topics for you to reflect on and include in your journal writing. For this chapter, consider these areas:

- Write about your main motives for wanting to become a helper. How do you expect your needs to be satisfied through your work?
- Write about factors that have influenced your conception of what it means to be a helper. Who are your role models? What kind of help did you receive?
- Spend some time thinking about the attributes of the ideal helper. What are your personal strengths that could enable you to become a more effective helper? How can you determine how realistic your expectations are about the profession you want to enter?
- What are your thoughts about selecting an educational and professional route to pursue? Write about your work values that you might consider in choosing a career path.

8. Attend a professional state, regional, or national conference offered by one of the various professional organizations. Attending as a student has numerous benefits, such as developing a network for jobs, field placements, and meeting colleagues with similar interests.

9. Bring your completed self-assessment inventory to class to compare your views with those of others in the class. Such a comparison might stimulate some debate and help get the class involved in the topics to be discussed. In choosing the issues you want to discuss in class, circle the numbers of those items that you felt most strongly about as you were responding. You may find it instructive to ask others how they responded to these items in particular.

10. At the end of each chapter we provide some suggestions for further reading. For the full bibliographic entry for each of the sources listed, consult the *References* section at the back of the book. For a discussion on a wide array of issues confronting those in the helping professions, see Kottler (1993, 1997, 2000a) and Kottler and Jones (2003). For comprehensive coverage of topics such as development of a professional identity, ethical standards, basic process skills, approaches to counseling, and the making of a professional counselor, see Hazler and Kottler (2005), Neukrug (2007), and Nystul (2006). For wisdom on a variety of topics for new counselors, see Gladding (2009) and Yalom (2003). For accounts of professional journeys of various counselor educators and practitioners, see Conyne and Bemak (2005).

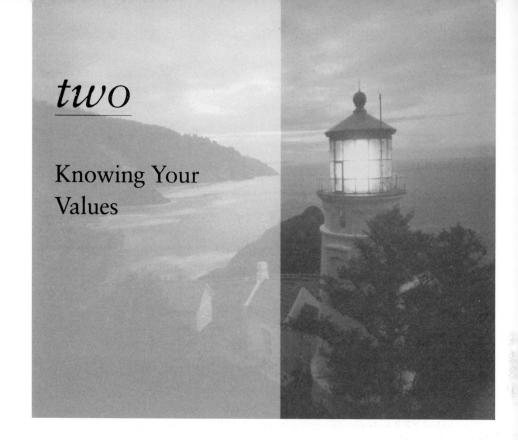

two

Knowing Your Values

Focus Questions

1. To what degree are you aware of your core values and how they could affect the way you work with clients?

2. Is it possible to interact with clients without making value judgments? Do you think it is ever appropriate to make value judgments? If so, when?

3. Can you be true to your own values and at the same time make allowances for your clients to make their own choices, even if they differ from yours?

4. Do you tend to try to influence your friends and family regarding "right" choices? If so, what are the implications for the way you are likely to function as a helper?

5. What distinctions do you see between exposing your values and imposing them?

6. To what extent can you give clients the latitude to make their own decisions, even if you believe they would be better served by following a different path?

7. How can you best determine whether a conflict between your values and those of a client dictates a referral to another professional?

8. When you become aware of difficulties in working with clients because of value differences, what course of action would you take?

9. What are the key values that you see as being an essential part of the helping process? How would you communicate such values to your clients?

Aim of the Chapter

This chapter is designed to help you clarify your values and identify how they are likely to influence your work as a helper. Toward this end, we explore how values operate in helping relationships. To assist you in clarifying your values and identifying ways in which they might interfere with effective helping, we describe practical situations in which you may find yourself.

Conflicts between clients and helpers often surface in discussions supported by values involving culture, sexual orientation, family, gender-role behaviors, religion and spirituality, abortion, sexuality, and end-of-life decisions. Value issues pertaining to multicultural populations are of special importance and we devote Chapter 7 to this subject.

The Role of Values in Helping

Values are embedded in therapeutic theory and practice. A national survey of the mental health values of practitioners found a consensus that certain basic values are important for maintaining mentally healthy lifestyles and for guiding and evaluating the course of treatment (Jensen & Bergin, 1988). These values include assuming responsibility for one's actions; developing effective strategies for coping with stress; developing the ability to give and receive affection; being sensitive to the feelings of others; practicing self-control; having a sense of purpose for living; being open, honest, and genuine; finding satisfaction in one's work; having a sense of identity and feelings of worth; being skilled in interpersonal relationships, sensitivity, and nurturance; being committed to marriage, family, and other relationships; having deepened self-awareness and motivation for growth; and practicing good habits of physical health. These are some of the values on which helping relationships are based.

Complete the following self-inventory as a way of focusing your thinking on the role your values will play in your work. As you read each statement, decide the degree to which it most closely identifies your attitudes and beliefs about *your role as a helper.* Use this code:

3 = This statement is true for me.
2 = This statement is not true for me.
1 = I am undecided.

____ 1. I believe it is my task to challenge a client's philosophy of life.
____ 2. I could work objectively and effectively with clients who have values that differ sharply from my own.
____ 3. I believe it is both possible and desirable for me to remain neutral with respect to values when working with clients.
____ 4. Although I have a clear set of values for myself, I feel quite certain that I could avoid unduly influencing my clients to adopt my beliefs.
____ 5. It is appropriate to express my views and expose my values as long as I don't impose them on clients.

____ 6. I might be inclined to subtly influence my clients to consider some of my values.

____ 7. If I discovered sharp value conflicts between a client and myself, I should refer the person.

____ 8. I have certain spiritual and religious views that would influence the way I work.

____ 9. I would not have any difficulty counseling a pregnant adolescent who wanted to explore abortion as one of her alternatives.

____ 10. I have certain views pertaining to gender roles that might affect the way I counsel.

____ 11. I would not have problems counseling a gay couple.

____ 12. I see the clarification of values as a crucial task in the helping process.

____ 13. My view of family life would influence the way I would counsel a couple considering divorce.

____ 14. I would have no trouble working with a woman (man) who wanted to leave her (his) children and live alone, if this is what my client decided.

____ 15. I have generally been willing to challenge my values.

____ 16. I might be willing to work in individual counseling with a client who is in a committed relationship and is having an affair, even if the client is not willing to disclose the relationship to his or her partner.

____ 17. I feel quite certain that my values will never interfere with my capacity to remain objective.

____ 18. I think I will work best with clients who have values similar to mine.

____ 19. I think it is appropriate to pray with my clients during a session if they request this of me.

____ 20. I could work effectively with a person with AIDS who contracted the disease through IV drug use or unprotected sex.

There are no "right" or "wrong" answers to these statements. The inventory is designed to help you think about how your values are likely to influence the way you carry out your functions as a helper. Select a few specific items that catch your attention, and talk with a fellow student about your views. As you read the rest of the chapter, assume an active stance, and think about your position on the value issues we raise.

Exposing Versus Imposing Values

The clients with whom you work ultimately have the responsibility of choosing what values to adopt, what values to modify or discard, and what direction their lives will take. Through the helping process, clients can learn to examine values before making choices. At times it may be appropriate to engage in a discussion with a client that includes revealing certain of your own values. Before you do so, ask yourself these questions: "Why am I disclosing and discussing my values with my client? How will doing so benefit my client? How vulnerable is my client to being unduly influenced by me? Is my client too eager to embrace my value system?" If you do disclose your values, it is critical that you assess the impact this might have on your client. It is important that you avoid disclosing a particular value you hold as a way to steer your client toward accepting a value orientation you hold. Reveal your values in a way that does not communicate, either directly or indirectly, that the client should adopt them.

At times, you may not agree with the values of your clients, but it is essential that you respect the rights of your clients to hold a different set of values and embrace a different worldview. Richards, Rector, and Tjeltveit (1999) do not think helpers should attempt to teach their clients specific moral rules and values because doing so violates clients' uniqueness and prevents clients from making their own choices.

Even if you think it is inappropriate to impose your values on clients, you may unintentionally influence them in subtle ways to subscribe to your values. If you are strongly opposed to abortion, for example, you may not respect your client's right to believe differently. On the basis of such convictions, you may subtly (or not so subtly) direct your client toward choices other than abortion. Indeed, some researchers have found evidence that clients tend to change in ways that are consistent with the values of their counselors, and clients often adopt the values of their counselors (Zinnbauer & Pargament, 2000). It is now generally recognized that the therapeutic endeavor is a value-laden process and that all counselors, to some degree, communicate their values to clients, whether intentionally or not (Richards & Bergin, 2005). Thus, it is essential that you take into consideration the ways you may influence your clients.

Some well-intentioned practitioners think their task is to help people conform to acceptable and absolute value standards. It is no easy task to avoid communicating your values to your clients, even if you do not explicitly share them. What you pay attention to during counseling sessions will direct what your clients choose to explore. The methods you use will provide them with clues to what you value. Your nonverbal messages give them indications of when you like or dislike what they are doing. Because your clients may feel a need to have your approval, they may respond to these clues by acting in ways to meet your expectations instead of developing their own inner direction.

There should be very few instances where you would have to tell clients that you could not work with them because you do not agree with their value system. Your task is not to judge your clients' values but to help them explore and clarify their beliefs and apply them to solving their own problems. The American Counseling Association (2005) states this clearly: "Counselors are aware of their own values, attitudes, beliefs, and behaviors and avoid imposing values that are inconsistent with counseling goals"(A.4.b.). Helpers need to be aware of how their personal values can influence many aspects of their professional work.

Our Perspective on Values in the Helping Relationship

In our view it is neither possible nor desirable for helpers to remain neutral or to keep their values separate from their professional relationships. From an ethical perspective, it is imperative that helpers recognize the impact their values have on the way they work with clients and that they learn the difference between imposing and exposing values. If you pay attention to your clients and why they are coming to see you, you will have a basis for inviting a discussion on how values influence your clients' behaviors.

There are certainly helpers who do not agree with our position about the role of values. At one extreme are those who see helping as very much a process of social influence. Some helpers, for example, have definite and absolute value systems, and they believe it is their function to influence their clients to adopt these values. At the other extreme are helpers who are so overly concerned about unduly influencing their clients that they strive for neutrality. Out of fear that their views might contaminate the client's decision making process, these helpers make it a practice never to verbally communicate their values to their clients.

Our position is that the helper's main task is to provide those who seek aid with the impetus needed to look at what they are doing, determine the degree to which what they are doing is consistent with their values, and consider whether their current behavior is meeting their needs. If clients conclude that their lives are not fulfilled, they can use the helping relationship to reexamine and modify their values or their actions, and they can explore a range of options that are open to them. Clients must determine what they are willing to change and the ways they may want to modify their behavior.

Dealing With Value Conflicts

When you find yourself struggling with an ethical dilemma over value differences, the best course to follow is to seek consultation. Supervision is a useful way to explore value clashes with clients. After exploring the issues in supervision, if you find that you are still not able to work effectively with a client, the ethical course of action could be to refer the client to another professional.

Although we may have a conflict of values with a client, this does not necessarily imply the need for a referral, for it is possible to work through a conflict successfully. You must determine what it is about a client or a particular value difference that prompts you to want to make the referral. Before making a referral, explore your part of the difficulty through consultation. What barriers within you would prevent you from working with a client who has a different value system? Why is it necessary that you and your client have a common set of values? Why is it a requirement that your clients accept your values in a particular area of living?

If you find it necessary to make a referral because of value conflicts, *how* the referral is discussed with the client is crucial. Make it clear to the client that it is *your* problem as the helper, not the client's problem. In short, if you feel a need to refer a client, the problem is likely to reside more in *you* than in a particular client. Do not be too quick to refer and consider a referral only as the last resort.

In the remainder of this chapter, we consider some value-laden issues that you might encounter in your work with a range of client populations. These areas include concerns of lesbian, gay, and bisexual individuals; family values issues; gender-role identity issues; religious and spiritual values; abortion; sexuality; and end-of-life decisions.

Lesbian, Gay, and Bisexual Issues

The concept of human diversity encompasses more than racial and ethnic factors; it encompasses all forms of oppression, discrimination, and prejudice, including those directed toward age, gender, religious affiliation, and sexual orientation. Working with lesbian, gay, and bisexual (LGB) individuals often presents a challenge to helpers who hold conservative values. Many helpers have blind spots, biases, negative attitudes, stereotypes, and misconceptions about lesbian, gay, and bisexual issues. Negative personal reactions, limited empathy, and lack of understanding are common characteristics in practitioners who work with LGB clients (Schreier, Davis, & Rodolfa, 2005). Helping professionals who have negative reactions to homosexuality are likely to impose their own values and attitudes, or at least to convey strong disapproval.

To work effectively with this client population, it is essential that you begin by critically examining your own attitudes, biases, and assumptions about specific sexual orientations. Identify and examine any myths and misconceptions you might hold, and understand how your values and possible biases regarding sexual orientation are likely to affect your work.

Imagine you are counseling a man who is gay and wants to talk about his relationship with his lover and the difficulties they have communicating with each other. As you work with him, you become aware that it is difficult for you to accept his sexual orientation. You find yourself challenging him about this rather than concentrating on what he wants to work on. You are so focused on his sexual orientation, which goes against what you think is morally right, that you and your client both recognize that you are not helping him. What steps could you take in addressing these value differences? Are you willing to explore the impact of your values on your interventions with this man who is gay?

Case example: Confronting loneliness and isolation. Consider how your values are likely to influence the way in which you would work with Art, a 33-year-old gay man. You are doing an intake interview with Art, who tells you that he is coming to counseling because he often feels lonely and isolated. He has difficulty in intimate relationships with both men and women. Once people get to know him, Art feels they will not accept him and somehow won't like him. During the interview, you discover that Art has a lot of pain regarding his father, with whom he has very little contact. He would like a closer relationship with his father, but being gay stands in the way. His father has let him know that he feels guilty that Art "turned out that way." He just cannot understand why Art is not "normal" and why he can't find a woman and get married like his brother. Art mainly wants to work on his relationship with his father, and he also wants to overcome his fear of rejection by others with whom he would like a close relationship. He tells you that he would like those he cares about to accept him as he is.

Your stance. What are your initial reactions to Art's situation? Considering your own values, do you expect that you would have any trouble establishing a therapeutic relationship with him? In light of the fact that he lets you know that he does not want to explore his sexual orientation, would you be able to respect this decision? As you think about how you would proceed with Art, reflect on your own attitudes toward gay men. Think especially about whether you might be inclined to impose any of your values, regardless of your stance. For example, if you have personal difficulty in accepting homosexuality on moral or other grounds, would you encourage Art to become heterosexual? Think about some of the issues you might focus on in your counseling sessions with Art: his fear of rejection, pain with his father, desire for his father to be different, difficulty in getting close to both men and women, sexual orientation, and values. With the information you have, which of these areas are you likely to emphasize? Are there other areas you would like to explore with Art?

Discussion. Lasser and Gottlieb (2004) identify sexual orientation as one of the most chronic and vexing moral debates plaguing our culture. They state that many people believe that homosexual or bisexual behavior is morally wrong. Many lesbian, gay, and bisexual (LGB) individuals have internalized such views, and some are significantly troubled regarding their sexual orientation. Lasser and Gottlieb add that therapists are faced with various clinical and ethical issues in working with LGB clients. One of these ethical issues involves therapists confronting their own values regarding homosexual-bisexual desire and behavior. Schreier, Davis, and Rodolfa (2005) remind us that no one is exempt from the influence of negative societal stereotyping, prejudice, and even hatefulness toward LGB people. Furthermore, many LGB people internalize these negative societal messages and experience psychological pain and conflict because of this. This is especially true of lesbian, gay, and bisexual people of color, who must cope with one or more forms of prejudice and discrimination from several places in their lives (Ferguson, 2009).

You may tell yourself and others that you accept the right of others to live their lives as they see fit, yet you may have trouble when you are in an actual encounter with a client. There could be a gap between what you can intellectually accept and what you can emotionally accept. If your value system is in conflict with accepting lesbian, gay, and bisexual people, you will likely find it difficult to work effectively with them.

Homosexuality and bisexuality were assumed to be a form of mental illness for more than a century. In 1973 the American Psychiatric Association stopped labeling **homosexuality**—a sexual orientation in which people seek emotional and sexual relationships with same-gendered individuals—as a form of mental illness. Today all major American mental health professional associations have affirmed that homosexuality is not a mental illness, and the American Psychological Association's Division 44 (2000) has developed a set of guidelines for working with lesbian, gay, and bisexual clients. But bias and misinformation about homosexuality and bisexuality continue to be widespread in society, and many lesbian, gay, and bisexual people face social stigmatization, discrimination, and violence, sometimes from therapists. Practitioners should familiarize themselves with the ways in which prejudice, discrimination, and multiple forms of oppression are manifested in society toward LGB people and explore with their clients how this affects their lives (Ferguson, 2009). Oftentimes families of origin are unprepared to accept a lesbian, gay, or bisexual family member because of familial, ethnic, cultural, societal, or religious beliefs. Families may need assistance in developing new understandings of sexual orientation (APA, Division 44, 2000).

Helpers who work with lesbian, gay, and bisexual people are ethically obligated not to allow their personal values to intrude into their professional work. Note that the ethics codes of the ACA (2005), the APA (2002), the AAMFT (2001a), the Canadian Counselling Association ([CCA], 2007), and the NASW (2008) clearly state that **discrimination,** or behaving differently and usually unfairly toward a specific group of people, is unethical and unacceptable. From an ethical perspective, practitioners must become aware of their personal prejudices and biases regarding sexual orientation. This is particularly important when a client discloses his or her sexual orientation after the helping relationship is firmly established. In such situations judgmental attitudes on the part of the helper can seriously harm the client.

The Association for Lesbian, Gay, Bisexual and Transgender Issues in Counseling (ALGBTIC, 2008) recognizes that helping professionals need to be well versed in understanding the unique needs of this diverse population. ALGBTIC has developed a set of specific competencies for trainees (available on their website) to help them examine their personal biases and values regarding lesbian, gay, bisexual, and transgender individuals. Helpers who acquire these competencies are in a position to implement appropriate intervention strategies that ensure effective service delivery to this client population.

If you do not have the knowledge and skills to work with lesbian, gay, and bisexual clients, take advantage of continuing-education workshops in acquiring competence in this area. If you do not possess knowledge and training about a specific group, ethically you are required to seek supervision and consultation before counseling these clients.

You might well be unaware of your client's sexual orientation until the therapeutic relationship develops. If you expect to provide services in a community agency with diverse client populations, you need to have a clear idea of your own values relative to issues associated with sexual orientation. As a way of clarifying your values pertaining to homosexuality, complete the following inventory, using this code:

3 = I agree, in most respects, with this statement.
2 = I am undecided in my opinion about this statement.
1 = I disagree, in most respects, with this statement.

_____ 1. Lesbian, gay, and bisexual clients are best served by lesbian, gay, and bisexual helpers.
_____ 2. A counselor who is homosexual or bisexual is likely to push his or her values on a heterosexual client.
_____ 3. I would have trouble working with either a gay male couple or a lesbian couple who wanted to adopt children.
_____ 4. Homosexuality and bisexuality are both abnormal and immoral.

_____ 5. A lesbian, gay, bisexual, or transgendered person can be as well adjusted (or poorly adjusted) as a heterosexual person.

_____ 6. I would have no difficulty being objective in counseling lesbian, gay, bisexual, or transgendered clients.

_____ 7. I have adequate information about referral sources in the local gay community.

_____ 8. I feel a need for specialized training and knowledge before I can effectively counsel lesbian, gay, bisexual, and transgendered clients.

_____ 9. I expect that I would have no difficulty conducting family therapy if the father were gay.

_____ 10. I think that lesbian, gay, bisexual, and transgendered people of color are subject to multiple forms of oppression.

After you finish the inventory, look over your responses to identify any patterns. Are there any attitudes that you want to change? Are there any areas of information or skills that you are willing to acquire?

Family Values

Values pertaining to marriage, the preservation of the family, divorce, traditional and nontraditional lifestyles, gender roles and the division of responsibility in the family, child rearing, and extramarital affairs can all influence the helper's interventions. The value system of helpers has a crucial influence on the formulation and definition of the problems they see in a family, the goals and plans for therapy, and the direction the therapy takes. Helpers may take sides with one member of the family against another; they may impose their values on family members; or they may be more committed to keeping the family intact than are the family members themselves. Helpers who, intentionally or unintentionally, impose their values on a couple or a family can do considerable harm. Consider the following case examples.

Case example: Counseling a dissatisfied mother. Veronika has lived a restricted life. She got married at 17, had four children by the age of 22, and is now going back to college at age 32. She is a good student—excited, eager to learn, and discovering all that she missed. She finds that she is attracted to a younger peer group and to professors. She is experiencing her "second adolescence," and she is getting a lot of affirmation that she did not have before. At home she feels unappreciated, and the members of her family are mostly interested in what she can do for them. At school she is special and is respected for her intellect.

Ultimately, Veronika becomes involved in an affair with a younger man. She is close to a decision to leave her husband and her four children, ages 10 to 15. Veronika comes to see you at the university counseling center and is in turmoil over what to do. She wants to find some way to deal with her guilt and ambivalence.

Your stance. How do you react to Veronika leaving her husband and her four children? Would you encourage her to follow her inclinations? If Veronika gave this matter considerable thought and then told you that, as painful as it would be for her, she needed to leave her family, would you be inclined to encourage her to bring her entire family in for some counseling sessions? For a moment, consider your own value system. What values might you impose, if any? If Veronika said that she was leaning toward staying married and at home, even though she would be resentful, what interventions might you make? If you had been left yourself, either as a child or by a spouse, how might this experience affect you in working with Veronika?

Case example: A family in crisis. A wife, husband, and three adolescent children come to your office. The family was referred by the youngest boy's child welfare and attendance officer. The boy is acting out by stealing and is viewed as the problem person in the family.

The husband is in your office reluctantly. He appears angry and resistant, and he lets you know that he doesn't believe in this "therapy stuff." He makes excuses for the boy and says he doesn't see that there is much of a problem, either in the marriage or in the family.

The wife tells you that she and her husband fight a lot, that there is much tension in the home, and that the children are suffering. She is fearful and says that she is afraid of what might happen to her family. She has no way of supporting herself and her three children and is willing to work on the relationship.

Your stance. How would you be affected by this family? What course of action would you take? How would your values pertaining to family life influence your interventions with this family? Would you expose your own values in this case, even if the family members did not ask you? If they asked you what you thought of their situation and what you thought they should do, what would you say?

Discussion. Even if you do not impose your values in working with this family in crisis, what you say to each family member is likely to be influenced by your core values. For instance, if you believe that the wife should be assertive with her husband in this situation, you might encourage her to challenge him and possibly risk losing the relationship.

Case example: Confronting infidelity. A couple seeks your services for marital counseling. The husband has confessed to his wife that he is having an affair, and the incident has precipitated the most recent crisis in their relationship. Although the wife is highly distraught, she wants to stay married. She realizes that their marriage needs work and that there is a lack of emotional connection between the two of them, but thinks it is worth saving. They have children, and the family is well respected and liked in the community.

The husband wants to leave, yet he is struggling with conflicting feelings and is not sure what to do. He is very confused and says he still loves his wife and children. He is aware that he is going through some kind of midlife crisis, and each day he comes up with a different decision. His wife is in great pain and feels desperate. She has been dependent on him and has no means of support for herself.

Your stance. What are your values pertaining to affairs in a marriage or a committed relationship? What would you want to say to the wife? to the husband? Should a helper counsel a couple to stay together or get divorced? In thinking about the direction you might pursue with this family, consider whether you have ever been in this situation yourself in your own family. If so, how do you think this experience would affect the way you worked with the couple? If the husband said he was confused, desperately wanted an answer, and was hoping that you would point him in some direction, would you be inclined to tell him what he should do?

Gender-Role Identity Issues

All helpers need to be aware of their values and beliefs about gender. Helpers who work with couples and families can practice more ethically if they are aware of the history and impact of gender stereotyping as it is reflected in the social-ization process in families, including their own. The way people perceive gender has a great deal to do with their cultural background. You can become a more effective practitioner if you are willing to evaluate your beliefs about appropri-ate family roles and responsibilities, child-rearing practices, multiple roles, and nontraditional careers for women and men. You will be challenged to be cultur-ally sensitive, gender sensitive, and to avoid imposing your personal values on individuals, couples, and families.

Case example: Working mother or homemaker? John and Emma recently entered couples therapy for help resolving conflict over Emma's recent return to work after several years as a full-time mother and homemaker. Both report that they "argue a lot about this issue." John states that he prefers to have Emma stay home full time and care for their two young children and the household responsibilities. Emma reports feeling happier when she works part time and contributes financially to the family. It also allows them to hire extra help for household tasks and child care. She loves her work and the social interactions with her colleagues and does not want to give it up. John believes mothers are better for children than babysitters, and because he has the greater earning capacity, Emma should be the one to stay home. Emma states her perception that it is more important for children to have a happy mother than a full-time mother, and her desire to have an outside work interest above and beyond her family should not be tied to income. Both John and Emma are very invested in their relationship, but they can't get past this hurdle.

Your stance. How would your own personal values regarding parenting and gender roles influence your assessment and approach to working with John and Emma? What are the ethical boundaries regarding the therapist's values in such a case? How do you avoid imposing your own beliefs and persuading or direct-ing this couple?

Discussion. If you had strong personal values about gender roles in mar-riage and family, it might be easy for you to impose your own values in this case. For instance, a belief that women should have choices and not be bound by tra-ditional family roles might lead you to align with Emma and try to persuade or convince John of this. Conversely, a view that children should have a mother at home versus another caregiver may lead you to try to convince Emma she needs to be home and to abandon her own personal goals, resulting in alignment with

John. As a couple's therapist, it is unethical for the therapist to determine the goals of the individuals involved, with the exceptions of abuse and danger. Alignment, collusion, and triangulation are all unhealthy possible outcomes when imposing our own values, and they could clearly cause more harm than good to the marriage in this case.

Case example: Parenting in a traditional family. Fernando and Elizabeth describe themselves as a "traditional couple." They are in marriage counseling with you to work on the strains in their relationship arising from rearing their two adolescent sons. The couple talk a lot about their sons. Both Elizabeth and Fernando work full time outside the home. Besides working as a school principal, Elizabeth has another full-time job as mother and homemaker. Fernando says he is not about to do any "women's work" around the house. Elizabeth has never really given much thought to the fact that she has a dual career. Neither Elizabeth nor Fernando shows a great deal of interest in examining the cultural values and stereotypes that they have incorporated. Each of them has a definite idea of what women and men "should be." Rather than talking about their relationship or the distribution of tasks at home, they focus their attention on troubles with their sons. Elizabeth wants advice on how to deal with their problems.

Your stance. If you become aware of the tension within this couple over traditional gender roles, will you call it to their attention in your counseling with them? Do you see it as your job to challenge Fernando on his traditional views? Do you see it as your job to encourage Elizabeth to want more balance of responsibilities in their relationship? If you were counseling this couple, what do you think you would say to each of them? How would your values influence the direction in which you might go? What bearing would your own gender-role conditioning and your own views have on what you did?

Discussion. If you will be working with couples and families, it is essential that you appreciate the fact that gender-role stereotypes serve a purpose and are not easily modified. As a helper, your role is to guide your clients in the process of examining their gender-role attitudes and behaviors if doing so is relevant to the problem for which they are seeking your services. Effective communication between you and your clients can be undermined by stereotypical views about how women and men think, feel, and behave. You need to be alert to the particular issues women and men struggle with and the ways their own views about gender keep them locked in traditional roles. You can offer assistance to both female and male clients in exploring and evaluating cultural messages they received about gender-role expectations. Without deciding what changes they should make, you can facilitate awareness on the part of your clients, which can open up new possibilities for making self-directed choices.

Margolin (1982) provides some recommendations on how to be a nonsexist family therapist and how to confront negative expectations and stereotyped roles in the family. One suggestion is that helpers should examine their own behavior and attitudes that would imply sex-differentiated roles and status. For example, helpers can show their bias in subtle ways by looking at the husband when talking about making decisions and looking at the wife when talking about home matters and rearing children. Margolin also contends that practitioners are especially vulnerable to the following biases: (1) assuming that remaining married would be the best choice for a woman, (2) demonstrating less interest in a woman's career than in a man's career, (3) encouraging couples to accept the belief that child rearing is solely the responsibility of the mother, (4) showing a different reaction to a wife's affair than to a husband's, and (5) giving more importance to satisfying the husband's needs than to satisfying the wife's needs. Margolin raises two critical questions for those who work with couples and families:

- How does the counselor respond when members of the family seem to agree that they want to work toward goals that (from the counselor's vantage point) are sexist in nature?
- To what extent does the helper accept the family's definition of gender-role identities rather than trying to challenge and eventually change these attitudes?

Religious and Spiritual Values

Effective helping addresses the body, mind, and spirit, but the helping professions have been slow to recognize spiritual and religious concerns. Helpers routinely address a range of sensitive topics in a client's life, including questions about race and sexuality, yet they may not inquire about the influence and meaning of spirituality and religion in an individual's life (Hage, 2006). Spirituality has received increasing attention in the literature since the 1970s, and these concerns are being addressed more often now in both assessment and treatment (Hall, Dixon, & Mauzey, 2004; Sperry & Shafranske, 2005). Religion and spirituality are oftentimes part of the client's problem, and they can also be part of the client's solution to a problem.

Religious faith or some form of personal spirituality is a critical source of strength for many clients. If helpers do not raise the issue of how spirituality influences clients, their clients may assume that such matters are not relevant in the helping relationship. However, religious faith can be a source for finding meaning in life and can be instrumental in promoting healing and well-being. For some, religion does not occupy a key place, yet personal spirituality may be a central force. Spiritual values help many people make sense out of the universe and the purpose of their lives. According to Francis (2009), spirituality can be viewed within the context of a person's search for an ultimate meaning and place in the world. This search may include a relationship that is developed with a transcendent or divine power beyond oneself. Because spiritual and religious values can play a major part in human life, these values should be viewed as a potential resource in the helping relationship rather than as something to be ignored (Harper & Gill, 2005). Exploring spiritual values with clients can be integrated with other therapeutic tools to enhance the helping process.

In clarifying your values pertaining to religion and counseling, consider these questions: Does an exploration of religion belong in formal helping relationships? Is the helping process complete without a spiritual dimension? If a client's religious needs arise in the therapeutic relationship, is it appropriate to deal with them? Are helpers pushing their values on their clients when they decide what topics can and cannot be discussed in counseling? Do you have to hold the same religious beliefs, or any beliefs at all, to work effectively with clients who have religious struggles?

Case example: Finding comfort in spirituality. Peter has definite ideas about right and wrong; sin, guilt, and damnation; and he has accepted the teachings of his fundamentalist faith. When he encountered difficulties and problems in the past, he was able to pray and find comfort in his relationship with his God. Lately, however, he has been suffering from chronic depression, an inability to sleep, extreme feelings of guilt, and an overwhelming sense of doom that God is going to punish him for his transgressions. He consulted his physician and asked for medication to help him sleep better. The physician and his minister both suggested that he seek counseling. At first Peter resisted this idea because he strongly felt that he should find comfort in his religion. With the continuation of his bouts of depression and sleeplessness, he hesitantly comes to you for counseling.

He requests that you open the session with a prayer so that he can get into a proper spiritual frame of mind. He also quotes you a verse from the Bible that has special meaning to him. He tells you about his doubts about seeing you for counseling, and he is concerned that you will not accept his religious convictions, which he sees as being at the center of his life. He inquires about your religious beliefs.

Your stance. Would you have any trouble counseling Peter? He is struggling with trusting you and with seeing the value in counseling. What are your reactions to some of his specific views, especially those pertaining to his fear of punishment? Do you have reactions to his strong fundamentalist beliefs? If you have definite disagreements with his beliefs, would that be an obstacle to working with him? Would you challenge him to think for himself and do what he thinks is right?

Assume that you have a religious orientation, yet you believe in a God who loves whereas Peter believes in a God he fears. You discuss the differences in the way the two of you perceive religion. Yet you also say that you want to explore with him how well his religious beliefs are serving him in his life and also examine possible connections between some of his beliefs and how they are contributing to his symptoms. With these assumptions, do you think you could be helpful to Peter? Would you accept him as a client? Now assume that you don't share any of Peter's religious values, that you are intolerant of fundamentalist beliefs, and that you see such beliefs as being the source of his problems. Given these values, would you accept a client like Peter? Would you be able to work with him objectively, or would you try to find ways to sway him to give up his view of the world?

Discussion. Counselors are increasingly recognizing the importance of incorporating a client's spiritual and religious beliefs into both assessment and treatment (Hall, Dixon, & Mauzey, 2004). Attention to spirituality can be part of an integrated and holistic effort to help clients resolve conflicts and improve health, as well as to find meaning in life (Shafranske & Sperry, 2005). A competent and thorough assessment of a client's spiritual domain can provide the necessary background to inform case conceptualization and treatment planning (Harper & Gill, 2005).

The beliefs, values, and faith systems of clients are often sources of support in difficult times, and they can be used by the counselor to help the client in the healing process (Francis, 2009). If helpers are to effectively give attention to a client's spiritual and religious concerns, however, it is essential for them to be clear about their own spiritual and religious beliefs, or lack thereof. Ethical practice requires that you avoid indoctrinating clients with a particular set of spiritual or religious values. You have an ethical responsibility to be aware of how your beliefs affect your work and to make sure you do not unduly influence your clients.

Even if spiritual and religious issues are not the focus of a client's concern, these values may enter into the sessions indirectly as the client explores moral conflicts or grapples with questions of meaning in life. Can you keep your spiritual and religious values out of these sessions? How do you think they will influence the way you counsel? If you have little belief in spirituality or are hostile to organized religions, can you be nonjudgmental? Can you empathize with clients who view themselves as being deeply spiritual or who feel committed to the teachings of a particular church?

As you think over your own position on the place of spiritual and religious values in the helping relationship, reflect on these questions:

- Is it appropriate to deal with religious issues in an open and forthright manner as clients' needs are presented in the helping process?
- Do clients have the right to explore their religious concerns in the context of the helping process?
- If you have no religious or spiritual commitment, how could this hinder or help you in working with diverse clients?
- Are you willing to refer a client to a rabbi, minister, or priest if it appears that the client has questions you are not qualified to answer?

Case study: Counseling and spirituality. Guiza is a student intern who feels deeply committed to spirituality and also claims that her religious faith guides her in finding meaning in life. She does not want to impose her values on her clients, but she does feel it is essential to at least make a general assessment of clients' spiritual/religious beliefs and experiences during the intake session. One of her clients, Alejandro, tells Guiza that he is depressed most of the time and feels a sense of emptiness. He wonders about the meaning of his life. In Guiza's assessment of Alejandro, she finds that he grew up without any kind of spiritual or religious guidance in his home, and he states that he is agnostic. He never has explored either religion or spirituality; these ideas seem too abstract to help with the practical problems of everyday living. Guiza becomes aware that she is strongly inclined to suggest to Alejandro that he open up to spiritual ways of thinking, especially because of his stated problem with finding meaning in his life. Guiza is tempted to suggest that Alejandro at least go to a few church services to see if he might find any meaning in doing so. She brings her struggle to her supervisor.

Your stance. Consider Guiza's situation as you reflect on how your values can influence your approach with clients. When, if ever, would you recommend to your client that he or she talk to a minister, priest, or rabbi? If you sought consultation from your supervisor, what key issues would you most want to explore and clarify? Could you maintain your objectivity? When would you consider suggesting a referral because of your problems with respect to the spiritual/religious beliefs and values of your client?

Discussion. You may experience conflicts in values with your clients in the spiritual realm. Holding a definite system of religious values is not a problem, but wanting your clients to adopt these values can be problematic. Without blatantly pushing your values, you might subtly persuade clients toward your religious beliefs or lead them in a direction you hope they will take. Conversely, if you do not place a high priority on spirituality and do not view religion as a salient force in your life, you may not be open to assessing your client's religious and spiritual beliefs.

In a national survey involving more than 1,000 clinical psychologists, Hathaway, Scott, and Garver (2004) found that the majority believes client religiousness and spirituality are important aspects of functioning. However, most of the clinical psychologists surveyed did not routinely incorporate spirituality into the assessment and treatment process. This omission could limit the effectiveness of the counseling venture.

Faiver and O'Brien (1993) have devised a form to assess the religious beliefs of clients for diagnostic, treatment, and referral purposes. They suggest that the assessment process can include questions pertaining to spiritual and religious issues as they are relevant to a client's presenting problems, questions about the roles religion and spirituality have played or currently play in a client's life, and questions about how spiritual/religious beliefs might be related to the client's cognitive, affective, and behavioral processes. Kelly (1995b) is in agreement with Faiver and O'Brien that a first step is to include the spiritual and religious dimensions as a regular part of the intake procedure and the early phase of the counseling process. Including questions pertaining to the client's spirituality and religion serves three purposes: (a) obtaining a preliminary indication of the relevance of spirituality and religion for the client, (b) gathering information that the helper might refer to at a later point in the helping process, and (c) indicating to the client that it is acceptable to talk about religious and spiritual concerns. If the client indicates concern about any religious beliefs or practices during the assessment process or later in counseling, this can be a useful focal point for exploration.

Case study: Resolving a value conflict. Yolanda is a devout Catholic. After a marriage of 25 years, her husband left her. She has now fallen in love with another man and very much wants a relationship with him. But because her religion does not recognize divorce, Yolanda feels guilty about her involvement with another man. She sees her situation as hopeless, and she cannot find a satisfactory solution. Living alone for the rest of her life scares her. But if she marries the man, she fears that her guilt feelings will eventually ruin the relationship.

Your stance. Consider these questions as a way to clarify how your values could affect your work with Yolanda. Do you know enough to inform Yolanda of the options available to her in terms of being remarried in a Catholic church? Would you recommend that Yolanda talk to a priest? Why or why not? If Yolanda asked you what she should do or what you think about her dilemma, how would you respond?

Discussion. There are many paths toward fulfilling spiritual needs, and it is not the helper's task to prescribe any particular pathway. However, we think it is the helper's responsibility to be aware that spirituality is a significant force for many clients. It is especially important for a practitioner to pursue spiritual concerns if the client initiates them. Practitioners need to be finely tuned to the client's story and to the purpose for which he or she sought professional assistance. It may also be important to have referral sources available for specific needs of clients.

Abortion

Helpers may experience a value clash with their clients on the issue of abortion. Clients who are exploring abortion as an option often present a challenge to helping professionals, both legally and ethically. From a legal perspective, mental health professionals are expected to exercise "reasonable care," and if they fail to do so, clients can take legal action against them for negligence. Millner and Hanks (2002) indicate that counselors can be charged with negligence when they (a) do not act with skill and withhold relevant information or provide inaccurate information, (b) do not refer a client, or (c) make an inadequate referral. For example, a counselor who makes a referral that supports his or her values rather than a referral in keeping with the client's values is vulnerable to a lawsuit. Stone (2002) takes the position that school counselors can discuss the topic of abortion with a student if the school board has not adopted a policy forbidding such a discussion. Stone adds that counselors who impose their values on a minor student are not acting in an appropriate, professional, or reasonable manner.

We suggest that you familiarize yourself with the legal requirements in your state that impinge on your work with clients, especially if you are in a position of working with minors who are considering an abortion. The matter of parental consent in working with minors varies from state to state. It is also important to know and apply the policies of the agency where you work.

Case study: Balancing contradictory advice. Connie, a 19-year-old college student, seeks your assistance because she is contemplating having an abortion. Some of the time she feels that abortion is the only answer; other times she feels that she wants to have the child. She is also considering the option of having her child and giving it up for adoption. Connie contemplates telling her parents but is afraid they would have a definite idea of what she should do. She is unable to sleep and feels guilty for putting herself into this situation. She has talked to friends and solicited their advice, and she has received many contradictory recommendations from them. Connie lets you know that she is not at all sure of what she should do and asks you to help her.

Your stance. With the information you have, what are some things you would say to Connie? Think about your values pertaining to abortion. Would you dissuade her from having an abortion and suggest other options? To what extent do you think you could keep your values out of this session? Sometimes we hear students say that they would refer a pregnant client who was considering an abortion to another professional because of their values. They would not like to sway the woman, and they fear that they could not remain objective. Does this apply to you? If a client in treatment with you for some time became pregnant and indicated she was considering getting an abortion, what would you do? Would you refer her at this point? What if she felt that you were abandoning her? Do you see any ethical or legal problems involved in your actions?

Sexuality

You may work with clients whose sexual values and behaviors differ sharply from your own. Ford and Hendrick (2003) conducted a study to assess therapists' sexual values for both themselves and their clients in the areas of premarital sex, casual sex, extramarital sex, open marriages, sexual orientation, and sex in adolescence and late adulthood. Their study also addressed how therapists deal with value conflicts as they arise in therapy.

Although helping professionals have personal values about sexual practices, the study found that when practitioners' beliefs conflict with those of clients, they appear to be able to avoid imposing their personal values on clients. However, 40% had to refer a client because of a value conflict. This research supports previous conclusions that the practice of therapy is not value free, particularly where sexual values are concerned. Those who participated in this survey indicated that they valued sex as an expression of love and commitment, fidelity, and monogamy in marital relationships and committed life partnerships.

Case study: Discussing sexuality in a sex-education program. You are working in a facility for adolescents and doing individual and group counseling. You discover that many young teenagers are sexually active and that a number of them have gotten pregnant. Abortion is common. Many of these young women keep their babies, whether they get married or do not. The agency director asks you to design a comprehensive education program for preventing unwanted pregnancy.

Your stance. In thinking about the kind of approach you would suggest, consider these questions: What are your values with respect to teenagers' being sexually active? What are your attitudes about providing detailed birth-control information to children and adolescents? How would your own values influence the design of your program?

Case study: Sex in a nursing home. You are working in a nursing home and discover that several of the unmarried older residents have sexual relationships.

At a staff meeting several workers complain that supervision is not tight enough and that sex between unmarried residents should not be permitted.

Your stance. What input would you want to have in this staff meeting? What are your thoughts about unmarried older people engaging in sex? How would your own values affect your recommendations to the staff?

Assessing your sexual values. Consider your values with respect to sexuality, as well as where you acquired them. How comfortable are you in discussing sexual issues with clients? Are you aware of any barriers that could prevent you from working with clients on sexual issues? How would your experiences in sexual relationships (or the lack of them) influence your work with clients in this area? Would you promote your sexual values? For example, if a teenage client was promiscuous and this behavior was in large part a form of rebellion against her parents, would you confront her behavior? If a teenage client took no birth-control precautions yet was sexually active with multiple partners, would you urge him or her to use birth control or would you encourage abstinence? Would you recommend that he or she be more selective in choosing sexual partners?

Although you may say that you are open-minded and that you can accept sexual attitudes and values that differ from your own, it may be that you are inclined to try to change clients who you believed are involved in self-destructive practices. Assess your attitudes toward casual sex, premarital sex, teen sexuality, and extramarital sex. What are your attitudes toward monogamy? What do you consider to be the physical and psychological hazards of sex with more than one partner? How would your views on this issue influence the direction you would take with clients in exploring sexual concerns?

When you have made this assessment, ask yourself whether you would be able to work objectively with a person who had sexual values sharply divergent from yours. If you have very conservative views about sexual behavior, for example, will you be able to accept the liberal views of some of your clients? If you think their moral values are contributing to the difficulties they are experiencing in their lives, will you be inclined to persuade them to adopt your conservative values?

From another perspective, if you see yourself as having liberal sexual attitudes, how do you think you would react to a person with conservative values? Assume your unmarried client says that he would like to have more sexual experiences but that his religious upbringing has instilled in him the belief that premarital sex is a sin. Whenever he has come close to having a sexual experience, his guilt prevents it from happening. He would like to learn to enjoy sex without feeling guilty, yet he does not want to betray his values. What would you say to him? Could you help him explore his own value conflict without contributing to his dilemma by imposing your own?

End-of-Life Decisions

Mental health professionals must be prepared to work with those who are dying and with their family members. Herlihy and Watson (2004) maintain that helpers will need to struggle with the ethical quandaries of how to balance the need to protect client rights to autonomy and self-determination with meeting responsibilities to the legal system and remaining true to their own moral and ethical values. Herlihy and Watson emphasize the willingness of counselors to examine their own values and beliefs to determine if they are able and willing to consider a request for aid in dying.

Psychological services are useful for healthy individuals who want to make plans about their own future care. Such services are also beneficial to individuals with life-limiting illnesses, families experiencing the demands of providing end-of-life care, bereaved individuals, and health care providers who are experiencing stress and burnout (Haley, Larson, Kasl-Godley, Neimeyer, & Kwilosz, 2003). Those in the helping professions need to acquire knowledge about the psychological, ethical, and legal considerations in end-of-life care. They can have a key role in helping people make choices regarding how they will die and about the ethical issues involved in making those choices (Kleespies, 2004). Bennett and Werth (2006) state that the functions of a counselor in cases pertaining to end-of-life decisions are "to help clients get their needs met, maximize client self-determination, help clients engage in informed decision making, and conduct an evaluation or refer clients to receive a thorough assessment regarding their capacity to make end-of-life decisions" (p. 227). Werth and Rogers (2005) suggest that the same kind of assessment can be conducted for those who are making end-of-life decisions as for people with suicidal ideation. Just as depression, hopelessness, and social isolation can contribute to an individual's suicidality, such conditions can also contribute to the decision process for people who are terminally ill (Bennett & Werth, 2006; Werth & Rogers, 2005).

Studies of attitudes toward suicide reveal sharp divisions of opinion regarding the meaning of the decision to end one's life. Some regard this as a basic personal right, and others consider it a sign of moral evil or societal pathology (Neimeyer, 2000). As a helper, you need to be willing to discuss end-of-life decisions when clients bring such concerns to you. If you are closed to any personal examination of this issue, you may interrupt these dialogues, cut off your clients' exploration of their feelings, or attempt to provide your clients with your own solutions based on your values and beliefs.

At this point in time, you might consider the following questions. What is your position on an individual's right to decide about matters pertaining to living and dying? What religious, ethical, and moral beliefs do you hold that would allow you to support a client's decision to hasten his or her death under certain circumstances? How might your beliefs get in the way of assisting your client in making his or her own decision? It is your responsibility to clarify your own beliefs and values pertaining to end-of-life decisions so you can assist your clients in making decisions within the framework of their own belief and value systems. Once you understand your own perspective on end-of-life decisions, you can focus on the needs of your clients.

Imagine yourself in a nursing home, growing more and more confused and demented. You are unable to read, to carry on meaningful conversation, or to go places, and you are partially paralyzed by a series of strokes. Do you think you would be able to find meaning through suffering in an extreme circumstance?

Would you want to be kept alive at all costs, or might you want to end your life? Would you feel justified in doing so? What would stop you?

Now apply this line of thought to other situations in life. Suppose you felt like ending your life even after trying various ways of making your life meaningful. Imagine you felt as if nothing worked and that nothing would change. What would you do? Would you continue to live until natural causes ended your life? Do you believe that any reason would justify you taking your own *life*?

Case study: The right to choose to die. A man in his 30s, Walfred discovers that he has tested positive for HIV. He says he wants to participate in a physician-assisted suicide before he gets to an intolerable state. Many of his friends have died from AIDS, and he vowed that he would take active measures to be sure that he would not die in the same way. Because he is rational and knows what he wants, he believes that taking this action is reasonable and in accord with his basic human rights. He has been your client for several months and has been successfully exploring other issues in his life. When he recently learned of his HIV status, he saw nothing ahead for him except a bleak future. He does want your help in making a decision, but he is clearly leaning in the direction of ending his life.

Your stance. What would you say to Walfred? Because Walfred is rational and able to make decisions that affect his life, should he be allowed to take measures to end his life before he becomes terminally ill? Because he is not yet seriously ill, should he be prevented from ending his life, even if it means taking away his freedom of choice? Given the fact that you have been working with Walfred for some time, would you respect his self-determination, or would you press him to search for alternatives to suicide at this stage in his life? As a mental health worker, if there were no legal mandate to report his intentions, would you feel justified in attempting to persuade Walfred to change his mind? What is the role of mental health professionals in working with people who are considering some form of hastened dying? Is it the proper role of the helper to steer the client in a particular direction? Should the helper's personal values enter the picture? What is the ethical course to follow when there is a conflict between the therapist's and the client's values on this matter? Is your role to prevent the person from taking actions that would hasten his or her death?

Case study: Confronting the right to die. Esmeralda, who is in her early 40s, is suffering from advanced rheumatoid arthritis. She is in constant pain, and many of the pain medications have serious side effects. This is a debilitating disease, and she sees no hope of improvement. She has lost her will to live and comes to you, her therapist of long-standing, and says: "I am in too much pain, and I don't want to suffer anymore. I don't want to involve you in it, but as my counselor, I would like you to know my last wishes." She tells you of her plan to take an overdose of pills, an action she sees as more humane than continuing to endure her suffering.

Your stance. Think about how your values might influence your interventions in this case. To what degree can you empathize with Esmeralda's desire to end her life? What role would your beliefs play in your counseling?

Do you see any conflict between ethics and the law in this case? Do you have an ethical and legal responsibility to prevent Esmeralda from carrying out her intended course of action? From previous counseling sessions, you know that Esmeralda's parents believe it is always wrong to take your own life. Should you inform Esmeralda's parents about her decision to end her life? If you were in full agreement with her wishes, how would this influence your intervention?

Case study: The counselor's legal and ethical duty to protect. Peter, a 65-year-old former client of Dr. Park's, returns to see him. He is now widowed, his only child is dead, and he has no living relatives. He has been diagnosed with a slow, painful, terminal cancer. Peter tells Dr. Park that he is contemplating ending his life but would like to explore this decision. Dr. Park fears being put in a bind because of the potential legal and ethical issues involved in protecting him if he decides to end his life. Peter comes weekly, discusses many things with his therapist, and talks lovingly of his deceased wife and daughter. He thanks Dr. Park for his kindness and his help throughout the years. He has made up his mind to end his life in the next few days, and after a last farewell he goes home.

Your stance. Do you think Dr. Park should make a report as a way to protect Peter? What would you do in this case? Explain your position in the context of your own values regarding end-of-life decisions.

Case study: Counseling an ill teenager contemplating suicide. Buford, a minor, cannot get along with his new stepfather, so he moves into his grandmother's apartment where she lives alone. Shortly thereafter, Buford develops an illness that attacks his nervous system, causing him to be too weak to attend school. The school assigns a home teacher who tells the school counselor that Buford is saying he does not want to live with this illness. The counselor visits Buford and is able to develop a relationship. Buford's mood seems to lift, but within 3 weeks he speaks again of suicide, indicating that he does not intend to die from this disease. He tells the counselor that he plans to take his grandmother's pills. Buford begs the counselor not to tell his grandmother or his parents.

Your stance. How would you deal with the situation? What are the most salient issues involved in this case? Does the counselor have a responsibility to inform Buford's parents? Why or why not?

Guidelines for dealing with end-of-life issues. Werth and Holdwick (2000) suggest that mental health professionals whose values preclude consideration of hastened death should not be obligated to provide professional services to clients who want to explore this issue. However, for helpers who do counsel these clients, Werth and Holdwick provide these guidelines for dealing with end-of-life issues:

- Assess your personal values and professional beliefs regarding the acceptability of rational suicide.
- As a part of the informed consent process, give prospective clients information about the limitations of confidentiality as it applies to assisted death, if applicable.
- Make full use of consultation throughout the process.
- Keep risk-management-oriented notes.

- Assess your clients' capacity to make reasoned decisions about their health care.
- Review clients' understanding of their condition, prognosis, and treatment options.
- Strive to include clients' significant others in the counseling process.
- Assess the impact of external coercion on clients' decision making.
- Determine the degree to which clients' decisions are congruent with their cultural and spiritual values.

Consider these guidelines as you contemplate your own position with respect to key questions on end-of-life decisions? Do individuals have a right to decide whether to live or die? If your personal or professional value system is not accepting of an individual ending his or her own life, is it ethical for you to work with clients who may be contemplating some form of hastened death? How might your beliefs get in the way of assisting your client in making his or her own decision? Are you aware of the laws of your state and the ethical standards of your professional organization concerning an individual's freedom to make end-of-life decisions?

By Way of Review

- Ethical practice dictates that helpers seriously consider the impact of their values on their clients and the conflicts that might arise if values are sharply different.

- Ultimately, it is the responsibility of clients to choose in which direction they will go, what values they will adopt, and what values they will modify or discard.

- It is neither possible nor desirable for helpers to remain neutral or to keep their values separate from their professional relationships.

- It is not the helper's role to push clients to adopt the value system of the helper.

- At times, it may be useful for helpers to expose their values to their clients, yet it is counterproductive and unethical to impose these values on them.

- Simply because you do not embrace a client's values does not mean that you cannot work effectively with the person. The key is that you be objective, nonjudgmental, and respect your client's right to autonomy.

- There are numerous areas in which your values can potentially conflict with the values of your clients. You may have to refer some clients because of such differences. However, a referral should be done with careful thought and is best considered as a measure of last resort.

What Will You Do Now?

1. Spend some time reflecting on the role you expect your values to play as you work with a range of clients. How might your values work for you? against you? Reflect on the source of your values. Are you clear about where you stand on the value issues raised in this chapter? In your journal, write some of your thoughts about these questions. Under what circumstances would you be inclined to share and perhaps explore your values and beliefs with your clients? Can you think of situations in which it might be counterproductive for you to do so?

2. Consider a personal value that could get in the way of your being objective when working with a client. Choose a value that you hold strongly, and challenge it. Do this by going to a source that holds values opposite to your own. If you are strongly convinced that abortion is immoral, for instance, consider going to an abortion clinic and talking with someone there. If you are uncomfortable with homosexuality because of your own values, go to a lesbian, gay, or bisexual organization on campus or in your community and talk with people there. If you think you may have difficulty with religious values of clients, find out more about a group that holds religious views different from yours.

3. For the full bibliographic entry for each of the sources listed here, consult the References at the back of the book. For books dealing with the role of spiritual values in the helping process, see Burke and Miranti (1995), Cashwell and Young (2005), Faiver, Ingersoll, O'Brien, and McNally (2001), Faiver and O'Brien (1993), Frame (2003), Kelly (1995b), Miller (1999), Miller and Thoresen (1999), Richards and Bergin (2005), and Shafranske and Sperry (2005). For an excellent treatment on end-of-life issues, see Werth, Welfel, and Benjamin (2009).

Ethics in Action *CD-ROM Exercises*

4. For supplemental activities that accompany this chapter, see Part Two [Values and the Helping Relationship] of the *Ethics in Action* CD-ROM. Before viewing role-play segments 4, 5, 6, and 7, complete the self-inventory provided in Part Two and bring your completed responses to class for discussion.

5. Complete the exercises and follow-up discussion questions after each of the role-play segments dealing with value conflicts in Part Two. To derive the maximum benefit, after viewing each role-play segment write out your reactions to the situation portrayed.

6. In role-play segment 4, The Divorce, it is clear that the counselor has an agenda for the client when she says that she has decided to leave her husband and get a divorce. The counselor's line of inquiry is about who will look after the welfare of her children. The client feels misunderstood and does not think the counselor is of help to her. Have one student role-play the counselor, using a different approach from the one that Gary used with this client. Have another student play the role of the client. After the role play, explore the issues you see

being played out. What are some other alternatives helpers could employ when dealing with a value conflict?

7. In role-play segment 5, Doing It My Way, Sally is attempting to influence her client to think about the effect of her behavior on her parents. The client (Charlae) is seeking increased independence and wants to break away from her parents and be "free." Her father wants her to stay at home, but she wants to live at college in the dorms. Sally suggests that Charlae talk with her parents about this, but she just wants to move out, without any discussion with her parents.

Sally is concerned about what Charlae's parents' reaction might be if she moves out without involving her parents in this decision. Charlae says, "I could really care less what they think." Sally wants Charlae to think about the consequences and the effect on her parents and the fact that they have made sacrifices for her. Have one student role-play Sally and another Sally's supervisor. Demonstrate how you might approach the counselor as her supervisor. What would you most want Sally to consider?

8. In role-play segment 6, The Promiscuous One, the client (Suzanne) is having indiscriminate sexual encounters. Richard expresses concern for his client, who reports meeting a guy in a bar and having sex with him, which she says is the best she has had in a week. He asks if she is protecting herself from pregnancy and/or HIV. She claims she has the greatest life as it is. Suzanne says, "I'm not going to get HIV. People are blowing it totally out of proportion." She says she doesn't know why he is so worried about it, for after all, it's her life. Richard then focuses on how Suzanne's behavior plays out the recurring theme of abandonment by her father. She thinks there is no connection.

If you were Suzanne's counselor, how would you deal with the situation as she presents it? Is it ethically appropriate for you to strongly influence your client to engage in safe sex practices? Demonstrate how you would approach Suzanne through role playing.

9. In role-play segment 7, The Affair, the client (Natalie) shares with her counselor that she is having a long-term affair. Natalie is struggling with her marriage and the fact that she is having a long-term affair. She feels alive, youthful, and beautiful when she is with this other person. At home she feels depressed and sees her purpose as being just to serve her husband. For years she has been there for others, but now she has to think about herself. The counselor (Janice) says, "Having an affair is not a good answer for someone—it just hurts everyone. I just don't think it is a good idea."

What are your values as they pertain to this issue, and how would your values influence your interventions? In a role play, show how you might work with Natalie.

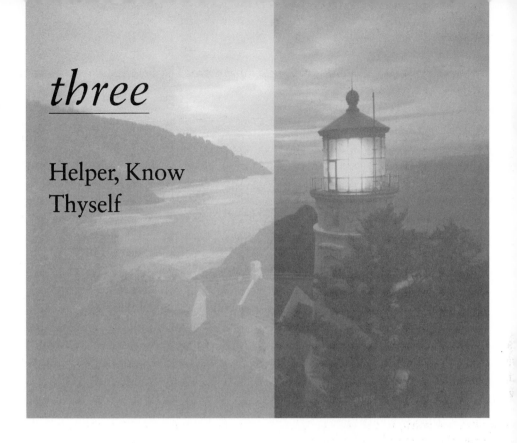

three

Helper, Know Thyself

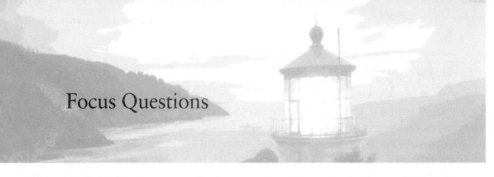

Focus Questions

1. Do you believe it is possible for people to change? What do you think the process of change has been like for you? What might it be like for people you want to help?

2. What importance do you place on self-exploration as part of the process of becoming a helper?

3. How much do you know about your family of origin's influence on your development? How familiar are you with the life experiences of your parents, your grandparents, and other relatives?

4. In what ways have the experiences within your family of origin affected your current relationships? How might these same experiences influence your role as a professional helper? Can you identify any unresolved issues between you and your family that might affect your professional work?

5. What unfinished business in your personal life could present difficulties for you in working with clients with a range of problems? What steps can you take to address these issues?

6. From which life experiences can you draw in an attempt to understand the diverse range of client problems you will encounter?

7. At this point in your life, how well have you dealt with the effects of key transition periods in your life? As you reflect on the developmental patterns in your life, what events have most influenced your present attitudes and behavior?

8. Your current life is largely a result of the earlier choices you have made. What earlier choices have particularly affected the kind of person you are today?

Aim of the Chapter

Most of us were raised in families that included at least one parent or parental figure, a certain amount of structure, and a set of rules designed to help us cope with life and meet the challenges we faced. Many problems your clients will bring to counseling are grounded in their experiences as children growing up in their families. To be an effective helper, you need to recognize the ways in which your own family of origin has influenced you and how your early background may influence your professional work. Whether you plan to work with individuals, groups, couples, or families, it is important for you to be familiar with your family-of-origin issues. Your perceptions and reactions to those whom you counsel are often influenced by your personal experiences with your own family. If you are unaware of these sensitive areas, you may misinterpret your clients or steer them in a direction that will not arouse your own anxieties. If you are aware of emotional issues that activate your defensiveness, however, you can avoid getting entangled in the problems of your clients.

When you work intensely with clients week after week, it is likely that you will be affected by their pain. When your pain surfaces and present struggles become overwhelming, you must seek help for yourself. There is a price to pay for numbing yourself to this pain, and you need to recognize that the nature of your work makes it difficult to hide from yourself. Your development as a helping professional will be intimately linked throughout your career to your development as a person.

The material we present in this chapter is personal and can assist you in examining many dimensions of your family experience. We ask you to unravel the mystery of your connection with your family of origin so you can develop an appreciation for the many ways you have been influenced by the patterns established during childhood. This knowledge will help you guard against countertransference in your practice. We cannot stress this message enough—helper, know thyself. If you want to be a therapeutic agent in the lives of others, you must know yourself and, when necessary, be able to heal yourself.

One way we train beginning helpers is to assist them in focusing on their own development as a person. We structure our training workshops for counselors around personal issues. We ask trainees to read about certain life themes, to think about their own development and turning points, and to recall key choices they have made. These themes include dealing with developmental transitions through childhood, adolescence, and adult life; struggles with friendships; love and intimate relationships; loneliness and solitude; death and loss; sexuality; work and recreation; and the meaning in life. These are some of the main themes clients will bring into counseling sessions. Helpers will be affected by the problems clients discuss in these areas. If helpers themselves have limited awareness of their own struggles, they may not be very effective. In training workshops, participants discover the impact their life experiences have on their clients and, in turn, how their clients' life experiences affect them.

The Impact of Therapeutic Work on Your Personal Life

In talking with mental health providers, we find that many are not able to separate themselves from their work. Both new and experienced practitioners may find it difficult to make a clear distinction between their personal life and their professional life. Helpers need to understand how they are personally affected by their professional work if they hope to maintain their own psychological health and continue to be effective in reaching those whom they serve. Self-knowledge is an essential place to begin. Jaffe (1986) argues that health professionals must see that they cannot simply give and remain detached from their feelings. Instead, they must look inward at their personal needs. Jaffe decries the mistaken notions that healers are not supposed to have needs, that personal feelings are not relevant, and that helpers should learn to ignore their own pain as they work with others' pain, much as in the Greek myth of the wounded healer. Such healers were supposed to possess the wisdom of life and death, yet they were not able to heal their own incurable wounds. According to Jaffe, helping professionals need to recognize the impact on their own life of working with suffering people. They must become aware of their inner responses and learn to work through their own pain in a constructive manner to be effective in their professional work.

Unless you have identified your own sources of vulnerability and to some extent worked through experiences that may have left you psychologically wounded, you may be constantly triggered by the stories of your clients. Old wounds can be opened, affecting both your personal and professional life. It is clear that therapeutic practice can reactivate your earlier experiences and reawaken unresolved needs and problems. It is important for you to be willing to deal with your personal issues when they are triggered through your work with others.

Case example: Therapy that triggers personal pain. Nancy, a beginning counselor working in an agency, is asked to co-lead a grief group for adults. Nancy believes there is a real need for this work, and she is enthusiastic in accepting the co-leadership role. She lost her husband in a tragic manner, yet she feels that she has allowed herself to fully experience the pain of his death and has accepted the loss. She works very well with the members in her group as the sessions begin. She can be compassionate, supportive, and empathic, and she is able to help them work through some of their pain. However, after a few weeks Nancy notices that she is no longer looking forward to going to the group. She feels somewhat depressed and finds herself becoming apathetic toward the members.

Your stance. If you found yourself dreading to meet with a group you had been enthusiastic about leading only a short time ago, what would you do? How would you get to the bottom of these feelings? Would you seek advice from colleagues or personal therapy? Would you continue to lead this group?

Discussion. Although some of Nancy's old wounds were healed, exposure to the intense pain of so many other people has reopened these wounds. Thus, the only way she could survive was to numb herself from feeling the others' pain. This numbing led to Nancy's depression and her inability to work effectively with her clients. She has ignored her vulnerability to the pain of her loss and her need to express and work through this pain as it is being reexperienced.

Simply because Nancy reexperiences her old pain does not necessarily mean that she will become ineffective in working with this type of group. Quite the contrary, if she accepts the fact that she is still wounded and explores these feelings, she can heal her own wounds at the same time that she is facilitating the healing process in others. She can model the ongoing nature of grief work and teach the members that although the pain will never be completely erased it can become less controlling. If it is appropriate, Nancy may share her present reactions and feelings. However, even if she chooses not to reveal her experiences to the group, she can use her experiences as a bridge to connect with the struggles of others.

Alternatively, Nancy can choose to seek personal therapy. If she repeatedly puts her own emotions "on hold," either in or out of the group, she is bound to become ineffectual as a helper, and if she continues this type of involvement over a long period, it is likely that she will experience burnout. The challenge for Nancy is to learn to listen to her inner experience and to use it as a road to her growth and as a way of making contact with others.

The Value of Self-Exploration for the Helper

You may discover that working with individuals or families resurrects themes in your life, some of which may previously have been outside your conscious awareness. If you are unaware of issues stemming from your family experiences, you are likely to find ways to avoid acknowledging and dealing with these potentially painful areas with your clients. As your clients confront events that trigger their pain, memories of your own pain may be stimulated. For instance, you may still have a great deal of hurt over your parents' divorce. At some level, you may believe the divorce was your fault or that you could have done something to keep your parents together. If you are counseling a couple considering divorce, you may want to steer them toward remaining married for the sake of the children. You are giving them solutions that originate from your reservoir of hurt. On some level, you could be protecting the children from the pain of your situation that you have yet to fully realize or appreciate. It is important to recognize that your capacity to facilitate the healing forces in others is based on your willingness to experience your own wounds and bring about healing for yourself.

Identifying and resolving unfinished business related to your family of origin allows you to establish relationships that do not repeat negative patterns of interaction. As you review your family history in this chapter, you will no doubt gain some insights into patterns that you have "adopted" from your family of origin. Your own therapy helps you to understand how these past conflicts are still affecting you.

As you begin to practice counseling, you might become aware that you are taking on a professional role that resembles the role you played in your family. For example, you may recognize a need to preserve peace by becoming the care-taker of others. During your childhood you may have assumed adult roles with your own parents by trying to take care of them. Now, as you begin your profes-sional work, it is possible that you could continue the pattern of taking more responsibility for the changes your clients make than they do.

Transference and countertransference are common in the therapeutic pro-cess. **Transference** generally has roots in a client's unresolved personal conflicts with significant others. Because of these unresolved concerns, the client may perceive the helping professional in a distorted way, bringing past relationships into the present relationship with the counselor. Transference can lead a client to gain insight into how he or she operates in a variety of relationships. The counterpart to the client's transference feelings toward a helper is the helping person's **countertransference;** that is, emotional-behavioral reactions toward a client that originate from some part of the helper's life. Consider your own pos-sible sources of countertransference. If you have fears about your dying or the aging and death of your parents, for example, it is quite possible for you to encounter difficulty in working with older people. The struggles of these clients can activate unconscious processes in you that, if left outside your awareness, can interfere with your ability to be truly helpful.

Many situations in a family can plant the seeds for potential countertransfer-ence: growing up in a home with the unpredictability of violence, conflicts that were never addressed, secrecy that was protected at all costs, fears surrounding incest, absence of any boundaries, and significant events (such as grave illness or the death of a family member) that were ignored on a psychological level. If you felt that no matter how much you did, it was never quite enough to win your mother's approval, for example, you may now be very finely attuned to the judg-ments of women who remind you of your mother. If you allowed your father to completely affirm or deny your value as a person, you may be very sensitive to what male authority figures think of you. You give them the power to make you feel either competent or incompetent. As a child, if you often felt rejected, you may now create situations in which you feel like the one who is left out and just does not fit. Conversely, you may always have been appreciated and now think this should continue in all situations and at all times. You can identify these kinds of situations in your own counseling sessions and get help in working through places where you may be psychologically stalled. (Transference and counter-transference are discussed in further detail in Chapter 4.)

Using Individual and Group Counseling for Self-Understanding

When you become aware of bringing patterns that originated from your personal experiences into your professional life, individual and group counseling can pro-vide a safe place to explore and talk about the sometimes painful memories that are often associated with these personal experiences. Ideally, you will consider participating in a combination of individual and group therapy, because the two approaches to therapy complement each other.

Individual therapy provides you with an opportunity to look at yourself in some depth. As a part of your internship experience, you may experience a reopening of old emotional wounds when you engage in intensive work with your clients. Your therapeutic work may bring to the surface feelings of unexpressed and unresolved grief over significant loss or challenge gender perspectives and cultural stereotypes with which you were raised. Personal counseling can support healthy growth and development as well as provide an avenue for remediation when needed. If you are in personal counseling while you are doing your internship, you can bring such problems to your therapy sessions. According to Norcross (2000), the majority of mental health professionals have participated in their own personal therapy, and the vast majority of mental health professionals rate the outcomes of personal therapy quite positively: "Our studies consistently find that psychotherapists regularly recommend, seek, and value episodic personal therapy as constructive self-care" (p. 712). Self-reported outcomes of personal therapy gathered by Norcross (2005) reveal positive gains in multiple areas, including self-esteem, work functioning, social life, emotional expression, intrapersonal conflicts, and symptom severity. When it comes to specific lasting lessons that practitioners learn from their personal therapy experiences, the most frequent responses pertain to interpersonal relationships and the dynamics of psychotherapy. Some of these lessons learned are the centrality of warmth, empathy, and the personal relationship; having a sense of what it is like to be a therapy client; and appreciating the importance of learning how to deal with transference and countertransference.

Dearing, Maddux, and Tangney (2005) conducted a study of factors that increase the chances that therapists-in-training will seek psychological help. They emphasize the responsibility of faculty, supervisors, and mentors in educating trainees about appropriate pathways to self-care and prevention of impairment. Dearing and colleagues recommend that trainees consider these potential benefits, both personally and professionally, of psychotherapy during their training: a way to alleviate personal distress, a means of gaining insight into being an effective therapist, and a means of developing healthy and enduring self-care practices. Norcross and Guy (2007) believe that self-care, which may include personal therapy, is a moral imperative for mental health practitioners. Foster and Black (2007) suggest that therapists often neglect self-care to their own detriment and to the detriment of their clients. Foster and Black add that "part of integral ethical practice involves the conscious attention of counselors to maintain their health and well-being" (p. 223).

In addition to individual or personal therapy, group counseling offers another pathway for self-awareness. Group therapy can offer you an opportunity to hear and consider feedback you receive from others. A group experience can help you become aware of your interpersonal style and give you a chance to experiment with new behaviors in a group setting. The reactions you receive from others can help you learn about personal attributes that could be either strengths or limitations in your work as a helper. Many of the patterns you acquired as a child may still be problematic for you today. You could do useful work in group therapy on any unresolved issues you have with your parents, with family rules that you have accepted, or in situations where you feel stuck.

Therapy—be it individual, group, or family—is not just for treatment purposes or for curing deeply rooted personality disturbances. We see therapy as an avenue for continuing to deepen your self-understanding and for looking at the ways in which your needs are related to your work. Becoming involved in some form of intensive self-exploration therapy can motivate you to assess your needs and motives for becoming a helper, which were outlined in Chapter 1. Therapy is not to be viewed as something that is finished when you complete your formal education. Committed helping professionals are open to engaging in lifelong self-exploration as the need presents itself. Baker (2003) advocates personal psychotherapy as being beneficial to both trainees and experienced practitioners, contending that therapy can serve different purposes at different stages of life. Even when therapy has ended, the process of paying attention to your behavior should not end.

Although both individual and group therapy are valuable routes to gaining a deeper knowledge of yourself, other less formal avenues to personal and professional development should also be explored. These include reflecting on the meaning of your life and work; remaining open to the reactions of significant people in your life; traveling and immersing yourself in different cultures; engaging in spiritual activities, such as meditating; participating in physical challenges; and spending time with your family and friends. By participating in various forms of self-exploration, you can gain firsthand knowledge of what your clients are likely to experience. This process will increase your respect for clients and their struggles. It may be difficult to teach others about the joys and pains of growth that result from a therapeutic relationship if you have not experienced it yourself. If you have not participated in the journey of self-exploration, how can you guide others?

We have found that some helpers would rather look at the dynamics of their clients than at themselves. Although there is nothing wrong in wanting to find better ways of working with clients, you can best learn how to do this by allowing yourself to be as open as possible to your own life experience. Thus, whenever you take measures to understand yourself more fully, you are at the same time preparing yourself to be of greater help to others in their quest for self-understanding.

Working With Your Family of Origin

Some programs in marital and family therapy require students to take a family-of-origin course. The assumption is that future practitioners need to know how their own **family of origin** influences them presently before they engage in professional work with individuals, couples, and families. Some states mandate such a course as a requirement for licensure as a couples and family therapist. Some writers suggest that training programs provide family-of-origin work for students as part of growth group experiences (Bitter, 2009; Lawson & Gaushell, 1991; Wilcoxon, Walker, & Hovestadt, 1989). Other authors discuss how family-of-origin work can be used for personal-growth training for couples and family therapists (Getz & Protinsky, 1994), ways that early childhood family influences are related to counselor effectiveness (Watts, Trusty, Canada, & Harvill, 1995), and explore ethical considerations when using the family autobiography in training counselors (Goodman & Carpenter-White, 1996). By exploring the dynamics of their own family of origin, helpers can relate more effectively to themes presented by families they encounter in clinical practice.

Lawson and Gaushell (1991) recommend that training programs address candidates' family issues before admitting them to a program. They suggest requiring a family autobiography as part of the application materials. This would yield useful information concerning intergenerational family characteristics that would have a relationship to a helper's ability to work with families. Lawson and Gaushell emphasize these intergenerational family characteristics of counselor trainees:

- Clinicians who have resolved negative family experiences are better able to assist their clients, especially those with whom they have issues in common.
- It is essential that trainees be given assistance in identifying and addressing their own problematic family issues to enhance their psychological functioning and their effectiveness as helpers.
- Unmet needs in early family experiences later manifest themselves in intense and conflicting ties with these family members.
- Helpers' early roles as peacemakers create later ambivalence regarding intimacy with significant others.
- Counselor trainees' experiences in their families of origin can lead to difficulties in their current relationships.

Identifying Your Issues in Your Family of Origin

Family therapists generally assume that it is inevitable that they will encounter some of the dynamics of their family of origin in the families they will treat. Virginia Satir, a pioneer in family therapy, used to say that if she walked into a room with 12 people she would meet everyone she ever knew. When you are counseling a couple or a family, many people are participating in this interaction. In other words, you do not always perceive individuals whom you meet with a fresh and unbiased perspective. The more you are aware of these patterns, the greater the benefit to your clients. It is crucial that you know to whom you are responding: to the individual in front of you or to a person from your past.

Try this exercise that Satir used to demonstrate that people are constantly revisiting friends and loved ones in their lives. Stand in front of someone (Person A) in your current life who interests you or with whom you are having some difficulty. This individual might be a client, an associate, a family member, or a friend. If the person is not present, you can imagine him or her. Take a good look at this person and form a picture on the screen of your mind. Now, let a picture of someone in your past come forward (Person B). Who comes to mind? How old are you, and how old is Person B? What relationship do you, or did you, have with this individual you are remembering? What feelings are linked with this relationship? What did you think about Person B? Now, reexamine your reactions to Person A. Do you see any connection between what Person A is evoking in you and the past feelings evoked by Person B? You can apply this exercise by yourself through the use of imagery when you have intense emotional reactions to other people, especially if you do not know them well. This exercise can help you begin to recognize the effects past relationships may have on your here-and-now responses (Satir, Banmen, Gerber, & Gomori, 1991). Perhaps what is most important is simply to be aware of ways in which you are carrying your past into present interactions.

In this section we invite you to identify as many family-of-origin experiences as possible and to reflect on how these life experiences are likely to have an influence on *who* and *what* you are at this point. Goldenberg and Goldenberg (2004) have written a workbook designed to provoke students into thinking about how their roles in their family of origin and their current family continue to play out in maintaining their attitudes, values, and behavior patterns. They write: "By learning more about yourself, especially by adopting a family perspective, we believe you can help others, future clients, see themselves within the contexts of their family lives" (Preface). You are not necessarily determined by your earlier experiences, and they do not have to serve as the template for your current significant relationships. You can shift your perspective, but only if you have recognized and dealt with your experiences. If you are working with a family, moreover, you will have an experiential starting point to invite them to look at their functioning as a system and as individuals within the family.

Much of the remainder of this section is based on our perspective on family history, which is a modification and integration of material taken from several sources: (1) Adlerian lifestyle assessment methods (Corey, 2009c; Mosak & Shulman, 1988; Powers & Griffith, 1986, 1987; Shulman & Mosak, 1988); (2) Satir's communication approach to working with families (Satir, 1983, 1989; Satir & Baldwin, 1983; Satir, Bitter, & Krestensen, 1988; see also Bitter, 1987, 1988); (3) concepts of family systems (Bitter, 2009; Goldenberg & Goldenberg, 2004, 2008; Nichols, 2008); (4) genogram methods (McGoldrick, Gerson, & Petry, 2008); and (5) family autobiography methods (Lawson & Gaushell, 1988). As you read the following material, try to personalize the information. We are primarily providing you with ways to understand and work with your own family material and secondarily offering you a basis for understanding the individuals and families in your professional work.

Your family structure. The many patterns of family life include nuclear, extended, single-parent, divorced, and blended families. The term **family structure** also refers to the social and psychological organization of the family system, including factors such as birth order and the individual's perception of self in the family context. Expand your awareness of your family of origin by thoughtfully answering these questions:

• In what type of family structure did you grow up? Did the structure of your family change over time? If so, what were these changes? What were some important family values? What stands out for you about your family life? How do these experiences affect you today?

• What is your current family structure? Are you still primarily involved in your family of origin, or do you have a different family structure? If you do, what roles do you play in your current family that you also enacted in your original family? Have you carried certain patterns from your original family into your current family? How do you see yourself as being different in the two families?

• Draw a picture of your family of origin. Include all the members, and identify their significant alliances. Identify the relationships with each person that you had as a child and your relationships with each member now.

• Make a list of the siblings, from oldest to youngest. Give a brief description of each (including yourself). What most stands out for each sibling? Which sibling is most different from you, and how? Which is most like you, and how?

• How would you describe yourself as a child in your birth family? What were some of your major fears? hopes? ambitions? What was school like for you? What was your role in your peer group? Identify any significant events in your physical, sexual, and social development during childhood.

• Identify a personal struggle of yours. How has your relationship with your family contributed to the development and perpetuation of this struggle? What options are open to you for making substantial changes? What are a few ways in which you can be different in your family?

• Make a list of strengths you have. How has your family contributed to the development of these strengths?

Parental figures and relationships with parents. Your parents were central figures in your development. A father or mother may have been absent from your early family life. If so, did any surrogate figures emerge? If you grew up in a single-parent family, did this one parent play the role of both mother and father? You may have grown up in a family with two parents of the same sex. What did you learn about yourself and the world? How did others react to you having same-sex parents? Did the discrimination that exists in society toward your parents have an effect on your life?

If you grew up in a heterosexual two-parent family, what did your parents teach you, mainly through the behavior they modeled, about marriage and about family life? Spend some time thinking about your parental figures and your relationships with them. Focus on what you learned from observing and interacting with your parents and on what you observed in their interactions with each other. How did they fight or solve problems? How did they express affection for one another? Who made the decisions and in what way? Who handled the money and family finances? How did each parent interact with each child? How did each of your siblings view and react to your parents?

Describe your father (or the person who substituted for him). What is he like? What were his ambitions for each of the children? How did you view him as a child? How do you view him now? How are you like him? How are you unlike him? What does your father say when he compliments you or when he criticizes you? What was his advice to you as a child? What is his advice to you now? What could you do to disappoint him now? What can you do to please him? What was his relationship to his children? What is his current relationship to your siblings? What sibling is the most like your father, and in what ways? What did your father tell you (either directly or indirectly) about yourself? life? death? love? sex? marriage? men? women? your birth? What is it about you or your behavior that you would not want him to know?

Now describe your mother. Use the same list of questions and ask each of them about your mother (or the person who substituted for her). Give a sketch of how you viewed your mother.

Your parents have been the "air-traffic controllers" of your life. They launched you, guided you, and helped you survive. They are the people on whom you depended for survival, and you may feel less than grown up in relation to them. You may find yourself acting the way you did as a child when you are with them as opposed to functioning as a psychological adult. It is important to remember that for many people the last relationships they work out are those with their parents.

Becoming your own person. A healthy person achieves both a psychological separateness from and a sense of intimacy with his or her family, which is known as **individuation**, or sometimes as a *differentiated self* (Bowen, 1978). This process of individuation involves the balance between belonging to and separating from your family of origin. The increasing differentiation from the family enables you to accept personal responsibility for your thoughts, feelings, perceptions, and actions. It decreases emotional reactivity or the experience of allowing others—both within and outside of the family—to push your buttons. Individuation, or psychological maturity, is not a fixed destination that you reach once and for all; rather, it is a lifelong developmental process achieved through reexamination and resolution of internal conflicts and intimacy issues with loved ones. You do not find yourself in isolation; rather, the process of self-discovery is bound up with the quality of your relationships to others in connection. Becoming your own person does not mean "doing your own thing" irrespective of your impact on those with whom you come in contact. Instead, being autonomous means that you have questioned the values you live by and made them your own; part of this process includes concern for the welfare of those people you love and associate with.

It is possible to assume responsibility by doing for yourself what you expected others to do for you as a child. If you are becoming a separate being, you still maintain connections, reach out to others, share with them, and give yourself in your relationships. Being an integrated person means that you recognize the many and varied aspects of your being, that you accept both positive and negative sides, and that you do not disown parts of yourself.

The notions of individuation, independence, autonomy, and self-determination are Western values, and not all cultures pay homage to such values. This emphasis on independence and self-determination tends to reduce the importance of the family of origin. Sue (1997) points out that in Chinese American families the notion of filial piety is a strong determinant of how children behave, even as they move to adulthood. Obedience, respect, obligation to parents, and duty leave little room for self-determination. For example, allegiance to one's parents is expected from a man, even after he marries and has his own family. The concept of individuation and separation from his family can easily lead to conflicts in his family relationships. For example, a son may have difficulty with the notion of being his own person beyond the limits of his family role. He may always think of himself as first a son and in the line of his family tree. For such a person, individuation is neither ideal nor particularly functional. He will discover who he is more easily within the family context than outside of it. It is quite clear that cultural values play a key role in adopting behaviors that reflect an individualistic or collectivistic spirit. At this point, reflect on these questions:

- What cultural values influenced the degree to which you have striven for autonomy? Which values stemming from your culture do you want to retain? Are there any of these values you want to challenge or modify?
- In what significant ways, if any, do you see yourself as having a distinct identity and as being psychologically separate from your family of origin? And in what ways, if any, are you psychologically fused with your family of origin? Are there any aspects of this relationship that you want to change?

Coping with conflict in the family. If you have difficulty dealing with conflict in your current relationships, one reason may be that conflict was not addressed in direct ways in your family of origin. You may have been taught that conflict was something to be avoided at all costs. If you observed that conflict had no resolution in your family or that people would simply not speak to each other for weeks after a conflict, you are probably fearful when conflicts emerge. Conflicts belong to the whole family, although parents often portray their children as the problem. The key to successful relationships lies not in the absence of conflict but in recognizing its source and being able to cope directly with the situations that lead to conflict. Conflicts that are denied tend to fester and strain relationships. Reflect on what you learned about conflict in your family. How was it expressed and dealt with? What were its sources? What was your role? Were you encouraged to resolve conflict directly with your antagonist? Did you feel safe in recognizing and dealing directly with disputes between you and members of your family?

The Family as a System

Families have certain rules governing interactions. These **family rules** are not simple commandments, such as what time children need to be home after a date. They also include unspoken rules, messages given by parents to children, injunctions, myths, and secrets. These rules are often couched in terms of "do's" or "don'ts." When parents feel worried or helpless, they tend to dictate rules in an attempt to control the situation. These family rules initially assist children in handling anger, helplessness, and fear. They are intended to provide a safety net for children as they venture into the world (Satir et al., 1988).

It is impossible for children to grow up without some rules or injunctions, and on the basis of them, children make early decisions. They decide either to accept family rules or to fight them. Here are some examples of family rules: "Never be angry with your father.""Always keep a smile on your face.""Don't confront your parents, but do what you can to please them.""Don't talk to outsiders about your family.""Children are to be seen but not heard.""Have fun only when all the work is finished."

Rules or messages that were delivered by our parents and parent substitutes might also have been couched in terms of "do this or that." Consider the following "do" messages: "Be obedient.""Be practical at all times.""Be the very best you can be.""Be appropriate.""Be perfect.""Be a credit to your family.""Be better than we are."

Consider some of the major do's and don'ts that you heard growing up in your family and your reactions to them.

- What are a few messages or rules that you accepted?
- What are some rules that you fought against?
- What early decisions do you deem most significant in your life today? In what family context did you make these decisions?
- Do you ever hear yourself giving the same messages to others that you heard from your parents?

Virginia Satir (1983) recognized that the family rules we learned were often in a form that lacked choice and were impossible to implement. "I must never get angry" is an example of this kind of family rule; so is "I must always be the best" or "I must always be kind." Cognitive therapists might want clients to challenge words like "must" and "always" and "never" as irrational, but Satir preferred to engage clients in a rules transformation process. This is how the transformation process goes:

1. Start with the rule as learned: "I must never get angry."
2. Change the "must" to "can": "I can never get angry." It's still a problematic statement, but at least it has *choice* in it.
3. Change the "never" or "always" to "sometimes": "I can sometimes get angry." Now, this rings with truth. The next step is to personalize it.
4. Think of at least three situations in which it would be OK for you to get angry. For example, I can get angry when I see and experience injustice toward others, or when other people presume to know what I think or feel and speak for me, or when I see cruelty to animals. Note that being angry at these times does not require you to be emotionally reactive or explosive. There are many ways to express anger without damaging your heart with explosiveness.

What rules did you learn in your family? You may not even have heard them out loud; rules often are enacted and controlled through family responses to behavior. See if you can identify three family rules that were part of your upbringing, and then go through Satir's rules transformation process for each one.

In healthy families there are fewer rules, and they are applied consistently. The rules are humanly possible, relevant, and flexible (Bitter, 1987). According to Satir and Baldwin (1983), the most important family rules are those that govern individuation (being unique) and sharing information (communication). These are the rules that influence the ability of a family to function in open ways and to allow all members the possibility for changing. Satir notes that many people develop a range of styles as a means for coping with stress resulting from the constrictions of family rules.

Bitter (1987) contrasts a functional family structure with one that is dysfunctional. In **functional families**, each member is allowed to have a separate life as well as a shared life with the family group. Different relationships are given room to grow. Change is expected and invited, not viewed as a threat. When differentiation leads to disagreements, the situation is viewed as an opportunity for growth rather than an attack on the family system. The structure of the functional family system is characterized by freedom, flexibility, and open communication. All the family members have a voice and can speak for themselves. In this atmosphere, individuals feel support for taking risks and venturing into the world.

By contrast, **dysfunctional families** are characterized by closed communication, by the poor self-esteem of one or both parents, and by rigid patterns. Rules serve the function of masking fears about differences. They are rigid and are frequently inappropriate for meeting a situation. In unhealthy families, the members are expected to think, feel, and act in the same way. Parents attempt to control the family by using fear, anger, punishment, guilt, or dominance. Eventually, the system breaks down because the rules are no longer able to keep the family structure intact. This can lead to intense stress.

When stress is exacerbated because of the breakdown of the family system, members tend to resort to defensive stances. Bitter (1987) describes how congruent people cope with stress. They do not sacrifice themselves to a singular style in dealing with it. Instead, they transform stress into a challenge that is met in a useful way. Such people are centered, and they avoid changing their colors like a chameleon. Their words match their inner experience, and they are able to make direct and clear statements. They face stress with confidence and courage because they know that they have the inner resources to cope effectively and to make sound choices. They feel a sense of belongingness and a connectedness with others. They are motivated by the principle of social interest, which means that they are not interested merely in self-enhancement but are aware of the need to contribute to the common good.

Think about this discussion of how family rules are manifested in both functional and dysfunctional family structures. Rather than labeling your own family as "functional" or "dysfunctional," think about specific aspects within your family system that may not have been as healthy as you wish. Also think about those aspects of your family life that were helpful, functional, and healthy. Apply the discussion of family structures and family rules to your own experiences. We recommend several books that will provide you with more detailed information on this topic: Satir (1983), Satir (1989), and Satir and Baldwin (1983).

Family secrets can also influence the structure and functioning of a family. Secrets can be particularly devastating because that which is hidden typically assumes greater power than that which is out in the open. Generally, it is not what is openly talked about that causes difficulty in families but what is kept hidden. If there are secrets in the family, children are left to figure out what is going on in the home. Did you suspect that there were secrets in your family? If so, what was it like for you to perpetuate the secrecy? to divulge the secrets? What do you think that secrecy did to the family atmosphere?

Significant developments in your family. You might find it useful to describe your family's life cycle. Chart significant turning points that have characterized your family's development. One way to do this is to look at family photo albums to see what the pictures reveal. Let them stimulate memories and reflections. As you view pictures of your parents, grandparents, siblings, and other relatives, look for patterns that can offer clues to family dynamics. In charting transitions in the development of your family, reflect on these questions:

- What were the crisis points for your family?
- Can you recall any unexpected events?
- Were there any periods of separation due to employment, military service, or imprisonment?
- Who tended to have problems within the family? How were these problems manifested? How did others in the family react to the person with problems?
- In what ways did births affect the family?
- Were there any serious illnesses, accidents, divorces, or deaths in your family? If so, how did they affect individual members in the family and the family as a whole?
- Was there a history of physical, sexual, or emotional abuse?

Looking into these areas can enable you to determine the forces that have changed you, and this in turn will help you work with clients.

Proceed With Caution

If there has not been severe trauma in your family, simply reflecting on the questions we have raised that deal with your family history can be therapeutic by itself, even though it may be accompanied by some turmoil. If there has been severe trauma in your family life, we recommend that you support any exploration of your family with personal counseling. If you decide to carry the process a step further and interview members of your family, being sensitive to their feelings and reactions will go a long way toward reducing the chances that you will alienate family members.

In Chapter 7 you will learn that it is essential to be sensitive to cultural themes in the lives of your clients and their families and that you might lose certain clients if you do not demonstrate an understanding of how their culture affects their choices and actions. Apply this general principle as you approach members of your family. Be sensitive to the cultural rules of your family structure, and consider how concepts such as roles, rules, myths, and rituals operate in your family. In some families, a mother or father would be offended if a child were to seek information from an aunt or uncle. A Japanese graduate student approached his father to interview him as part of his family autobiography assignment. The father was reluctant to engage in any significant sharing of family material despite the student's insistence that getting this knowledge was important for him. Explain to family members your reasons for asking these questions.

In doing a review of your family history, be prepared for the possibility of a crisis developing, either for you or within your family. Doing this level of work may lead to a number of surprises and discoveries for which you are not prepared. One student discovered that she had been adopted. She was faced with dealing with anger and disappointment over not having been told. You may learn of family secrets, or you may learn that your "ideal family" is not as perfect as you thought. You may well find that your family has both functional and dysfunctional aspects. Many of the students who were enrolled in a personal-growth group with one of us (Marianne) became anxious or depressed by what they were learning about both themselves and their family system in their other classes and felt a need to talk about how they were being affected.

You may well discover that the sources of information are scarce, even about your grandparents. For example, I (Jerry) know precious little about my father's life before he and my mother married. From my father, I have some knowledge about his difficult beginnings in this country. At the age of 7, he and his brother came from Italy to New York. His father (whom I know almost nothing about) brought the two children to this country after his wife died. Again, there is scant information about my father's mother. I don't even know how she died. Apparently, my grandfather's intentions were to have a relative in this country care for his boys, yet this relative was unable to do so because of other family responsibilities. This led to my father's placement in an orphanage. I recall some stories he told me about the loneliness of his childhood in the institution and how difficult it was coming to this country not being able to speak a word of English. What is striking to me is how little I do know about my father's side of the family, and this in itself reveals how much material was denied and was kept secret. Because my father died over 40 years ago, I have had to look for bits of information from my mother about my father's history and also to relatives who knew something about his life.

In contrast, Marianne's family history is easily traced back to the early 1600s. For many years, I (Marianne) have heard rich stories that formed the tapestry of my family's history. As I grew up in an extended family in a German village, many relatives and townspeople revealed information about several generations. I did become aware of one pattern from my father's side. Someone in the family would typically get angry, and an emotional cutoff would result in which certain people would never speak to each other again. It saddens me to see how this pattern unfolds even with one of my brothers, who, in spite of my efforts to form a closer relationship, seems to be following the tendency of keeping himself distant. This experience is teaching me that family patterns repeat themselves and that we cannot change another person. But we do have power over how we allow ourselves to be affected by the actions and decisions of others.

Doing this level of self-exploration is a must if you intend to work with families. Committing yourself to this task will better enable you to appreciate what client family members go through when they are in therapy with you. We encourage you to stick with the process of discovery, preferably under supervision. It helps to be able to talk to someone about what you are learning.

Change does not come about without some pain and anxiety. Your commitment to exploration and change may bring discomfort to significant people in your life. Being involved in a training program as a helper involves some risks to your current relationships. Your parents, siblings, husband, wife, children, or other relatives may be threatened by some of your changes. You may believe in the value of recognizing pain and dealing with it, and as a result of your changed perspective you may want your parents or siblings also to adopt a new outlook and change their ways. Perhaps they have avoided pain and are not interested in disturbing this pattern. Even if facing their situation could lead to basic changes and a fuller existence, it is not for you to decide that they should be any different than they are.

As a result of what you are learning about human relationships in your program, along with positive changes you are making in your life, it can be difficult for you to see family members who seem to settle for a limited existence, if not a destructive lifestyle. You might ask, "How can I help other families in trouble if I cannot help my own family?" If you burden yourself with the thought that it is your task to change members of your family, you will end up feeling frustrated.

A graduate student in a counseling program approached one of us and said he felt burdened in putting to use in his own family what he was learning in his courses. Asked what he hoped to accomplish for a weekend therapeutic group aimed at self-exploration, he said: "I feel an urgency to clean up all my problems with my family by the end of this weekend workshop. After all, how can I help my future clients solve their problems if I have problems within my family?" Although this student was to be encouraged in his attempt to deal with his problems, he was setting himself up for failure by trying to meet an unrealistic expectation. Even more of a burden was his belief that it was his place to get significant people in his life to change. If people within his family were not motivated to make certain changes, he needed to realize that he would never be able to do it for them—no matter how talented he was. What he could do was to focus on himself and be true to himself, which in itself could be an invitation for them to change. He could talk about the changes he had made. He could also let others know how he was affected by some of their behaviors and, as well, what kind of relationship he would like with them.

The point is to avoid adopting an attitude that others should change. Patience and respect are critical. We can never be counselors for our own family members, and our parents are generally the last people in our lives we come to accept as peers in the human race (Jim Bitter, personal communication, March 17, 2009).

To make changes in your life, you probably had to get through layers of your own defenses. It took both time and patience for you to allow yourself to become more vulnerable and open to new possibilities. Allow this same space for others in your life to consider their changes.

Understanding Life Transitions

In this section we discuss major life themes at the various stages of human development from infancy through old age. **Personal transformation** demands an awareness of how you dealt with developmental tasks in the past and how you are now addressing these issues. By drawing on your own life experiences, both past and present, you are in a better position to appreciate the struggles of your clients, which enables you to intervene more effectively with them.

Our goal is for you to reflect on your life transitions, along with significant decisions that you have made at those junctures. It is a major challenge to work through an upheaval such as marriage or divorce, the birth or death of a child, losing a job, or retiring. All of these transition points test your ability to handle uncertainty, to leave what is known and secure, and to take a new direction in life. This kind of growth entails a willingness to suffer and a learning of life-giving lessons through that suffering. If your goal is comfort at all costs, you are likely to miss rich opportunities to become more of the person you are capable of becoming.

By understanding the challenges at each period of life, you will understand how earlier stages of personality development influence the choices you continue to make in life. There is a great variability among individuals within a given developmental phase. Your family of origin, culture, race, gender, sexual orientation, and socioeconomic status all have a great deal to do with the manner in which you experience the developmental process. Chronological age is only one index in considering emotional, physical, and social age.

A Theoretical Basis for Understanding Life Stages

There are many theoretical approaches to understanding human development, each of which provides a somewhat different conceptualization of the stages from infancy to old age. These theories provide a road map to understanding how people develop in all areas of personal functioning. We address three alternative perspectives on lifelong personality development in this section: we describe a model that draws on Erik Erikson's (1963, 1982) psychosocial theory of human development; incorporate Thomas Armstrong's (2007) "gifts" of each of the stages of life; and highlight some major ideas about development from the self-in-context approach, which emphasizes the individual life cycle in a systemic perspective (McGoldrick & Carter, 2005). The **systemic perspective** is grounded on the assumption that how we develop can best be understood through learning about our role and place in our family of origin. The systemic view is that individuals cannot really be understood apart from the family system of which they are a part.

We describe nine stages of development from infancy to old age by pointing out the psychosocial tasks for each phase. We also briefly describe potential problems in personality development if these tasks are not mastered. Acute and chronic illness during any period of life can disrupt the transition through the different life stages. For example, juvenile diabetes may disrupt normal childhood experiences; spinal cord injury, cancer, and HIV/AIDS can disrupt midcareer and social development. It is essential to recognize how your own development can be either an asset or a liability in your efforts to help others. As you read and reflect on these stages of development, ask yourself how well you have mastered some of the major **psychosocial tasks** at each period of your development.

Erikson's model is holistic, addressing humans inclusively as biological, social, and psychological beings. **Psychosocial theory** provides a conceptual framework for understanding trends in development; major developmental tasks at each stage of life; critical needs and their satisfaction or frustration; potentials for choice at each stage of life; critical turning points or developmental crises; and the origins of faulty personality development, which lead to later personality conflicts. Erikson's theory holds that we face the task of establishing equilibrium between ourselves and our social world at each stage of life.

Erikson describes human development over the entire life span in terms of various stages, each marked by a particular crisis to be resolved. For Erikson, **crisis** means a turning point in life, a moment of transition characterized by the potential to go either forward or backward in development. Critical turning points in our lives are influenced by a variety of biological, psychological, and social factors. Although we may not have direct control of some key elements of our development, such as early experiences and genetics, we have choices about how we interpret these experiences and use them to further our growth. At key turning points in our life, we can either successfully resolve the basic conflict or get stuck on the road to development. These turning points represent both dangers and opportunities: crises can be viewed as challenges to be met or as catastrophic events that simply happen to you. Each developmental stage builds on the psychological outcomes of earlier stages, and individuals sometimes fail to resolve the conflicts and thus regress. To a very large extent, an individual's current life is the result of earlier choices; life has continuity.

In *The Human Odyssey: Navigating the Twelve Stages of Life,* Thomas Armstrong (2007) maintains that every stage of life is equally significant and necessary for the welfare of humanity. Each stage of life has its own unique *gift* to contribute to the world. Armstrong believes that we should take the same attitude toward nurturing the human life cycle as we do toward protecting the environment from global warming and other threats. He argues that by supporting each of the developmental stages, we are helping to ensure that people are given care and helped to develop to their fullest potential.

McGoldrick and Carter (2005) have criticized Erikson's theory of individual development for underplaying the importance of the interpersonal realm and connection to others. Contextual factors have a critical bearing on our ability to formulate a clear identity as an individual and also to be able to connect to others. The **self-in-context perspective**, as described by McGoldrick and Carter, takes into account race, socioeconomic class, gender, ethnicity, and culture as central factors that influence the course of development throughout the individual's life cycle. These factors influence a child's beliefs about self and ways of being emotionally connected with others. For healthy development to occur, it is necessary to establish a clear sense of our unique selves in the context of our connection with others at each stage of life.

Infancy

In **infancy**, birth to age 1, the basic task is to develop a sense of trust in self, others, and the environment. The infant is a vibrant and seemingly unlimited source of energy (Armstrong, 2007). The core struggle at this time is for **trust versus mistrust**. If the significant persons in an infant's life provide the needed warmth and attention, the child develops a sense of trust. This sense of being loved is the best safeguard against fear, insecurity, and feelings of inadequacy.

If there is an absence of security in the home, personality problems tend to occur later. Insecure children come to view the world as a potentially frightening and dangerous place. They have a fear of reaching out to others, a fear of loving and trusting, and an inability to form or maintain intimate relationships. Rejected children learn to mistrust the world and view it largely in terms of its ability to do them harm. Some of the effects of rejection in infancy include tendencies in later childhood to be fearful, insecure, jealous, aggressive, hostile, and isolated.

Daniel Goleman (1995) believes that infancy is the beginning point for establishing **emotional intelligence**, which he defines as the ability to control impulses, empathize with others, form responsible interpersonal relationships, and develop intimate relationships. He identifies the most crucial factor in teaching emotional competence as timing, especially in our family of origin and in our culture of origin during infancy. He adds that childhood and adolescence expand on the foundation for learning a range of human competencies. Later development offers the critical windows of opportunity for acquiring the basic emotional patterns that will govern the rest of our lives.

Reflections and application. As you reflect on the developmental tasks during this stage, think about the foundation you had during your earliest years and how these experiences either prepared you or handicapped you for the tasks you now face in your life. Consider these questions: What did you learn from your family of origin about how to be in the world? Do you have difficulty trusting others? Are you able to trust yourself and your ability to make it in the world? Do you have fears that others will let you down and that you have to be very careful about how much you show of yourself?

Early Childhood

The most critical task of **early childhood**, ages 1 to 3, is to begin the journey toward autonomy. The core struggle at this time is for **autonomy versus shame and doubt**. By progressing from being taken care of by others to being able to care for one's own needs, children increase their understanding of interdependence and develop a sense of emotional competence, which involves delaying gratification.

Children who fail to master the task of establishing some control over themselves and coping with the world around them develop a sense of shame and feelings of doubt about their capabilities. Parents who do too much for children hamper their development. If parents insist on keeping children dependent, these children will begin to doubt the value of their own abilities. During this period it is essential that feelings such as hostility, anger, and hatred be accepted rather than judged. If these feelings are not accepted, children may not be able to accept their negative feelings later on. They will become adults who feel they must deny all of their "unacceptable" feelings.

Reflections and application. Some helpers have trouble recognizing or expressing angry feelings. Thus, they also have trouble allowing their clients to have these "unacceptable" feelings and may steer clients away from these feelings. If this description fits you, are you able to see any alternatives other than withdrawing from anger? One way you could behave differently is to remain in the room physically and psychologically as a client directs his anger toward you. Later, during a supervision session, you can deal with the fears that were evoked in you. If these feelings and attitudes get in the way of dealing with your clients, you may need to address this in your personal therapy.

Preschool

During the **preschool** years, ages 3 to 6, children seek to find out what they are able to do. The core struggle at this time is for **initiative versus guilt.** Preschoolers begin to learn to give and receive love and affection, learn basic attitudes regarding sexuality, and learn more complex social skills. According to Armstrong (2007), the gift of this stage of life is *playfulness.* When young children play, they re-create the world anew. They take *what is* and combine it with *what is possible* to fashion new events. According to Erikson, the basic task of the preschool years is to establish a sense of competence and initiative. If children are allowed realistic freedom to choose their own activities and make some of their own decisions, they tend to develop a positive orientation characterized by confidence in their ability to initiate and follow through. According to the self-in-context perspective, this stage ushers in the awareness of "otherness" in terms of gender, race, and disability. A key task is to increase trust in others (McGoldrick & Carter, 2005).

If children are unduly restricted or not allowed to make decisions for themselves, they develop a sense of guilt and ultimately withdraw from taking an active stance toward life. Parental attitudes toward children are communicated both verbally and nonverbally, and children often develop feelings of guilt based on negative messages from their parents. Children may pick up subtle messages that their body and their impulses are unacceptable, for example, and thus they soon begin to feel guilty about their natural impulses and feelings. Carried into adult life, these attitudes can prevent them from enjoying sexual intimacy.

During this period the foundations of gender-role identity are laid, and children begin to form a picture of appropriate masculine and feminine behavior. At some point both women and men may want to broaden their conception of what kind of person they want to be. However, early conditioning often makes the expansion of the self-concept somewhat difficult. Many people seek counseling because of problems they experience in regard to their gender-role identity.

Reflections and application. As you read and apply the developmental tasks of this stage to your own life, look for patterns in your present attitudes and behavior that could be traced to your preschool years. Consider some of these questions: Have you become the kind of woman or man you want to be? Where did you acquire your standards of appropriate gender-role behavior? What conflicts from your childhood affect you today? Do your present behaviors and current conflicts indicate areas of unfinished business?

Middle Childhood

Erikson states that the major struggle of **middle childhood**, ages 6 to 12, is for **industry versus inferiority.** The central task is to achieve a sense of industry; failure to do so results in a sense of inadequacy. Children need to expand their understanding of the world and continue to develop an appropriate gender-role identity. The development of a sense of industry includes focusing on creating goals, such as meeting challenges and finding success in school. According to Armstrong (2007), *imagination* is a key gift during the first half of this stage. The sense of an inner subjective self develops, and this sense of self is alive with images taken from the environment. During the second half of this stage, *ingenuity* is a key characteristic. Older children acquire a range of social and technical skills that enable them to deal with the increasing pressures they are facing.

From the self-in-context view, this is a time when children increase their understanding of self in terms of gender, race, culture, and abilities. There is an increased understanding of self in relation to family, peers, and community. A key task is developing empathy, or being able to take the perspective of others (McGoldrick & Carter, 2005).

Children who encounter failure in their early schooling often experience major handicaps later in life. Those children with early learning problems may begin to feel worthless. Such feelings often dramatically affect their relationships with their peers, which are also vital at this time. Problems that can originate during middle childhood include a negative self-concept, feelings of inferiority in establishing and maintaining social relationships, conflicts over values, a confused gender-role identity, dependency, a fear of new challenges, and a lack of initiative.

Reflections and application. What were some of the highlights of the first few years in school for you? Did you feel competent or incompetent as a learner? Did you see school as an exciting place to be or as a place that you wanted to avoid? What were some of the specific ways in which you felt that you were successful or that you were a failure? What attitudes did you form about your competence as a person during your early school years? Think of some significant people in your life at this time who affected you either positively or negatively. Attempt to recall some of their expectations for you, and remember the messages they gave you about your worth and potential. How might this be influencing you today?

Adolescence

Adolescence, ages 12 to 20, is a period of searching for an identity, continuing to find one's voice, and balancing caring of self with caring about others. The core struggle is for **identity versus identity confusion.** Armstrong (2007) describes the unique gift of this stage of life as *passion.* A powerful set of changes in the adolescent body is reflected in sexual, emotional, cultural, and spiritual passion and a deep inner zeal for life. From the self-in-context perspective, key developmental tasks include dealing with rapid body changes and body image issues, learning self-management, developing one's sexual identity, developing a philosophy of life and a spiritual identity, learning to deal with intimate relationships, and an expanded understanding of self in relation to others (McGoldrick & Carter, 2005).

For Erikson, the major developmental conflicts of adolescence center on the clarification of who you are, where you are going, and how you are getting there. The struggle involves integrating physical and social changes. Adolescents may feel pressured to make career choices early, to compete in the job market or in college, to become financially independent, and to commit themselves to physically and emotionally intimate relationships. Peer-group pressure is a major force, and it is easy to lose oneself by conforming to the expectations of friends. With the increasing stress experienced by many adolescents, suicidal ideation is not uncommon.

During the adolescent period, a major part of the identity-formation process consists of separation from the family system and establishment of an identity based on one's own experiences. The process of separating from parents can be an agonizing part of the struggle toward individuation. Although adolescents may adopt many of their parents' values, to individuate they must choose these values freely as opposed to accepting them without thought.

Reflections and application. Take a few moments to review some of your adolescent experiences. How did you feel about yourself during this time? In reviewing these years, how might your experiences work for or against you in dealing with your clients? Think about your degree of independence and interdependence during your adolescence. Focus on what gave meaning to your life. Also ask yourself these questions: At this time in my life, did I have a clear sense of who I was and where I was going? What major choices did I struggle with during my adolescent years? As you review this period, focus on how your adolescent experiences affected the person you are today.

Early Adulthood

According to Erikson, we enter **early adulthood,** ages 20 to 35, after we master the adolescent conflicts over identity. Our sense of identity is tested anew in adulthood, however, by the core struggle for **intimacy versus isolation.** The ability to form intimate relationships depends largely on having a clear sense of self. One cannot give to another if one has a weak ego or an unclear sense of identity. Intimacy involves sharing, giving ourselves, relating to another based on our strength, and a desire to grow with that person. If we think very little of ourselves, the chances are not good that we will be able to give meaningfully to others. The failure to achieve intimacy often results in feelings of isolation from others and a sense of alienation.

Armstrong (2007) identifies the principle of *enterprise* as a key characteristic of this stage of life. For young adults to accomplish the tasks facing them (such as finding a home and a partner or establishing a career), enterprise is required. This characteristic serves us well at any stage of life when we go into the world to make our mark.

Erikson and other early developmental psychologists thought adolescence ended around 18 to 20 years of age, but current research suggests that the adolescent brain keeps growing and developing well into our 20s. Boys and girls develop different capacities at different times, and one of the last capacities to develop in young men is the capacity for commitment—usually in their late 20s (Strauch, 2003).

The major aim of early adulthood is being able to engage in intimate relationships and find satisfying work. Some developmental issues include caring for self and others, focusing on long-range goals, nurturing others physically and emotionally, finding meaning in life, and developing tolerance for delaying gratification to meet long-range goals (McGoldrick & Carter, 2005).

As we leave adolescence and enter early adulthood, our central task is to assume increased responsibility and independence. Although most of us have moved away from our parents physically, not all of us have done so psychologically. To a greater or lesser degree, our parents will have a continuing influence on our lives. Cultural factors play a significant role in determining the degree to which our parents influence our lives. For example, in some cultures developing a spirit of independence is not encouraged. Instead, these cultures place a prime value on cooperation with others and on a spirit of interdependence. In some cultures, parents continue to have a significant impact and influence on their children even after they reach adulthood. Respect and honor for parents may be values that are extolled above individual freedom by the adult children. In these cultures the struggle for autonomy may be to define one's place in the family rather than to separate from it.

Autonomy, a key developmental task of early adulthood, refers to mature self-governance. If you are an autonomous person, you are able to function without constant approval and reassurance, are sensitive to the needs of others, can effectively meet the demands of daily living, are willing to ask for help when it is needed, and can provide support to others. You are at home with both your inner world and your outer world. Although you are concerned with meeting your needs, you do not do so at the expense of those around you. You are aware of the impact your behavior may have on others, and you consider the welfare of others as well as your own self-development. Making decisions about the quality of life you want for yourself and affirming these choices are partly what autonomy is about. Autonomy also entails your willingness to accept responsibility for the consequences of your choices rather than placing the responsibility on others if you are not satisfied with the way your life is going. Furthermore, achieving a healthy balance between independence and interdependence is not something you do at a given time once and for all. The struggle toward autonomy and interdependence begins in early childhood and continues throughout life.

In writing about genuine maturity from the self-in-context perspective, McGoldrick and Carter (2005) remind us that the ultimate goal in Western societies is to develop a mature, interdependent self. We are challenged to establish a solid sense of our unique self in the context of our connection to others. This systemic perspective is based on the assumption that maturity requires the ability to empathize, communicate, collaborate, connect, trust, and respect others. McGoldrick and Carter maintain that the degree to which we are able to form meaningful connections with people who differ from us in terms of gender, class, race, and culture "will depend on how these differences and connections were dealt with within our family of origin, within our communities, within our culture of origin, and within our society as a whole" (p. 28).

Reflections and application. If you are a middle-aged or older person, what decisions did you make in early adulthood, and how do you think those decisions would influence the way you might work with clients? Do you have any regrets about the choices you made? How do you think your own struggles or lack of them would affect you in working with clients who have problems deciding for themselves what they want to do personally and vocationally?

Middle Adulthood

Middle adulthood, between ages 35 and 55, is characterized by a "going outside of ourselves." The core struggle at this time is for **generativity versus stagnation.** It is a time for learning how to live creatively with ourselves and with others, and it can be the time of greatest productivity in our lives. This is a period when people are likely to engage in a philosophical reexamination of their lives, which may result in reinventing themselves in their work and in their involvement in the community (McGoldrick & Carter, 2005). Armstrong (2007) refers to *contemplation* as the gift of middle adulthood. People in midlife reflect on the deeper meaning of their lives, which is an important resource that can be drawn on to enrich life at any age. Other tasks include nurturing and supporting one's children, partner, and older family members. A challenge is to recognize accomplishments and accept limitations. Generativity includes more than fostering children. It includes being creative in one's career, finding meaningful leisure activities, and establishing significant relationships in which there is giving and receiving.

As is true with any stage, there are both dangers and opportunities during this time. Some of the dangers include slipping into secure but stale ways of being and failing to take advantage of opportunities for enriching life. Many individuals experience a midlife crisis, when their whole world seems to be unstable. During middle age there is sometimes a period of depression. When people begin to see that some of their visions have not materialized, they may give up hope for a better future. A problem of this period is the failure to achieve a sense of productivity, which then leads to feelings of stagnation. What is important is that individuals realize the choices they have in their life and see the changes they can make rather than giving in to the feeling that they are victims of life's circumstances.

Reflections and application. If you have reached middle adulthood, what struggles and decisions could you draw on as a resource? If you have not yet reached middle age, what would you most want to have accomplished in your life by this time? What would be your expectations for your relationships? What would you want from your work? How might you go about keeping yourself alive and avoiding predictable ruts?

Late Middle Age

Erikson does not differentiate between middle age and late middle age, but instead has one general stage that spans the period from the mid-30s to the mid-60s. For Armstrong (2007), the gift of this period is *benevolence.* Through their example, others are able to learn ways of striving to make the world a better place. McGoldrick and Carter (2005) differentiate between these two phases of middle age. For them, **late middle age,** ages 55 to 70, is a time when many adults are beginning to consider retirement, pursuing new interests, and thinking more about what they want to do with the rest of their lives. It is a period for taking up new interests, which may be increasingly possible as child rearing or financial responsibilities fade in importance. During this time, people become more aware of the reality of death, and they may reflect more on whether they are living well. It is a time for reevaluation and a time when people are at the crossroads of life. They may begin to question what else is left, and they may establish new priorities or renew their commitments. Late middle age is a period when people reach the top of the mountain and become aware that they must begin the downhill journey. They might painfully experience the discrepancy between the dreams of their younger years and the harsh reality of what they have actually accomplished with their life so far. A challenge during this period of life is coming to terms with the reality that not everything could be done. People must let go of some of their dreams, accept their limitations, stop dwelling on what they cannot do, and focus on what they *can* do (McGoldrick & Carter, 2005).

When people reach their mid-50s, they often begin the process of preparing for older age. Many are at their peak in terms of status and personal power, and this can be a satisfying time of life. Adults at this stage often do a lot of reflecting, contemplating, refocusing, and evaluating of themselves so they can continue to discover new directions.

Reflections and application. For a moment, reflect on a few personal and professional accomplishments you would most want to realize by the time you reach late middle age. If you could create a new direction at this time in your life, what might it look like?

Late Adulthood

Late adulthood, age 70 onward, is characterized by the core struggle for **integrity versus despair.** Encountering the death of parents and losses of friends and relatives confronts us with the reality of preparing ourselves for our own death.

A basic task of late adulthood is to complete a life review in which we put our life into perspective and come to accept who we are and what we have done. From Armstrong's (2007) perspective, people in late adulthood give the gift of *wisdom.* Older adults represent the source of wisdom that exists in each of us, which helps us avoid the mistakes of the past and reap the benefits of life's lessons. This is also a time in life when spirituality may take on a new meaning and provide us with a sense of purpose, even as we face a growing dependence on others (McGoldrick & Carter, 2005). Prevalent themes for people during late adulthood include loss; loneliness and social isolation; feelings of rejection; the struggle to find meaning in life; dependency; feelings of uselessness, hopelessness, and despair; fears of death and dying; grief over others' deaths; sadness over physical and mental deterioration; and regrets over past events. Today, many of these themes characterize people in their mid-80s more than people in their 60s and even 70s.

People who succeed in achieving ego integrity are able to accept that they have been productive and that they have coped with whatever failures they faced. Such people are able to accept the course of their lives, and they do not endlessly ruminate on all that they could have done, might have done, and should have done. In contrast, some older persons fail to achieve ego integration. They are able to see all that they have not done, and they often yearn for another chance to live in a different way.

Late adulthood has changed just as dramatically as the earlier middle-age stages. As is the case for each of these developmental stages, there is a great deal of individual variance. Many 70-year-olds have as much energy as many middle-aged people. How people look and feel during late adulthood is more than a matter of physical age; it is largely a matter of attitude. To a great degree, vitality is influenced by state of mind more than by mere chronological years lived.

Reflections and application.   If you have not reached old age, imagine yourself at that time of life. What would you like to be able to say about your life? What kind of relationships would you most hope to be able to have established at this time in your life? Focus especially on your fears of aging and also on what you hope you could accomplish by this time. What do you expect in these later years? What are you doing now that might have an effect on the kind of person you will be when you are old? Can you think of any regrets you will be likely to express? As you anticipate growing older, think about what you can do today to increase the chances that you will be able to achieve a sense of integrity as an older person. Are you cultivating interests and relationships that can become a source of satisfaction in later years?

If you find yourself postponing many things that you would like to do now, ask yourself why. Assess the degree to which you are satisfied with the person you are becoming today. Finally, assess your present ability to work with older clients. If you yourself have not reached this age, what experiences could you draw on as a way of understanding the world of an older client? Even though you might not have had some of the same experiences, do you see how you can relate to some of their feelings that are very much like your own?

Most of us can look back in our lives and remember enough to reflect effectively on our past transitions and experience, but we are able to look forward only about 10 years beyond our current age. If you are in late adolescence or early adulthood, interview older people at different developmental stages to gain a better understanding of what lies ahead. Listen with your heart. What can these people teach you about life and about what is yet to come?

It is critical to understand and reflect on the turning points in your own life so you will have a framework for working with clients. Self-exploration and self-understanding is a continuous process. You will need to know yourself if you hope to become a therapeutic agent in the lives of others. As we tell our own students, "You won't be able to take clients any further than you have been willing to go in your own life."

By Way of Review

• Some training programs offer family-of-origin work for students as a way for them to come to a fuller appreciation of how their family experiences have influenced who and what they are. This training enables helpers to relate more effectively to the families they will meet in their clinical practice.

• To increase your effectiveness when working with families, it is essential that you unravel the mystery of your connection with your family of origin and that you become aware of ways you continue to play out patterns established during childhood.

• When interpreting the meaning of your experiences growing up in your family, it is useful to think about the structure of your family, your relationships with your parents and siblings, key turning points for your family, and the messages your parents conveyed.

• Being a professional helper often reopens your own psychological wounds. If you are not willing to work on your unfinished business, you might reconsider whether you want to accompany clients on their journey of dealing with their past wounds.

• Personal counseling, both individual and group work, is of value in increasing your self-awareness and providing you with an opportunity to explore your unresolved conflicts. By becoming involved in your own counseling, you can gain increased insight into personal issues that could intrude in your work.

• Family therapy and personal therapy can illuminate your own areas of transference and countertransference and broaden your vision of how your family-of-origin experiences have served as a template for later interpersonal relationships. Your experience with the therapeutic process can increase your awareness of certain patterns of thinking, feeling, and behaving.

- Each of the nine stages of life represents a turning point when individuals are challenged with the fulfillment of their destinies. Both helpers and clients need to realize that personal transformation entails the willingness to tolerate pain and uncertainty. Growth is not generally a smooth process but involves a degree of turmoil.

- At each stage of life there are choices to be made. Your earlier choices have an impact on the kind of person you are now.

- Specific tasks and specific crises can occur from infancy through old age. Review your own developmental history so that you have a perspective in working with the developmental struggles of your clients. You will be in a better position to understand your clients' problems and to work with them if you have an understanding of your own life experiences and vulnerabilities.

- How you cope with crises in your own life is a good indication of your ability to help your clients work through theirs. If you face and deal with your problems with all the resources available to you, you can be present for clients who are in crisis. Your understanding of ways to tap internal resources can serve you as you guide clients in discovering their resources for change.

What Will You Do Now?

1. As a basis for discovering more about your family of origin, interview your parents and any others who knew you well as you were growing up. You can ask each of these people a specific list of questions about yourself. The point of this exercise is for you to gather events or situations that can assist you in getting a fuller picture of your childhood. What does each person remember the most about you? Are you able to detect any themes in what the people you interview recall about you?

2. Develop a list of questions to help you understand what it was like for your parents as they were growing up. For example, you might ask your parents what their relationships with their parents were like at ages 6, 14, or 21. The aim of the exercise is not to put them on the spot or to get them to divulge secrets, but to better understand the hopes, goals, concerns, fears, and dreams your parents had as children, adolescents, and young adults. You might talk with your parents about how their early experiences influenced them as parents. Discuss with them any patterns you see between them and yourself.

3. If possible, consider interviewing your grandparents. Again, in thinking about questions you would like them to address, be sensitive to how they might respond to sharing personal facets of their lives. You might simply ask them to share any events or memories that they would feel comfortable disclosing. Rather than simply asking them questions, consider sharing with them

significant memories you have of them as you were growing up. What did they teach you? What similar patterns do you see that have been handed down from your grandparents, to your parents, to you, and to your children, if any?

4. Consider making a personal journal that will compile significant information about your family of origin. In putting this journal together, focus on the self-exploration questions raised in this chapter. You might even have short chapters illustrating turning points in your life. In doing this project, it would be useful to include pictures of you and your parents, siblings, grandparents, other relatives, and friends. Include any input from your parents, grandparents, and other relatives that will provide details of your family-of-origin experiences. Look for themes and patterns that will give you a clearer picture of the forces that still influence you today.

5. Much of this chapter provides you with material for reflection about how your family-of-origin experiences influence the person you are today. Spend some time thinking about what you learned about yourself *personally* by reading this chapter. Are there any personal issues that you see as being unresolved and that you are committed to exploring? If so, write about this unfinished business in your journal. How might your own unresolved personal issues affect your ability to work with individuals who are struggling with concerns pertaining to their family?

6. Write down a list of resources for personal growth and ways of increasing your self-awareness. Think of some avenues that would promote self-exploration on your part. Are you willing to do something that will encourage you to reflect on the quality of your life?

7. Remember a time in your life that was either the most difficult (painful) or the most exciting (joyful). What did you learn from these experiences? If this time occurred during childhood, talk with someone you knew well as a child about what he or she remembers of you. What are the implications of these experiences in your own life for you as a helper? How might some of your life experiences affect you as you work with others who are like you? different from you?

8. Reflect on some of your life experiences that you think will facilitate your work with clients. Use your journal to record a few key turning points in your life. Can you think of one or two times when you were faced with making a major decision? If so, how might this turning point still have an influence on your life? What lessons did you learn from making this decision, and how might this experience better enable you to identify with the struggles of clients?

9. In small groups, spend some time exploring how your experiences with your family are likely to influence your work with families and with individuals as well. What are some of your attitudes about family life that will show up in your professional work?

10. For the full bibliographic entry for each of these sources, consult the References at the back of the book. Thomlison (2002) is a good source as a family assessment workbook. For a self-in-context developmental approach that emphasizes an individual life cycle in a systemic perspective, see McGoldrick and Carter (2005). See Armstrong (2007) for a discussion of the stages of development in the life cycle. For an overview of development through life from a psychosocial perspective, see Newman and Newman (2009). For a comprehensive and well-written book on family therapy, see Bitter (2009). For themes and choices dealing with childhood, adolescence, and adulthood, refer to G. Corey and Corey (2010).

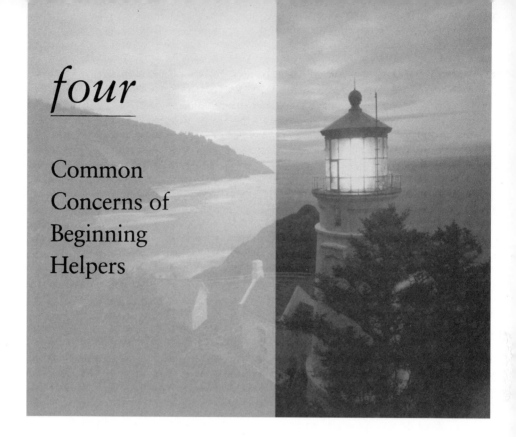

four

Common Concerns of Beginning Helpers

Focus Questions

1. As a helper, how can you best deal with clients exhibiting difficult behavior? angry clients? unmotivated clients? quiet or withdrawn clients?

2. How can you handle your fear of angering clients when you confront them about problematic behaviors? How would you deal therapeutically with clients' resistance so they are more likely to look at their behavior than defend themselves?

3. How can you avoid bringing the problems of clients home with you? How can you remain open and sensitive to your clients' struggles yet at the same time acquire some appropriate distance from their problems?

4. How can you deal with your reactions that are stimulated by working with a wide range of clients?

5. What client behaviors do you find most problematic? Why?

6. What do you generally do when you are faced with working with "difficult clients" (or difficult friends)?

7. What aspects from your past are likely to affect your ability to work with certain types of clients? What have you done to heal your own psychological wounds?

8. What kind of clients would you most likely refer to another professional? What might this tell you about yourself?

9. How do you respond when you feel personally threatened? How open are you to recognizing your patterns of resistance? What do you think your job would be like if you had a caseload composed of clients like yourself?

10. How willing are you to examine your own personal issues as part of your professional development?

Aim of the Chapter

Chapter 3 stressed the importance of helper self-knowledge and how helpers can use their own life experiences as a way to better understand those with whom they will work. In this chapter we look at ways that you are likely to be personally affected by your work as a helper. Your capacity and willingness to be open to what is emerging inside of you as you confront defensive behavior in your clients is the theme of this chapter.

As a helper you will encounter a range of special concerns throughout your career, but some problems will be particularly pressing for you. It is critical that you understand and learn how to deal effectively with the feelings that some of your clients have toward you and the corresponding feelings that they evoke in you. Even experienced helpers show an interest in learning creative ways to deal with difficult clients, especially people who are highly defensive. In this chapter we address the important issues of transference, countertransference, resistance, and understanding and managing your own feelings and actions as you work with clients with whom you have difficulty.

Some helpers become too invested in getting well-defended clients to change, and they fail to be aware of their own dynamics and reactions as they interact with clients they perceive as being difficult. It can be productive to pay as much attention to yourself as you do to your clients. Don't think that you should know exactly what to do in every complex situation. In your program you will have many opportunities to learn and practice the skills that can be applied to demanding situations. Your supervised field placement activities and your supervisory sessions are ideal places to talk about the concerns raised in this chapter as well as to practice various intervention skills. If you are beginning your training program, you are not expected to have the knowledge or skills to cope effectively with some of the cases we present in this chapter, but at least these cases can get you thinking.

This chapter will probably raise more questions than it answers. There are no simple solutions to the many complex situations that you can encounter in your helping relationships. Our purpose is to introduce you to a range of common concerns that beginning helpers typically face.

Exploring Self-Doubts and Fears

Students in human services programs sometimes bring up fears, perfectionist strivings, and other personal concerns. Students often express their anxiety over the prospect of facing clients. They ask themselves: "What will my clients want? Will I be able to help them? What if I don't know what to say? Will they want to come back?" Realize that anxiety can be a normal reaction to facing a new or threatening situation. Too much anxiety can render an intern unable to pay attention to the client, however; so it is critical for helpers to learn how to manage their anxiety. Another concern of many students and practitioners is their expectation that they must be able to help all clients. They often burden themselves with the belief that they cannot afford to be less than perfect, lest they make a mistake and hurt a client.

In practicum and internship courses we frequently hear statements of self-doubt from those who are beginning to help others. Apply these statements to yourself, and decide to what degree you see them as your concerns. If a statement is more true than false for you, place a "T" in front of it; if it is more false than true for you, mark it with an "F."

_____ 1. I am afraid my clients will suffer from my mistakes and my uncertainty in knowing what to do.

_____ 2. I often feel I should know more than I do.

_____ 3. I feel uncomfortable with silences in counseling situations.

_____ 4. It is important for me to know that my clients are making continuous improvement.

_____ 5. It would be difficult for me to deal with overly demanding clients.

_____ 6. I am likely to have trouble working with clients who are not motivated to change or who are mandated to come to me for counseling.

_____ 7. I have trouble deciding how much of the responsibility for change is mine and how much is my client's.

_____ 8. I feel very responsible for my clients.

_____ 9. I am concerned that I may have trouble being myself and trusting my intuition when I practice counseling.

_____ 10. I am afraid of confrontation, and I think this might be a problem when helping others.

_____ 11. I worry that my clients will think I am incompetent because I am a beginner.

_____ 12. I am not sure how much of my personal reactions I should reveal in counseling sessions.

_____ 13. I tend to worry about making the proper intervention.

_____ 14. I worry that I may overidentify with my client's problems to the extent that they become *my* problems.

_____ 15. During a counseling session, I might find myself wanting to give advice.

_____ 16. I am afraid that I might say or do something that would greatly disturb a client.

_____ 17. I'm concerned about working with clients whose values and culture are different from my own.

_____ 18. I am apprehensive about whether my clients like and approve of me.

_____ 19. I am nervous about videotaping my sessions.

_____ 20. I am concerned about the ending of a counseling session or a counseling relationship.

Now go back and select the issues that represent your greatest concerns. What negative messages are you telling yourself, and how might you begin to critically evaluate them if they are not serving you well?

Transference and Countertransference

In the questionnaire that you just took, you may have pinpointed concerns and fears that could influence your ability to work effectively with clients. Certainly a major concern of many helpers, both personally and professionally, is being able to deal constructively with clients' reactions to them. A central task is to know when your reactions are being triggered by your own internal conflicts rather than resulting from the dynamics of your clients.

Various Forms of Transference

The previous chapter introduced the concepts of transference and countertransference, and this chapter addresses these topics in more detail. You will recall that your experiences with your family of origin may influence the manner in which you will be able to manage feelings a client may project onto you. **Transference** often operates on the unconscious level and involves clients projecting onto a helper past feelings or attitudes they had toward significant people in their lives.

Transference typically has its origins in early childhood and constitutes a repetition of past material in the present. "It reflects the deep patterning of old experiences in relationships as they emerge in current life" (Luborsky, O'Reilly-Landry, & Arlow, 2008, p. 46). This pattern causes a distortion in the way clients perceive and react to the counselor. Clients may have a multitude of feelings and reactions to you. A client may view you with a mixture of positive and negative feelings. At different times the same individual may express love, affection, resentment, rage, dependency, and ambivalence. Transference feelings take place even in the practice of brief counseling. It is essential to understand what transference means and how to deal with it skillfully.

In our training workshops for students and mental health practitioners, we explore examples of difficult client behavior that participants present to us. We stress the importance of understanding the functions that these behaviors serve for individuals, examining the payoffs of a client's defensive style and understanding how it is an attempt to cope with anxiety. Rather than focusing on the dynamics of difficult clients and ways of dealing with them, we devote attention to assisting helpers in becoming aware of, understanding, and exploring their own reactions. We encourage those whom we teach to approach defensive behaviors with interest and respect rather than with impatience and judgment.

Here are some examples of transference situations that you are likely to encounter. Ask yourself what your response might be to a client's feelings toward you and what feelings are likely to be evoked in you.

🌑 ***Clients who perceive you in distorted ways.*** Some clients will perceive you as an idealized parent. They may have an expectation that you will take care of them in ways that their parents never did. In considering clients who make you into a parent and want you to adopt them, ask yourself these questions: How comfortable or uncomfortable am I with clients who attribute to me unrealistic traits and attributes? How do I feel when clients have unrealistic expectations of me? How tempting would it be for me to accept clients' idealized version of me?

Other clients may immediately distrust you because you remind them of a former spouse, a critical parent, or some other important figure in their life. For example, consider the female client who is assigned to a male therapist and lets him know that she has little regard for men. The men in her life have been untrustworthy, and because her therapist is male, he, too, might well betray her. If you had a client who prejudged you on the basis of earlier experiences, how would you react? Are you able to recognize your client's behavior as a transference reaction and deal with it nondefensively? How would you show this client that you are a different person than people in her past? How would you respond if no matter how positive your interactions are with her, she continues to tell you that you will eventually let her down?

Some clients will not let themselves get emotionally close to you because they experienced abandonment in early childhood. They are taking past experiences and superimposing them on you. Assume that a client of yours comes from a divorced family. She is somehow convinced that she caused her parents to separate. Because she was abandoned in the past and remembers the pain of that time in her life, she is wary of letting you into her life. If she gets too close to you, she fears that she will not know what to do and that you may also abandon her. In working with such a client, consider these questions: What can I do to convince her that I do not intend to abandon her? What are my reactions to being told that I am going to be like her parents? How would I handle such a situation?

● **Clients who see you as perfect.**   Consider this male client: He uses superlative adjectives to describe you. He sees you as always understanding and supportive. He is sure that you have the ideal family and cannot imagine that you might have any personal difficulties. He credits you with the changes he is making in his counseling with you. How would you deal with this client and all the adulation he heaps on you?

●**Clients who make unrealistic demands on you.**   Some clients make no decisions without first finding out what you think. They may want to know if they can call you at any time. They may request that you extend the allotted time for their sessions. They talk about how close they feel to you and would like to be your friend. They want you to affirm them and tell them that they are special. Even though you may intellectually understand the nature of these unrealistic demands, how do you imagine such demands would affect you emotionally? In what ways could you help such clients see the connection between how they are treating you and how they treated some significant person in their past?

● **Clients who displace anger onto you.**   Some clients will lash out at you with displaced anger. They will be annoyed with you if you confront them. These clients let you know that they resent you when you give them your observations and reactions to their behavior. Recognize that you are probably getting more of this client's anger than you deserve, and avoid getting into a debate with the person. If you take the client's reactions to you too personally, you are bound to react defensively. As a helper, how do you deal with your feelings toward a person who behaves in this way? How can you express your reactions to clients in a way that does not cause them to become increasingly defensive? With this kind of client, you may need to express and deal with your own feelings with a supervisor or a trusted colleague.

● *Clients who fall in love with you.* Some clients will make you the object of their affection. They may tell you that there is nobody in the world whom they feel as much affection for as you. They are convinced that they would not have the problems they are faced with now if they could find a person like you who would love and accept them. How would you respond to this kind of adulation? Could your client's reactions distort or enhance your self-perceptions?

Understanding and Working With Transference Therapeutically

These illustrations of transference behaviors demonstrate how essential it is for you to gain awareness of your own needs and motivations. If you are unaware of your own dynamics, you will tie into your clients' projections and get lost in their distortions. You are likely to avoid focusing on key issues and instead attempt to defend yourself. Paying attention to your own feelings about a client who imposes on you and makes unreasonable demands of you will give you a sense of how significant people in this client's life are affected by his or her behavior.

When clients appear to work very hard at getting the counselor to reject them, it can be useful to explore what they are getting from this self-defeating behavior or how what they are doing serves them. Handled properly, clients can experience and express feelings toward you that more properly belong to others who have been significant in their lives. When these feelings are therapeutically explored, clients become aware of how they are keeping old patterns functional in many of their current relationships. By paying attention to how your clients behave and react to you, you can begin to understand how they react to significant others in their lives.

It is a mistake to think that all feelings your clients have toward you are simply transference. At times clients may be realistically angry with you because of something you have done or said or not done. Their anger does not have to be an irrational response triggered from past situations. If you answer your phone during a session with a client, for example, she may become angry with you over the interruptions and your lack of presence. Her anger could be a justifiable reaction and not one that should be "explained away" as a mere expression of transference.

Likewise, clients' affection for you does not always indicate transference. It could be that they genuinely like some of your traits and enjoy being with you. Of course, some helpers are quick to interpret positive feelings as realistic and negative feelings as distortions. You can err both by being too willing to accept unconditionally whatever clients tell you and by interpreting everything they tell you as a sign of transference.

In a group setting we have found it useful to have the participants gradually become aware of their transference reactions to each other and to the group leaders. At the beginning of a group, we ask members to pay particular attention to people in the room whom they notice most. We facilitate the process of members' increasing their awareness of others by asking these questions:

- Whom in this group are you most aware of?
- Are you finding yourself drawn to some people more than to others?
- Do some people seem especially threatening to you?
- Are you finding yourself making quick assumptions about others? For example, "He looks judgmental." "She's intimidating me." "I think I can trust him." "I definitely want to stay away from her." "It looks as if these three people are a clique."

We pay particular attention to group members who have strong reactions to a person whom they hardly know. It is common for people to "see" in others some of the very traits they disown in themselves. This process of projection forms the basis of transference. Although we ask the participants to become aware of their first reactions to others, we do not ask them to reveal these thoughts or to respond to others too quickly. Instead, we suggest that participants share their reactions after they have had some chances for interaction. By disclosing such persistent positive or negative responses, they have opportunities to come to a deeper understanding of aspects of themselves that they are unaware of. A therapeutic group provides a context for increasing awareness of certain patterns of psychological vulnerability. Members of a group can gain insight into the ways their unresolved conflicts create certain patterns of dysfunctional behavior. By focusing on what is going on within a group session, the group provides a dynamic understanding of how people function in out-of-group situations. This insight may include coming to an understanding of how they were impacted by important figures in their childhood and how they now act around people who are significant to them. With this new insight, people are able to catch themselves when old patterns become evident in their daily interactions. Rather than responding automatically, they are now able to respond in different ways. Thus, a man who treats most women in authority roles with deference can stop himself from making them into representations of his mother. He can then respond to different women more as they really are.

Some writers take a dim view of the concept of transference. One such person is Carl Rogers, the founder of the person-centered approach to counseling and therapy. In describing Rogers's perspective on transference, Thorne (2002) states: "Essentially he [Rogers] sees the notion of transference as a hugely sophisticated device for preventing true relationship and for defending the therapist against real involvement where the exploration of the actual feelings between two persons can take place" (p. 56). Erving Polster (1995), a pioneer in Gestalt therapy, believes the concept of transference can have depersonalizing effects by taking the therapist out of the here-and-now relationship. This tends to minimize what is actually going on in the therapeutic encounter and diminishes connectedness. Instead, Polster emphasizes the experience of genuine contact between client and therapist.

Understanding and Dealing With Countertransference

Transference tends to evoke reactions in the helper, and these reactions can become problematic if they result in **countertransference:** the therapist's unconscious emotional responses to a client that result in a distorted perception of the client's behavior. This phenomenon occurs when there is inappropriate affect, when counselors respond in highly defensive ways, or when they lose their objectivity in a relationship because their own conflicts are triggered. It is important to be alert to the possibility of countertransference and to guard against unrealistic reactions helpers may have toward their clients that interfere with their objectivity. If you want to be effective in your helping efforts, it is essential that you consider countertransference as a potential source of difficulties. You do not have to be problem free, but it is crucial that you understand how your own problems and countertransference can affect the quality of your relationships with clients.

Countertransference is not always harmful. You can use all of your reactions in therapeutic ways, assuming that you eventually become aware of the sources of your countertransference. Remember that we are considering countertransference from a broader perspective than the psychoanalytic view of countertransference as being merely a reflection of an individual's unresolved internal conflicts that need to be overcome as a prerequisite to working effectively with a client. Brockett and Gleckman (1991) conceptualize countertransference broadly to encompass all of the counselor's thoughts and feelings in reaction to clients, whether prompted by the clients themselves or by events in the helper's own life. Ainslie (2007) states that the contemporary understanding of countertransference "has broadened significantly to include a range of feelings, reactions, and responses to the client's material that are not seen as problematic but, on the contrary, are viewed as vital tools to understanding the client's experience" (p. 17). Countertransference reactions can provide powerful information for both the client and the practitioner.

The helper's task is to attend to the feelings he or she is experiencing in relationship to the client and then to identify the sources of these emotional reactions. It is essential that counselors monitor their feelings during their sessions with clients, and that they use their responses as a source for understanding clients and helping them to understand themselves. When counselors' personal issues are brought into awareness, the chances increase that their countertransference will be managed appropriately, which means that their reactions are less likely to interfere with the helping relationship. Brockett and Gleckman (1991) believe that supervision, honest introspection, and involvement in one's own therapy as a client are particularly useful ways of achieving understanding of countertransference phenomena.

Simply having feelings toward a client does not automatically mean that you are having countertransference reactions. You may feel deep empathy and compassion for some of your clients as a function of their life situations. Countertransference occurs when your needs become too much a part of the relationship or when your clients trigger old wounds of yours. Just as your clients will have some unrealistic reactions to you and will project onto you some of their unresolved personal matters, so too can you have unrealistic reactions to them.

As you reflect on ways that you may be emotionally triggered in working with certain clients, think about how you are affected by those you perceive as being especially difficult. How do you respond to the different forms of transference? What kind of client tends to elicit your countertransference? Do you take the guarded behavior of a client in a personal way? Do you blame yourself for not being skillful enough? Do you tend to become combative with clients who you perceive as being difficult?

We ask you to look at how your own attitudes, behaviors, and reactions to clients may, at times, actually foster defensiveness in them. Without being overly self-critical or blaming yourself, examine your reactions to those with whom you work to determine how what you are doing can either decrease or escalate the problematic behaviors your clients manifest. As a helper, it is crucial that you be willing to look at the part you may play in contributing to problematic behaviors in clients.

If you use your own feelings as a way of understanding yourself, your client, and the relationship between the two of you, these feelings can be a positive and healing force. Even though you may be insightful and self-aware, the demands of the helping profession are great. The emotionally intense relationships that develop with your clients can be expected to bring your unresolved conflicts to the surface. Because countertransference may be a form of identification with your client, you can easily get lost in the client's world, and thus your ability to be helpful is limited. Below are some illustrations of countertransference:

• *"Let me help you."* Your client has had a very difficult life. No matter how hard he tries, things don't work out, in spite of his best efforts. You find yourself going out of your way to be helpful to this client to the extent that he becomes dependent on you.

• *"I hope he cancels."* You are intimidated by a client's anger directed at you or others. When you are in the presence of this client, you are not yourself but are self-conscious and guarded. When he cancels a session, you find yourself relieved.

• *"You remind me of someone I know."* Your clients will often remind you of significant people in your own life. Put yourself in each of these situations, and imagine how you would respond and to whom you are responding when you have reactions to a client.

1. You are a middle-aged therapist, and your husband has left you for a younger woman. You are faced with a female client who is having an affair with a middle-aged married man. Now, consider that your client is the middle-aged man who is having an affair with the much younger woman.
2. You have been a rape victim, and your client discloses that she has been raped. Or your client informs you that he has raped a woman years ago.

3. You were abused as a child, and your client tells you, after several months, that he has abused his own children.
4. You have just dealt at home with a rebellious teenage daughter, and your first client for the day is a hostile, acting-out boy.
5. You lost a grandfather, but you have never really gone through a mourning process and come to terms with his death. One of your older male clients is in poor health and almost dies. As he talks about his feelings, you are extremely uncomfortable and find yourself unable to respond to him. You attempt to reassure him that he will be all right.

• *"You are too much like me."* Some of your clients are bound to remind you of some of the traits that you would rather not acknowledge in yourself. Even if you do recognize certain traits, you may find it disconcerting to work with clients who talk about problems and situations that are very much like your own. A client may be a compulsive workaholic, for example, and you may see yourself as working too hard. You might find yourself spending a lot of energy getting this client to slow down and take it easy.

• *"My own reactions are getting in my way."* Sometimes your clients will express pain and show tears. This anguish may make you anxious because it reminds you of some past or present situation in your life that you would rather avoid. You may intervene, asking questions in an attempt to stop the client's feelings. It is important to realize that such interventions are motivated by bringing comfort to the helper, not by doing what is in the best interest of the client.

No one is immune to countertransference, and it is crucial that you be alert to its subtle signs. You may find that certain clients evoke a parental response in you. Their behavior can bring out your own critical responses to them. Knowing this about yourself enables you to work through some of your own projections or places where you are strongly affected.

Among the most vulnerable to the effects of countertransference may be those caregivers who work with the seriously ill or dying. These caregivers are continually confronted with the reality of death. In their work they watch people around them die. Unless these caregivers are able to process their reactions, this work will take an emotional toll on them. Unless you have explored your feelings about death, loss, separation, and grief, your feelings will continue to be activated as you work with clients. In our experience in training students, we find that many of them have difficulty working with people who are terminally ill or with older persons because of the constant reminder of their own mortality. Working with these clients can be very rewarding, but it can sometimes be anxiety provoking and stressful as well (Brockett & Gleckman, 1991).

Empathy fatigue, a form of countertransference, can result from helpers being exposed to the pain that clients express, especially if counselors are not aware of their own unresolved personal issues (Stebnicki, 2008). Stebnicki notes that counselors can easily experience intense feelings of being overwhelmed by listening to multiple client stories of grief, stress, loss, and trauma. Counselors can get lost in clients' themes of trauma and pain. As a defense, helpers may dissociate and distance themselves from their clients' overwhelming feelings of grief and helplessness.

You probably will not be able to eliminate countertransference altogether, but you can learn to recognize manifestations of countertransference and deal with them as *your problem* rather than your client's problem. Countertransference becomes problematic when it is not recognized, understood, monitored, and managed. Recognizing countertransference is the most important first step in learning how to manage it. Here are some additional signs to watch for in recognizing your own countertransference:

- You become intensely irritated by certain clients.
- With some clients you continually run overtime.
- You find yourself wanting to lend money to some unfortunate clients.
- You feel like adopting an abused child.
- You quickly take away pain from a grieving client.
- You usually feel depressed after seeing a particular client.
- You are developing sexual feelings toward a client.
- You tend to become bored with some clients.
- You often work much harder than your client.
- You frequently get overly emotional with certain clients.
- You give a great deal of advice and want your clients to do what you think they should do.
- You are quick not to accept a certain type of client, or you suggest a referral even though you have little information about the client.
- You find yourself lecturing or debating with some clients.
- You need approval or admiration from certain clients.

Remember that it is not the feelings that are the problem; rather, it is the behavior generated by certain feelings that we need to be concerned about. To manage countertransference, you must have a receptive attitude and welcome self-awareness, be self-disciplined, and be willing to share your responses in a timely and therapeutic manner (Brockett & Gleckman, 1991). Accept whatever feelings you are experiencing without feeling guilty or judgmental.

When you begin to realize that certain topics or issues stimulate heightened feelings or specific reactions on your part, it is essential that you strive to understand what is contributing to your excessive or inappropriate responses. Self-exploration and consultation are excellent paths toward gaining this self-understanding (Brems, 2001).

Your own supervision will be a central factor in learning how to deal effectively with both transference and countertransference reactions. You can become more aware of your own manifestations of countertransference by focusing on yourself in your supervision sessions. Rather than talking exclusively about a client's problem, spend some time talking about how you feel when you are in a session with a client. A good way to expand your awareness of potential countertransference is by talking with colleagues and supervisors about your feelings toward clients.

Ongoing supervision will enable you to accept responsibility for your reactions and at the same time prevent you from taking full responsibility for directions that your clients take. Self-knowledge is your most basic tool in dealing effectively with transference and countertransference. It is well to remember that helping others change will certainly also change you. If you are unwilling to resolve your own personal problems and conflicts, you will not have much credibility when you ask your clients to explore their deeper concerns.

Understanding and Dealing With Difficult Clients

Professional helpers and students alike are concerned with how to handle difficult clients. They hope to learn techniques for making these clients less troublesome, for such clients tax them personally and professionally. There are no simple techniques. In our workshops we help participants become aware of and understand their own reactions to behavior they view as being problematic, and we teach ways of constructively sharing their reactions with clients.

Attitude Questionnaire on Understanding and Working With Problematic Behavior and Difficult Clients

Take a few minutes to complete this self-inventory to examine your attitudes toward resistance and problematic behaviors exhibited by clients. Indicate your position on each statement using the following scale:

1 = strongly agree
2 = slightly agree
3 = slightly disagree
4 = strongly disagree

_____ 1. Difficult clients force me to reflect on and explore my own unresolved problems that get in the way of being an effective helper.
_____ 2. Problematic behavior is best approached with a sense of interest.
_____ 3. Resistance on the part of clients generally leads to ineffective results in the helping process.
_____ 4. When I encounter clients' reluctance, it generally gets me to question my part in contributing to this behavior.
_____ 5. Involuntary clients will rarely benefit from professional helping relationships.
_____ 6. When clients are silent, this is almost always a lack of willingness to cooperate with treatment.
_____ 7. Client defensiveness is often a sign of handling a transference relationship poorly.

_____ 8. The most effective way of dealing with client defensiveness is to be highly confrontational with clients.

_____ 9. One way of working with difficult clients is to pay attention to my own feelings.

_____ 10. Labeling or judging clients who exhibit difficult behavior tends to entrench this behavior.

Now look over your responses and try to identify patterns in your perceptions of defensiveness and difficult behavior. At this point, how does problematic behavior from clients generally affect you, and how can you effectively deal with this?

Handling Resistance With Understanding and Respect

Most people with whom you work will test you in some way to determine if the relationship with you will be a safe one. It is essential that you encourage openness on the part of your clients so that they are able to express their hesitations and anxieties. Most clients will experience ambivalence and defensiveness at various times in the helping process. Clients are likely to have mixed feelings regarding staying in a safe zone versus taking the risk of letting you know them. Both you and your clients need to understand the meaning of resistance and defensiveness and come to view these behaviors as something to explore in the helping relationship.

From a psychoanalytic perspective, **resistance** is defined as the individual's reluctance to bring into conscious awareness threatening material that has been previously repressed or denied. It can also be viewed as anything that prevents individuals from dealing with unconscious material. From a broader perspective, resistance can be viewed as behavior that keeps us from exploring personal conflicts or painful feelings. Resistance can be thought of as ways we attempt to protect ourselves from anxiety and defend ourselves from pain, and thus it serves a function.

Clients may manifest resistance in a variety of problematic behaviors. Learn to respect resistance and various forms of avoidance, and strive to understand the meaning of these behaviors. Teyber (2006) suggests that counselors can understand the client's reluctance as an outdated coping strategy that at one time served a self-preservative and adaptive function. Teyber asserts that by honoring clients' resistance, helpers are able to appreciate the fact that a particular coping strategy was the best possible response to a difficult situation. By viewing clients' symptoms and problematic behaviors as survival mechanisms, both helpers and clients can recognize that some resistance is perfectly normal and makes good sense. According to Teyber, it is inaccurate to view client resistance as manifestations of lying or lacking motivation. He views resistance as a natural part of the therapeutic process, which needs to be explored and understood: "Resistance occurs when clients are simply unaware of the multiple and often contradictory feelings that have been activated by seeking help, exploring difficult topics, or successfully making changes and getting better" (p. 100). Teyber encourages helpers to explore with clients how they are experiencing each session, beginning at the initial meeting. Unless helpers ask clients about any potential problems with the helping process, their concerns will likely remain unspoken.

You don't get clients' respect immediately, nor do credentials alone really earn you genuine regard. Instead, your clients will come to trust you, and thus let down some of their guard, if you approach their reluctance with compassion, regard, and respect. Part of respecting resistance means that you appreciate the functions these defenses serve. If you succeed in helping clients to surrender some of their defenses, are you able to assist them in developing better ways of coping with life's demands? There are times when people need their defenses to survive a crisis situation. At such times, you need to be supportive rather than insist that your clients surrender their protection.

Perhaps the key to understanding clients' various forms of defensive behavior is in paying attention to your countertransference, which is evoked by behaviors on the part of the client. You cannot afford to have a fragile ego as a professional helper. Give your clients some rope, and strive not to respond defensively to any problematic behavior they might display. If you keep in mind that your clients are coming to you for help, you may be able to be more patient with them.

In dealing with difficult clients, monitor your responses to their behavior. If you respond in an aggressive or harsh way, a tense situation is likely to worsen. If clients exhibit initial distrust, view this as a sign of strength and recognize ways you can utilize clients' cautiousness in the helping process. This is an example of how a perceived weakness can actually be reconceptualized as a strength. Clients have their own reasons for lack of cooperation and for refusing the help that they have sought. The helper and the client need to know what these reasons are, and they need to address these in the helping relationship. Your task is to approach difficult clients in a different way and work cooperatively with them so that they might learn new and more effective ways of coping.

Clients whom you perceive as being difficult or challenging may contribute to your own feelings of self-doubt and incompetence and bring out your feelings of inadequacy and anger. If you too quickly become annoyed with clients who are challenging, you are likely to cut off avenues of reaching them. We hope you would avoid labeling clients as "resistant" and instead describe the behaviors you are observing. When you view clients as being scared, overwhelmed with grief, cautious, or hurt, you can reframe any problematic behavior pattern they may manifest. By simply changing the word "resistant" to more descriptive and nonjudgmental terminology, your own attitude toward clients who appear to be "difficult" may change. As you change the lens by which you perceive clients' behaviors, it will be easier for you to adopt an understanding attitude and to encourage clients to explore the meaning of their reluctance. Instead of viewing their behavior as something designed to make your work impossible, try to approach such behavior with a genuine sense of interest and curiosity.

If your client, Enrique, exhibits hostile behavior, consider reframing this experience: "It's interesting how hard Enrique is trying to get me to be angry with him. I wonder how his behavior is serving a purpose and whether he could find another way to get what he wants more directly." As another example, consider Maribel, a client who sits silent for much of each session. "Maribel seems scared. Her silence during the sessions may be due to her lack of understanding of how to ask for help with her problems." Describe how you see your clients behaving toward you and invite them to explore the meaning of their behavior. It may be appropriate to let them know how certain of their behaviors are affecting you. After this declaration of your personal reactions, clients are more likely to explore alternative ways of getting what they want from you and from others.

Types of Challenging Clients

Albert Ellis (2002) has described the many forms that resistance takes as counselors work with what he calls "difficult customers." Rational emotive behavior therapy (REBT) acknowledges that some resistance is a normal reaction because fears are attached to the process of change. From the REBT perspective, resistance is caused by a variety of factors within the client (such as irrational thinking), but the counselor's attitudes and behavior can also produce much client resistance. Ellis has written about how to deal with the resistance of your most difficult client—*you*. His main point is that therapists are human and very fallible. Therapists, like their clients, all too often incorporate irrational beliefs and accept assumptions that they have not questioned. When helpers encounter clients who display resistance, for example, helpers often take full responsibility for this, believing that if they were competent helpers their clients would be cooperative.

If you want to be effective with difficult clients, develop patience and give clients room to maneuver. Establish whether clients' are interested in changing patterns of behavior that they perceive as problematic. If clients assert that they do not want to change a certain behavior, or that this behavior is not a problem in their outside life, your efforts to facilitate change may be in vain.

While working with clients whom you perceive as being problematic, do not put the exclusive focus on them. Rather than constantly paying attention to the problematic behaviors manifested by your clients, reflect on your reactions to your clients. See what these reactions tell you, both about yourself and about your client. Regardless of which specific behavior a client exhibits, it is essential that you understand your own countertransference. Certain clients are more difficult for you because they evoke your countertransference reactions. Think about which of the characteristics of difficult clients described in the following pages would provide the greatest challenge to you.

Involuntary clients. You may not always be able to work with clients who freely come to you for your help. Some will be sent by the court, others will be sent by their parents, others will come in under duress with a spouse, and some will be referred to you by another helper. Involuntary clients may have little motivation for change and may see little value in the help that you offer. For example, Herman attends a class for those found guilty of driving under the influence. His main motivation in coming to this class is to satisfy the judge's order. He figures that attending class is better than going to jail. Although he is willing to come to the sessions, he tells you that he doesn't believe that he has a problem. Rather, his intoxication was due to a series of unfortunate circumstances. He does not see much that he needs to change.

In your role as a helper, you could become either defensive or apologetic. We see it as a mistake to apologize for the fact that an involuntary client is sitting in your office. A client who is not seeing you voluntarily can be difficult to engage. Sometimes clients are reluctant to seek help because of their misconceptions about what the helping process entails, or they may have had negative experiences with counseling. How you approach such clients will determine the degree to which they will become more or less cooperative. For example, by exploring Herman's resistance and showing your willingness to provide information about the services you offer, his resistance may be reduced, increasing the likelihood that Herman will become more interested in the help you have to offer. Together you can make a contract specifying the willingness you both have to work productively.

Clients who are silent and withdrawn. Clients who say very little almost always evoke anxiety. Imagine this client sitting in your office: He looks down at the floor much of the time, responds politely and briefly to your questions, and does not volunteer any information. For you the session seems to last forever, and you feel as though you are getting nowhere. You might ask, "Do you want to be here?" He will reply, "Sure, why not?" If you ask him what he wants to change in his life and what he wants to talk about, he will say that he doesn't know.

Is it your responsibility to get this client talking? Are you taking his silence personally? Are you thinking of ways to draw him out? Before you assume an inordinate amount of responsibility, or before you judge his silence unfavorably, attempt to put his silence in some context. You might ask yourself, and even at times your client, what the silence means. His silence could have any one of the following meanings: He is frightened. He sees you as the expert and is waiting for you to ask a question or tell him what to do. He feels dumb; he may be rehearsing every thought and critically judging his every reaction. He feels shame over asking for help. He is responding to past conditioning of "being seen but not heard." His culture may put a value on silence. He may have been taught to listen respectfully and merely to answer questions. Furthermore, your client may be quiet and invisible because this pattern served to protect him as a child. In other words, all forms of silence should not be interpreted as a refusal to cooperate with your attempts to help.

Silent clients in a group counseling situation can affect you and the other members in many ways. You may judge yourself, thinking that if you knew the right things to say and do, your client would open up and talk fully. You could do the talking for your client or constantly draw him out. It might be helpful to say something like this: "I notice that you are very quiet in this group. You seem to pay attention to what other group members are saying, yet I rarely hear from you. I'd like to know more about how it is for you to be in this group." If this client does not interpret his silence as a problem, maybe you will be working in vain in trying to change him. This silent group member will have many reasons for being quiet. If he does see his silence as a problem, you can explore with him the ways in which this behavior is problematic. If you assume full responsibility for bringing him out, he never has to struggle with the reasons underlying his silence.

Clients who talk excessively. The opposite of the client who very rarely talks is the person who talks incessantly. Some clients tend to get lost in telling stories. They provide you with every detail so they won't be misunderstood. However, you may be left wondering what the point of the story is. Instead of talking about how they are affected by a particular situation, they overwhelm people with information that is not relevant.

Consider the case of Bertha, who inundates you with detailed information. Any attempt you make to slow her down results in her telling you that she wants to be sure that you understand what she is saying. She gets very involved in "he-said" and "she-said" monologues. Bertha keeps talking because if she slows down and experiences some of the things she is talking about, she is likely to feel anxious.

In working with Bertha, you might feel overwhelmed and not know how to intervene. Although she is talking about painful situations, she is doing so in a very detached and rehearsed style. You might have reservations about interrupting her, out of fear of cutting her off. One of your functions is to help Bertha gain awareness into how her behavior might serve as a defense. Here are a few examples of some helpful comments you might make:

- I notice that when you speak of your relationship with your mother you tear up. Then you quickly change the subject and talk about another matter.
- I have trouble following what you're saying. I wonder what it is you are trying to tell me.
- Would you be willing to stop right here, and tell me what you are feeling at this moment?
- You are making a real effort to give me a lot of details so that I can understand you better. I want to understand you, yet the many details you provide make it difficult for me to hear what you are trying to tell me.
- If you had to express in one sentence all that you have been trying to tell me, what would you say?

If you are having reactions to a client like Bertha who overwhelms you with words, such as noticing that you have a hard time staying with her, it could be therapeutic to deal with your own reactions. Chances are that Bertha is affecting many people in her life in much the same way as she is affecting you. This is an opportunity for her to get feedback on how she comes across and for her to determine if she wants to do anything different. If you chronically suppress your reactions and pretend that you are listening with unconditional positive regard, you are reinforcing her talkativeness.

Clients who overwhelm themselves. Some of your clients have an abundance of problems, which chronically overwhelm them. They may overwhelm you as well. Such clients often have an endless reserve of problems. They come in each week and excitedly begin with "Just wait until I tell you what happened to me this week." Although some of the situations they describe are painful, you suspect that they get some sense of excitement out of reporting these long lists of problems. You need to intervene actively and sensitively, or they will overwhelm both themselves and you! You may not know where to begin, and you are likely to feel burdened with all of these problems, especially if you think that you must solve them.

As with other forms of unsuccessful communication, you need to explore with clients who overwhelm themselves the ways in which they contribute to their problems by what they are doing. It can be helpful to say something like this: "I know there are many things that you feel are pressing on you today. I suggest you sit quietly for a moment and reflect on what it is that you most want from this session? Select the one concern that is most pressing to you at this time." By focusing the client, you may be a catalyst in helping the person avoid being drowned in a sea of problems.

Clients who often say "Yes, but . . ." You will encounter clients who are exceptionally talented at inventing reasons your interventions just won't work. As a helper faced with such clients, you will quickly feel depleted. No matter what insights or hunches you share or what suggestions you make, the end result is the same: the client quickly retorts with an objection. Some illustrations of the "yes, but" syndrome follow:

HELPER: I recommend that you bring your wife to one of your counseling sessions.
CLIENT: "Yes, but you don't know my wife." "I agree that it might help, but my wife would be very threatened." "But my wife will never change!" "I'm willing to talk to her, but I don't think it would help."
HELPER: Every time I suggest something, you come back with reasons why my suggestion wouldn't work. I wonder if you really want to change.
CLIENT: "Yes, but you just don't understand my situation." "You expect so much of me. I try, but things just don't work out." "Of course I want to change, but there are just so many things that keep me from changing."

When you are trying to help such clients, there is a tendency to become easily discouraged. It doesn't take much to get irritated. Even though you are willing to help this client, he is convinced that he cannot be helped. Eventually you may feel helpless and be inclined to give up. When you sense that you are working harder than your client is working, it may be time to renegotiate with him what he wants and why he is coming to see you.

Clients who blame others. Some clients adopt a style of blaming circumstances and other people for most of what happens to them. Carrie is a good illustration of a client who is quick to find fault outside of herself for her unhappiness but slow to recognize her part in contributing to her unhappiness. She views herself as having no control over her life. She does not consider her role in creating her own unhappiness, largely because she is attuned to looking outside of herself. Here are just a few of the outside factors that she sees as being responsible for her unhappy life: her husband does not understand her; her children are selfish and inconsiderate; she has severe allergies, which keep her from doing what she wants; she really can't lose weight because she is too depressed.

As long as Carrie puts the focus of her problems outside of herself, no change is possible in her life unless others change. It is possible for you to work with her to change, but you cannot work with all of the variables apart from her, nor can you change the people in her life.

It would not be surprising if Carrie were to annoy you. You might engage in a lot of argumentation with her, challenging her on all of the ways in which she makes her life unhappy. If she continually refused to look at her own role, you might be tempted to refer her. As with most of these forms of problematic behaviors, you can confront her on certain behaviors, share your reactions with her, listen to her, and ask her what she is willing to do to get what she says she wants.

Clients who deny needing help. Some people do not see that they have a problem. They may come to a couples counseling session wanting to help their spouse but be unwilling to see their part in the troubled relationship. It is not likely to be productive for you to attempt to convince these clients that they have a problem when they insist otherwise.

For example, if you ask Roy what he wants from you, he will probably reply: "My wife wanted me to come to counseling, and I'm here for her sake." You may be able to get through to Roy if you take his word for it and accept his view that he is problem free. By asking him how he is being affected by his wife's problems, you may eventually get to problems that he wants to deny. Another alternative is to ask him how it is for him to come to your office. If he replies by saying, "Oh, it's fine," you could respond, "What were you thinking as you approached the office?" Or you could ask: "You say you're here to help your wife. What are some of the areas that you think she needs help with?" Or you could say: "You tell me that you don't have any problems and that your wife made you come here today. Could this be a problem for you?"

Some of the students we work with talk about how much they want to help others, but they are less able to identify personal issues in their own lives. We have heard such students talk about their problems in the past tense. They are ready to admit that they had problems, but they maintain that they have dealt with and solved these problems. In some of your classes you have probably had opportunities for experiential and personal-growth activities. Think about how open you were to exploring any facets of your life with others. How defended were you? How motivated were you to listen to and reflect on feedback given you by others? If you find it difficult to own up to potential problems in your life, do you think you will be able to effectively challenge clients to make an honest assessment of what troubles them?

Clients who manifest passive-aggressive behavior. Certain clients have learned to defend themselves from hurt by dealing with people indirectly. They use hostility and sarcasm as a part of their style of avoiding. They are highly evasive when they are confronted. If you give your reactions, they are likely to say: "Well, you really shouldn't feel this way. When I made that remark, I was just kidding. You take me too seriously."

Some common signs of clients who exhibit **passive-aggressive behavior** are as follows: They often arrive late. They say little. You see reactions on their faces, yet they assure you that everything is fine. They giggle when you talk. They raise eyebrows, frown, sigh, shake their head, look bored, and show other non-verbal reactions yet deny that anything is going on with them. They chronically draw attention to themselves, and when they have the attention, they do little with it.

Clients who behave in passive-aggressive ways may be hard to deal with. It is not helpful to label them and to interpret their behavior by saying, "You are passive-aggressive." It is hard to deal directly with such behavior because of its elusive quality. However, you will certainly have reactions to clients who make hostile remarks, who offer sarcasm, and who seem to engage in hit-and-run behavior. One way of cutting through this indirect behavior is to be aware of what it brings up in you and to give your reactions. Avoid making judgments, but describe the behavior you see and tell the clients how their behavior is affecting you. It is also useful to ask them if they are aware of their behavior and to tell you what it means. For example, you might say something like this: "I have noticed that when I talk, you sometimes smile, or roll your eyes, or turn around. I find myself reacting to you and wonder if there is something you want to say to me." This comment gives the client an opportunity to be more direct and to interpret his or her own behavior.

Here are some possible questions to consider: Do certain clients who display hostility remind me of any people in my life? What do I feel like when people are not direct and I sense that there are some things they are not telling me? Is it timely and appropriate for me to give my reactions to the hostility I perceive from my clients?

Clients who rely primarily on their intellect. Individuals who block out feelings and present themselves in intellectual ways are another type of difficult client. Any time they get close to an emotion, they find a way to evade the feelings and turn them into a safer cognitive zone. They constantly try to figure out why they have a problem. They are adept at self-diagnosis and theorizing abstractly about the nature of their dysfunctions. They know that as long as they function primarily on an intellectual level they are safe. If they allow themselves to feel jealousy, pain, depression, anger, or any other emotion, they do not feel safe. To avoid experiencing anxiety, they have learned to insulate themselves from feelings.

Don't attack such clients and insist that they get to a feeling level. You can let them know how it is for you to be with them when they show little affect, but it is not helpful to try to strip away their defense. When they feel ready to let go of it, they will do so. Think about the ways in which you are affected in dealing with a woman who remains very cerebral. If you are successful in getting her to give up her protection, will you be able to help her? Will you be able to be present for this person when she lowers her defenses and gets in touch with years of repressed feelings? Will you be overwhelmed by her pain? If you are not able to be present when she expresses her fear, will this prove to her that people are not to be trusted with her emotions?

Clients who use emotions as a defense. The opposite of clients who use their intellect as a defense are clients who often emote. Their behavior may put you in a bind. You may have trouble trusting their emotions. You may become annoyed, feel manipulated, or suspect that they are not sincere.

We are not suggesting that clients who genuinely express emotions are resisting. We are talking about clients who use their emotions as a defense. When you are with such clients, reflect on what they bring out in you. It is possible that some of your highly emotional clients could remind you of people in your life who manipulated you with their emotions. For example, a sister might have succeeded in making you feel guilty when she cried and stormed out of the room. Now, as you work with clients who exhibit some of these behaviors, you may feel a lack of compassion for them and, in turn, wonder whether you have a problem with empathy.

Dealing Effectively With Defensive Behavior

Learn to listen attentively and with respect as clients express their fears, reservations, ambivalences, and reluctances. Think about ways you can intervene when clients exhibit problematic behavior or give signs of defensiveness. Here are some guidelines for you to consider:

- Express your reactions to clients respectfully.
- Avoid responding to sarcastic remarks with sarcasm or to hostile comments with hostility.
- Provide clients with necessary information so they can get the most from the helping process.
- Encourage clients to explore their fears and hesitations rather than expecting immediate trust.
- Avoid judging a client; instead, describe the behavior you are observing that tends to be self-defeating.
- State observations and hunches in a tentative way as opposed to being dogmatic.
- Be sensitive to clients who are culturally different from you without stereotyping a client because of his or her culture.
- Monitor your own countertransference reactions.
- Avoid using your knowledge, expertise, and power to intimidate those seeking help.
- Do not take clients' reactions in an overly personal way.

When we talk about dealing with difficult client behaviors in workshops, participants are always interested in learning specific strategies for dealing with the type of client behavior they find most frustrating. In our discussion here, we have avoided suggesting techniques that might change clients. Instead, we put the focus on you, as a person and as a helper. You cannot directly change clients who are manifesting defensive behaviors, but you can learn significant lessons about the dynamics of their behavior as well as better understand your own defenses.

Focus on why your clients have come to you, what they hope to get, and how you can teach them better ways of fulfilling their needs. If you respond in a negative manner to clients who exhibit negative behaviors, it will hamper your effectiveness with them. If you resist the temptation to attack their defenses, and if you avoid labeling or judging them, the chances of their defenses being lowered increase. If you can acknowledge your reactions to these clients, you are more likely to be effective with them. For a useful treatment of the subject of understanding and working with difficult clients, we recommend Fred Hanna's (2002) book, *Therapy With Difficult Clients*.

Recognizing Competence and Learning to Refer

It is common for beginning helpers to have doubts about their general level of competence. In fact, it is not at all unusual for even experienced mental health practitioners to wonder seriously at times whether they have the personal and professional abilities, knowledge, and skills needed to work with some of their clients. It is more troubling to think of helpers who rarely question the adequacy of their skills. In thinking about the matter, you may range from one extreme to the other, at times being plagued with self-doubts and at other times thinking that you can deal with any problem a client presents.

Striving for competence is a lifelong endeavor (Barnett, Doll, Younggren, & Rubin, 2007), and it is best to think of competence as a process rather than as something we achieve once and for all. You may achieve competence in a particular field, but you need to take steps to maintain this level of knowledge and skills throughout your career. One of the most important steps toward maintaining our competence is to engage in regular consultation with other professionals throughout our career (Bennett et al., 2006).

Assessing Your Competence

All of the professional codes of ethics spell out that you should not practice beyond the limits of your competence. Here is one example of a standard pertaining to competence:

> Counselors practice only within the boundaries of their competence, based on their education, training, supervised experience, state and national professional credentials, and appropriate professional experience. Counselors gain knowledge, personal awareness, sensitivity, and skills pertinent to working with a diverse client population. (ACA, 2005, C.2.a.)

Assessing competence is not an easy task. Many people who complete a doctoral program lack the skills or knowledge needed to carry out certain therapeutic tasks. Obviously, a degree alone does not guarantee competence for any and all helping services. In your role as a helper, you will work with a wide spectrum of clients in very diverse settings, which requires different skills and competencies. You need to assess how far you can safely go with clients, when to seek consultation, and when to refer clients to other professionals. Careful self-monitoring is an effective way to ensure that you are providing quality services. It is important to learn when to consult another professional if you have not had extensive experience working with a particular problem.

Knowing When and How to Make Referrals

When faced with difficult clients like those described in this chapter, you might well doubt your competence and be inclined to make a referral. We hope you will not see the answer for working with difficult clients, on a routine basis, as referring them to another professional.

The ethics codes of most professional organizations stipulate that making referrals, when appropriate, is a responsibility of the professional helper. For example, the National Association of Social Workers (2008) provides this guideline:

> Social workers should refer clients to other professionals when other professionals' specialized knowledge or expertise is needed to serve clients fully or when social workers believe they are not being effective or making reasonable progress with clients and additional service is required. (2.06.a.)

How do you know when and how to refer? How will the client be affected? Why would you want to refer? What kind of referral might be the most appropriate? What if few referral resources are available? It is crucial for you to refer clients to other resources when working with them is beyond your ability. A client's failure to make progress with you is another reason to consider a referral. Other circumstances may also lead you to wonder if a referral is in order. You and a client may decide that because of value conflicts or for some other reason your relationship is not productive, and the client may want to work with another helper. For these and other reasons you will need to develop a framework for evaluating when to refer a client, and you will need to learn how to make this referral in such a manner that your client will be open to accepting your suggestion rather than be harmed by it.

Clients can be negatively affected when you too quickly refer them. If you follow the practice of referring all clients with whom you have difficulty, you might soon have very few clients! It is a good idea to think about the reasons that motivate you to suggest a referral. If you recognize a pattern of frequent referrals, then you may need to examine your reasons for doing so.

In cases where you have limited experience, it is especially important to be open to consulting another professional as a way to acquire or upgrade your skills. We hope that you can say to a client, "I don't know what to do, but I know where we can get some help." Beginning helpers sometimes believe that they must always know what to do, and they hesitate to let their clients know that they might not be sure how best to proceed. Although we do not expect you to know everything, we certainly expect that you can learn much under supervision.

Keeping Current

Your academic program will provide some basic training, yet it is essential to find ways of extending your education beyond graduation. Your knowledge and skills will soon be outdated unless you take steps to keep abreast of new developments.

Some current issues in the helping professions that are receiving increased attention are methods of dealing with substance abuse; eating disorders; gay, lesbian, bisexual, and transgender issues; traumatic stress; survivors of natural disasters; people with physical disabilities; domestic violence; physical, psychological, and sexual abuse of children; abuse of older persons and spouses; addictions recovery; HIV/AIDS; conflict resolution skills; parent education; adolescent suicide; school violence; culturally diverse client populations; and legal and ethical issues. Many professions have mandatory continuing-education requirements for relicensing or recertification of their members. Take advantage of in-service and continuing-education programs to learn about emerging trends. You can keep abreast of developments by taking specialized courses and workshops that deal with particular client groups and newer interventions. Another way of keeping current of developments in your field is through reading. In addition to professional journals and books dealing with your specific subject of interest, novels and nonfiction works about other cultures can contribute to your continuing education.

Perhaps the best way of keeping yourself up to date is to be involved in a professional network with colleagues who are willing to learn from one another as well as assume a teaching role. Colleagues can offer both the challenge and the support for practitioners to adopt a fresh perspective on problems they encounter in professional practice. Networking among professionals can also provide a consistent means of identifying and addressing sources of negative feelings and loss of objectivity. An excellent way to develop this network is by joining the professional organization that most interests you and by attending the state, regional, and national conferences offered by this organization (see Chapter 1).

By Way of Review

- Effective helpers must become aware of clients' transference and of their own countertransference. Neither of these factors is to be eliminated but is to be understood and dealt with therapeutically.

- Countertransference refers to the unrealistic reactions that therapists have toward clients, which are likely to interfere with their objectivity. One way of becoming more aware of your potential for countertransference is by being willing to seek your own therapy. Another way is by focusing in your supervisory sessions on yourself and your reactions to clients.

- Defensive behavior and reluctance take many forms, and it is necessary to understand the ways in which they protect clients. Not all cautiousness or reluctance stems from stubbornness on the part of the client. Some can be caused, or at least contributed to, by the attitudes and behaviors of helpers.

• The goal in a helping relationship is not to eliminate resistance but to understand what functions it serves and to use it as a focus for exploration.

• There are many types of difficult clients. Some of them will evoke your own countertransference reactions. When this happens, you are now part of the problem.

• Ethics codes explicitly state that it is unethical to practice outside the boundaries of your competence. It is essential that you be able to make an accurate assessment of your knowledge and skills to determine your ability to effectively work with a particular client. You need to learn what clients you can best work with and to know when a referral is appropriate.

• Either as an intern or on your job, you may be asked to take on clients or to provide therapeutic strategies that are beyond the scope of your training and experience. Learn to be assertive in staying within your limits.

• Referral resources are sometimes limited. This is particularly true in some less-populated areas where mental health facilities are scant. To make good referrals, become knowledgeable about the resources that might be available for your clients.

• Graduation from a training program does not signal the end of learning but merely the beginning of a process of professional growth and development. To maintain your effectiveness, continuing education is a necessity.

• One of the best ways of keeping on the cutting edge of one's profession is to become involved in a peer-consultation group that affords professionals opportunities to share their concerns and learn from one another. Through peer groups, helpers can actively contribute to their own personal and professional development and that of their colleagues.

What Will You Do Now?

1. Select the most difficult client whom you can imagine working with, and reflect on the ways this client could present problems for you. What makes this client a difficult one for you? What do you think you would do if you actually had this person as a client? What might you do if you felt that you could not work with him or her?

2. Reflect on the kinds of defensive behavior that you see within yourself. How open are you to accepting your limitations? If you were a client in counseling, what defenses to changing do you imagine that you might develop? What

do you think it would be like if your clients were very much like you? Talk with a friend about this subject as a way of confirming (or contradicting) your views.

3. Look over the descriptive list of difficult client behaviors and identify specific kinds of client behaviors you would find it most difficult to deal with in a helping relationship. In your journal write down what you can learn about yourself from your reactions to certain behaviors displayed by clients.

4. In small groups explore what you think the criteria should be for determining whether a therapist is competent. Make a list of specific criteria, and share it with the rest of the class. Are you able as a class to identify some common criteria for determining competence?

5. In small groups explore the topic of when and how you might make a referral. Role-play a referral, with one student playing the client and another playing the counselor. After a few minutes the "client" and the other students can give the "counselor" feedback on how he or she handled the situation.

6. Look again at the inventory at the beginning of the chapter that helped you identify your self-doubts and fears pertaining to your role as a helper. Select one or two of these concerns and write about them. What are some steps you might take in dealing with your greatest concerns?

7. Review the attitude questionnaire on working with resistance and difficult clients. Write down your ideas about how you might become more therapeutic in dealing with resistance and difficult clients.

8. For the full bibliographic entry for each of the sources listed here, consult the References at the back of the book. For a treatment of transference and countertransference, see Luborsky, O'Reilly-Landry, and Arlow (2008). See Ellis (1999, 2002) and Ellis and MacLaren (2005) for a discussion of cognitive, emotive, and behavioral approaches in dealing with resistance. For ways of confronting and dealing with resistances, see Kottler (2005), and for an excellent treatment of what makes clients difficult and how to manage difficult cases, see Kottler (1992). For an in-depth discussion of honoring the client's resistance, see Teyber (2006). For a discussion of what makes a client difficult and for working therapeutically with difficult clients, see Hanna (2002).

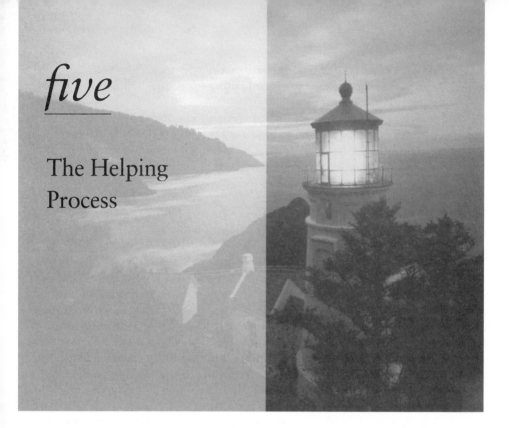

five

The Helping Process

Focus Questions

1. What beliefs do you have about the capacity of people to change? How can change best be facilitated? What constitutes effective helping? What is the best way to evaluate the degree of change in clients?

2. How is your philosophy of human nature related to your approach to working with people who seek your help?

3. What basic beliefs do you hold about the helping process? How do you think these beliefs influence your practice?

4. Which of your assets and resources can you draw on in establishing helping relationships? What liabilities or limitations do you have that might interfere with forming working relationships with certain clients?

5. If a client appeared to be getting little from a helping relationship with you, what questions could you ask yourself and your client?

6. How does knowledge about the stages of helping influence what you do with a client?

7. What guidelines would you use in confronting (or challenging) clients? What is the purpose of confrontation? What difficulties do you anticipate when confronting clients?

8. How important is helper self-disclosure in the helping relationship? What guidelines would you use to determine when self-disclosure is appropriate? Can you think of any difficulties involved in self-disclosure?

9. How would you work with clients to formulate goals for the helping relationship? How do you develop action plans with your clients?

10. What guidelines would you use for effective termination? Can you think of any factors that would make it difficult for you to end therapy with clients?

Aim of the Chapter

The purpose of this chapter is to help you clarify your role at various stages in the helping process. We look at the skills and knowledge you need and the personal characteristics that are required to apply your skills. We identify specific skills that are especially relevant for the various stages in a helping relationship and ask you to assess your current level of skill development. Our basic assumption is that the kind of person you are and the attitudes you bring to the helping relationship are the major determinants of its quality.

In our view you need to integrate knowledge, skills, and the person you are to be an effective helper. Knowledge alone is not sufficient, yet without it you cannot become an effective helper. If you focus mainly on acquiring skills and neglect theory and knowledge, these skills will have little value. Effective helpers must be sensitive to the interpersonal dimension of the helping process to productively apply their skills and knowledge in each situation. Helpers who have little self-awareness are at best skilled technicians with a limited ability to make a difference in the lives of clients. Helping is more than technique; it is also an expression of who the helper is. The helping professions are based on scientific knowledge that practitioners are able to use in creative and personal ways. In short, helping is both an art and a science.

In this chapter we assist you in clarifying your thinking about helping by raising these questions: Who is responsible for change in the helping relationship? What is the helper's role at various stages in the helping process? What is the role of clients in identifying personal goals and in achieving these goals? How can you best determine the appropriate balance of focusing on feeling, thoughts, and behaviors? What is the best balance between providing a great deal of structure and providing only minimal structure? What is an appropriate balance between challenge and support? Do you believe clients are capable of finding their own solutions to problems? How can you best create and maintain a collaborative working relationship with your clients?

Your View of the Helping Process

Your view of the helping process is largely a function of your beliefs about human nature and about how people change. Before you accept a position in any setting, it is essential that you understand the philosophy of the agency because this influences the manner in which the agency functions. Sometimes a particular perspective will be imposed on you. For example, you might work in a state facility that employs behavior-modification strategies. Or an agency may make extensive use of a diagnostic framework, and you will be expected to conduct initial interviews and arrive at a specific diagnostic category for each client you see. If what an agency expects of you in your role as a helper is not compatible with your views of your role, you will experience conflict. A good starting point is to identify and clarify your views pertaining to how helping can best occur.

The Impact of Your Beliefs on Your Work

Your views and beliefs about human nature are very much related to the helping strategies you will employ with your clients. If you see people as basically good, for example, you will trust that your clients can assume responsibility for the direction of their lives. If you see human nature through a negative lens, you will most likely adopt a role as a helper who attempts to correct people's flawed nature. To clarify your views about human nature, use this scale as you reflect on these statements:

5 = strongly agree
4 = agree
3 = undecided
2 = disagree
1 = strongly disagree

_____ 1. People need direction to resolve their problems.
_____ 2. People have the capacity to find answers within themselves.
_____ 3. People create their own unhappiness.
_____ 4. People are victims of outside circumstances.
_____ 5. People are basically good and are therefore trustworthy.
_____ 6. People are inclined to flounder and therefore need a great deal of direction.
_____ 7. People are the product of their choices; that is, they are the architects of their lives.
_____ 8. People are shaped by fate.
_____ 9. People won't change unless they are in pain.
_____ 10. People are motivated by their goals.
_____ 11. People's behavior is determined by their early childhood experiences.

Review your choices and determine how your view of human nature could influence your style of helping. If you expect the best in people, they are likely to give you their best. If you treat people as though they have the capacity to understand and resolve their problems, they are more likely to find answers within themselves. By developing a collaborative partnership with your clients, you are telling them that they can use the helping relationship as a pathway to re-creating their lives.

Effective helpers hold positive beliefs about people, have a healthy self-concept; ground their interventions in values; are respectful of cultural differences; are able to fully listen and understand; and possess empathy, congruence, warmth, compassion, genuineness, and positive regard. They test their beliefs and examine whether their interventions are expressions of their core beliefs and assumptions about how people change. In contrast, ineffective helpers tend to be rigid and judgmental, telling clients how to think and how to solve their problems. They do not see their clients as having the means to control their own lives. Ineffective helpers are not willing to challenge their own assumptions and tend to look for client behaviors to support their biases and convictions.

If you worked with a difficult client population over a period of years, you might begin to assume that people generally resist change. If you generalized this attitude and applied it to all the clients you saw, you might increasingly see behavior that confirmed your expectations. You would be fostering a self-fulfilling prophecy in your clients that reinforced your assumptions. Ask yourself these questions: How rigidly do I hold certain assumptions? Am I quick to generalize on the basis of limited experience? Do I tend to form quick judgments about people and make generalizations? Am I willing to seriously examine the assumptions that I make, and am I open to changing some of them? Have my assumptions changed over time? Being willing to question the origin of your assumptions and modify them, if necessary, enhances your growth as a helper.

Learning to Critically Evaluate Your Assumptions

We provided a series of in-service training workshops at a state institution. Although we had the good fortune to meet and work with some dedicated and effective helpers, we also encountered some judgmental and ineffective helpers who seemed to think that their patients could do no right. A few workers at the institution were quite outspoken in their beliefs that these patients were resistant to therapy, were not motivated to change, and were only putting in their time as ordered by the court. If the clients did not talk during the sessions, they were labeled "resistant"; if they did talk, they were often viewed as "manipulative."

In our training workshops we urged the staff members to suspend their judgments at least during the time they were providing therapy. We encouraged them to give their patients a chance to show something more of themselves than the problem with which they had become identified. If staff members are open to discovering other facets of the patient's personality, they might discover struggles in the patient's life with which they could identify. We asked these helpers to carefully assess their assumptions that seemed nontherapeutic and to be open to the possibility that they could begin to see clients and the helping process in a different light.

If you are making some of the assumptions we have described, think about how they determine the way you approach clients. Your beliefs about yourself, the people with whom you work, and the nature of the helping process are often more subtle than the assumptions we have highlighted. Whether your beliefs are subtle or extreme, however, you tend to behave on the basis of them. If you do not trust your clients to understand and deal with their problems, you will use strategies to get them to accept your assessment and to follow your prescriptions.

After becoming aware of the attitudes and assumptions you hold, you can begin to see how your attitudes are being expressed in your behavior. Then you can assess how well such attitudes and behaviors are working for you and are helping your clients. We suggest that you examine the source of your beliefs regarding an individual's capacity to make substantial change and your beliefs regarding the role of the helper–client relationship in bringing about change. Think through, clarify, and question these beliefs, and make it an ongoing process of self-examination.

You may not have clear beliefs about the helping process. You may have incorporated your beliefs in an uncritical and unconscious manner. It is possible that your beliefs are narrow and have not been tested to determine whether they are valid or functional. If you have lived in a sheltered environment and have rarely stepped outside of your social and cultural group, you may not even be aware of how narrow your belief system is. It is possible to live in an encapsulated environment that only allows you to see what confirms your existing belief system. This is known as **confirmatory bias.**

One good way to identify and clarify your beliefs is to put yourself in situations that may enable you to question your beliefs. If you have limited contact with alcoholics, consider learning more about programs such as Alcoholics Anonymous. If you have limited experience with certain cultural and ethnic groups, volunteer or do fieldwork placements with a culturally diverse population. If you are aware that you hold stereotypes about old people, volunteer to work in a board and care home for older persons. Direct contact with populations that are unfamiliar to you is the best way to learn about people whom you might have stereotyped. It is important that you approach these situations with an open mind and that you avoid simply looking for evidence to support your prior judgments. A stance of openness will enable you to develop a different orientation toward helping.

Our Beliefs About the Helping Process

It took us some time to learn that there is no one right way to approach clients. Instead of looking for the right thing to do or say, we strive to follow what we think is a productive path to pursue with a client. In this process we trust our intuition and develop our own ways of working. If our hunches about a client are incorrect, that quickly becomes apparent if we pay attention to the relationship. We continually relearn that it is important to talk with clients about what we think is going on between us, which is known as the skill of **immediacy.** At times, when we have trouble relating to a particular client, this person is reflecting some dimension within ourselves that we are reluctant to accept. Perhaps it can be helpful to consider our clients as mirrors that reflect some aspect of our being. We do not necessarily need to change anything, but it does help to recognize patterns that we have in common with our clients.

We do not accept the full responsibility for deciding what the focus of a helping relationship will be. Rather than working very hard to figure out what clients should want, we ask them frequently what it is they want. We often ask: "Is what you are doing working for you? If not, what are you willing to do to change it?" If their current behavior is generally serving them well, they may not feel a strong need to change a particular style. We encourage them to look at the price they could be paying for being the way they are, and then the decision whether to change is up to them. We do not see it as our task to decide for our clients how they should live their lives; rather, our role is to encourage them in making a self-assessment and then deciding for themselves what they most want to explore in the professional relationship with us.

If clients appear to be getting little from the helping relationship, we still examine our part in this outcome by asking ourselves about our involvement and willingness to risk with this client. We may ask a client, "Is something I am doing making it difficult for you to make progress?" We also explore with the client his or her part in the lack of progress. We recognize that we cannot make clients want to change, yet we can create a climate where together we look at the advantages and disadvantages of making certain changes. We see the helping process as a collaborative endeavor in which both parties share the responsibility for making change happen.

The Impact of Managed Care on the Helping Process

Managed care refers to the contemporary health care delivery system in which third-party payers regulate and control the duration, quality, cost, and terms of helping services rendered. In large measure, failure within the professional ranks to control rising costs has contributed to external control by the managed care industry. Those who support managed care assert that it aims to provide services that are as brief as possible to ameliorate presenting problems. In a managed care environment, the emphasis is on making relatively quick assessments of clients' problems and designing brief interventions geared more to relief of problematic symptoms than to intensive self-exploration aimed at long-term behavioral change.

This change in the focus of helping will have an impact on your role as a helper. You will be expected to work with clients in very few sessions. You will be required to develop interventions tailored to short-term and specific behavioral change. **Brief interventions** emphasize time-limited, solution-focused, structured, effective strategies that empower clients by enabling them to make specific behavioral changes they desire. In addition to short-term interventions aimed at a variety of client problems, you may be expected to participate in prevention programs such as assertiveness training, stress management, parent education, vocational counseling, couples counseling, and wellness programs. Miller and Marini (2009) describe some of the main characteristics of the brief therapy model. Emphasis is on discovering the immediate concerns clients describe at the first session. The therapist attempts to answer this question: "Why has this client decided to seek counseling at this time?" Practitioners who operate from a brief therapy model are actively involved from the beginning, establish a collaborative relationship with clients, are ever mindful of termination, summarize each session, and with clients devise homework to be carried out in between the sessions. Clients are invited to consider returning to counseling months or even years after termination if they want assistance in dealing with future life adjustment or developmental challenges.

There are many critics of managed care, but others view managed care as an effective way to serve consumers. Koocher and Keith-Spiegel (2008) list the following benefits to society in managed care: reductions in the cost of services and insurance, decreasing the moral hazards of insurance, and putting increased pressure on practitioners to critically evaluate all aspects of their treatment planning. Bobbitt (2006) contends that managed care has contributed significantly to the development and implementation of "quality improvement processes" and to the overall assessment of the health care system.

Consider how you can maximize short-term strategies aimed at teaching clients problem-solving skills they can apply to their current and future problems. Ask yourself how you can best balance quality care with cost-containment requirements in an agency where you work. As you read about the stages of helping in the next section, reflect on how you would apply the range of skills described if you were to work in a setting that required you to think in terms of brief interventions.

The Stages of the Helping Process

This section is designed to help you determine your assets and liabilities as a potential helper. We present a conceptualization of approaches to skills development based on a number of authors who devote books to this subject. Some of these authors include Brammer and MacDonald (2003), Brems (2001), Cochran and Cochran (2006), Cormier and Hackney (2005), DeJong and Berg (2008), Egan (2010), Hackney and Cormier (2005), Ivey, Ivey, and Zalaquett (2010), James (2008), Moursund and Erskine (2004), Murphy and Dillon (2008), Okun and Kantrowitz (2008), Shulman (2009), Teyber (2006), and Welfel and Patterson (2005). Our focus is on presenting a model that describes the stages in the helping process and the major tasks facing helpers at each of these stages. The skills development model offers a general framework of the phases of the helping process and is not linked to any particular theoretical approach. You can apply any of the current theories of counseling (see Chapter 6) to this model of helping.

Egan (2010) describes the stages of the helping model by framing these stages in the context of four basic client questions:

1. *What is going on?* What are the problems or concerns that I most want to work on?
2. *What do I need or want?* In what ways do I want my life to be different? What are the changes I most want to make?
3. *What do I have to do to get what I need or want?* What kind of plan will help me get what I want?
4. *How can I get results?* How can I put my plan into action and accomplish my goals? What are some ways to get moving and keep the momentum going?

These four questions form the focus of each of the stages of helping. Each stage consists of a set of themes that helps clients move forward in coping with their personal concerns and in developing opportunities for change.

The model of the helping process we discuss has five major stages, each with particular tasks to be accomplished. At each stage in this process, helpers have different roles and tasks requiring specific skills. There is considerable overlap among the functions at each of these stages. Rather than thinking of this model as discrete steps that flow in linear order, it is best to think of it as a circular process of decision making. Ivey, Ivey, and Zalaquett (2010) point out that a circle has no beginning and no end and can be used as a symbol of an egalitarian relationship in which the client and the helper form a partnership in working on commonly agreed-upon concerns.

The helper's theoretical orientation greatly influences what occurs at the various stages. Not all clients will feel comfortable with the stages as presented, regardless of cultural background, nor will all clients progress through all of the stages. Issues of rapport, structuring, defining problems, establishing goals, and assessing progress will be important for the duration of the helping relationship. The framework we provide will help you assess your ability to engage others in a helping relationship.

As we describe each of these stages, we focus on *you as a helper*. Assess your own qualities to determine your interest and ability in helping others. Realize that the helping relationship is not just a technical process, but a deeply personal human endeavor. As a helper you will be actively involved with those with whom you are working by drawing on what you know, by applying skills and interventions in a timely and appropriate manner, and by using yourself as a person in creating meaningful relationships with clients or others you help. This is true whether you are involved in the counseling or the administrative aspects of the human services. The human relations skills we describe are crucial for all helpers in all settings. If you are unable to apply some basic human relations skills, the chances are slim that you will be able to create and maintain adequate rapport with those whom you are supposed to be helping. Although the main emphasis of our discussion is on these skills as they apply to counseling relationships, you can also apply them to a variety of other interpersonal situations besides counseling.

Stage 1: Establishing a Working Relationship

The main task of this first stage of helping is to work toward building the therapeutic relationship, which is created through open communication, honesty, and trust as a way to promote client self-exploration (Welfel & Patterson, 2005). This is a time for establishing and structuring the helping relationship. During this stage of relationship building, the emphasis is on preparing the client for the helping process, stating and clarifying the concerns of the client, formulating a contract, and providing structure (Okun & Kantrowitz, 2008). This initial phase sets the foundation upon which all other interventions are able to take root in later phases of helping.

People often seek professional assistance when they realize they are not dealing with problem situations satisfactorily. Helpers are expected to create a relationship in which clients can reveal their story, identify what they want to change, and attain a new method of dealing with their problems. Some people seek counseling because they struggle with self-doubt, feel trapped by their fears, and suffer from some form of loss. Others seek help not because they feel plagued by major problems but because they are not living as effectively as they would like or because something is missing in their lives. They may feel caught in a meaningless job, experience frustration because they are not living up to their own goals and ideals, or feel dissatisfied in their personal lives. In short, they are not managing their lives as well as they might. They are not dealing effectively with life problems, and they are not using the full range of their potential or taking advantage of those opportunities that are available to them. Two general goals of helping arise from these assumptions: one goal relates to clients' managing their lives more effectively and the other relates to clients' abilities to deal realistically with problems and develop opportunities (Egan, 2010).

Not all clients come to you voluntarily. Involuntary clients may be unwilling to accept help, and they may not even believe that you can help them. Working with involuntary clients can be extremely difficult because of the degree of minimization and denial clients bring with them. Your task is to get through the initial intimidation such clients can present and to work in a way that will increase the chances of their acknowledging their problems. A good place to begin is to ascertain why they are seeing you *now,* and what they expect from you. Dealing with their hesitation and doubts, rather than ignoring these feelings and attitudes, is one of the best ways to begin with a reluctant client.

To address any barriers to creating a working relationship, you must be able to recognize the signs of defensiveness and resistance (see Chapter 4), both in your client and in yourself. It is important to understand the many meanings of client resistance and not to interpret it as a sign of failure on the client's part or as your failure as a helper. If you are primarily concerned with defending yourself against the various forms of difficult behaviors you will encounter with clients, you deprive these clients of opportunities to explore the real meanings of their behavior.

One way of not reacting defensively to a client's problematic behavior and of exploring its meaning is illustrated by the following example. You are seeing an involuntary client for the first time. She is extremely hostile and lets you know that she neither wants nor needs your help. She attacks your abilities as a counselor. As an effective helper, you cannot indulge yourself in feelings of rejection. However, in a nondefensive way you can explore with this client her unwillingness and her difficulty in seeing you. If you are patient, you may discover that this client has some very good reasons not to trust a professional like you. She may have felt betrayed by a counselor, and she may fear that the information she gives you will be used against her at some future time. For an excellent discussion on working nondefensively with client reluctance and resistance, see Egan (2010) and Teyber (2006).

Creating a climate for change. In your work with both voluntary and involuntary client populations, your clients' willingness to engage in self-exploration will have a lot to do with the kind of climate you establish during the initial sessions. If you work too hard, ask too many questions, and offer quick solutions, clients will have little incentive to participate. Your role is to create a collaborative partnership with your clients, which means that they assume a fair share of the responsibility for what takes place both inside and outside the session. During the early sessions, you can greatly assist clients by teaching them how to assess their own problems and search for their own solutions. In *The Elements of*

Counseling, Meier and Davis (2008) suggest the following guidelines for the first session with clients:

- Make personal contact.
- Develop a working alliance.
- Explain the helping process to the client.
- Talk about what is happening in the session.
- Pace and lead the client.
- Speak briefly; at times silence is golden.
- Find a balance between confronting and supporting.
- Individualize your helping approach.
- Pay attention to resistance.
- When in doubt, focus on feelings.
- Plan for termination at the beginning of the helping relationship.

Establishing the relationship. To create an effective helping relationship, it is essential for you to assist clients in becoming aware of their assets and strengths rather than concentrating on their problems, deficits, and liabilities. For clients to feel free to talk about themselves, you need to provide attention, active listening, and empathy. Clients must sense your respect for them, which you can demonstrate by your attitudes and behaviors. You reveal an attitude of respect for your clients when you are concerned about their well-being, view them as able to exercise control over their own destiny, and treat them as individuals rather than stereotyping them. You actually show clients that you respect them through your behavior, such as actively listening to and understanding them, suspending critical judgment, expressing appropriate warmth and acceptance, communicating to them that you understand their world as they experience it, providing a combination of support and challenge, assisting them in cultivating their inner resources for change, and helping them consider the specific steps needed to bring change about.

In addition to demonstrating respect, you help clients tell their story through your own genuineness. Being genuine does not mean acting on any impulse or saying everything that you think or feel. You can be genuine with your clients when you avoid hiding yourself in a professional role; are open and nondefensive, even if you feel threatened; and show a consistency between what you are thinking, feeling, and valuing and what you reveal through your words and actions. These questions are typically asked at the initial session:

- What brings you here?
- What has been going on in your life recently that prompted you to seek professional help at this time?
- What did you do when you faced problems before this time?
- What expectations do you have regarding the helping process?
- What are your hopes, fears, and reservations?
- What would you most like to accomplish in these sessions?

James (2008) describes the early stages involved in crisis intervention under the general framework of being able to listen. In crisis intervention work, the first step is to define and understand the problem from the client's point of view.

To do this, helpers must possess listening and attending skills. Their capacity to understand and to respond with empathy, genuineness, respect, acceptance, and caring greatly influences their ability to help their clients clearly identify their problems. The next step involves ensuring the safety of clients who are experiencing a crisis. This involves making an assessment of lethality by determining the seriousness of the threat to the client's physical, emotional, and psychological safety. Another step consists of providing support for clients in crisis. Helpers demonstrate their support by their words but even more so by their voice and body language.

In establishing a therapeutic relationship, it is essential to be able to give your full attention to the other person. If you are preoccupied with your own agenda, it will be difficult to understand the experiential world of another person. Your presence is truly a gift to a client. Ask yourself how well you are able to pay attention to others, to fully listen to them, and to empathize with their struggle. Assess the qualities you possess that will either help or hinder you in doing what is needed to assume the client's internal and subjective frame of reference. Consider these questions:

• Are you able to attend to what clients are telling you both verbally and nonverbally? Do you pay attention mainly to *what* (content) people tell you, or do you also notice *how* (process) they deliver their messages?

• Are you able to set aside your own biases for a time and attempt to enter the client's world? For example, are you willing to accept the client who tells you that she is satisfied in her traditional role as a housewife, even if you do not agree with her gender-role values?

• As your client speaks, are you able to listen to and detect the core messages? How do you check with your client to confirm that you understand him or her?

• Are you able to keep your clients focused on issues they want to explore? Are you able to keep your own centeredness, even when your clients may seem very fragmented or are making demands on you?

• Are you able to communicate your understanding and acceptance to your clients?

• Are you able to work nondefensively with signs of guardedness from your clients? Can you use any reluctance on the part of your clients as a way of helping them explore their issues more deeply?

Although it may seem deceptively simple to merely listen to others, the attempt to understand the world as others see it is demanding. Respect, genuineness, and empathy are best considered as a "way of being," not as techniques to be used on clients. You might interfere with clients' willingness to express themselves if you put forth too much effort in trying to be real. For example, you may want to prove to clients that you are a real person and that you struggle with your own problems. To demonstrate your "realness," you may take the focus away from your clients and put it on yourself by telling detailed stories about your life. Ask yourself why you are making this kind of self-disclosure and the degree to which it may or may not be benefiting your clients.

Establishing a working relationship with clients implies that you are genuine and respectful in behavioral ways, that the relationship is a two-way process, and that the clients' interests are supreme. This means that you avoid doing for clients what they are capable of doing for themselves. For example, assume that an adolescent client tells you that he wants more time with his father but feels intimidated and shy around him. He is afraid to approach his father. You show respect for this client when you encourage him to risk approaching his father and teach him ways of taking this initiative. You demonstrate a lack of trust in his ability if you take it upon yourself to talk to his father, even if your client has asked you to intervene.

In establishing rapport and a collaborative relationship with clients, the helper needs to master basic helping skills such as attending, listening, reflecting, clarifying, formulating questions, getting significant details, asking open questions, summarizing, paraphrasing, noticing nonverbal behavior, and attending to the evolving process. A number of books provide useful discussion of these basic interviewing and counseling skills, a few of which are Brems (2001), Cochran and Cochran (2006), Cormier and Hackney (2005), DeJong and Berg (2008), Egan (2010), Ivey et al. (2010), and Welfel and Patterson (2005).

Educating clients and obtaining informed consent. The process of educating clients about how to get the most from the helping relationship, addressing their questions, and clarifying their expectations are routes to ethical and effective practice. Create a balance between giving clients too much and not enough information. Provide clients with the opportunity to talk about what they hope to gain from being in counseling. For clients to feel trusting enough to meaningfully express themselves, they need to have at least some minimal information about the nature of the helping relationship. During the early sessions, discussion should be guided by clients' concerns, interests, and questions. Therapists may want to explore with clients questions such as these: How is confidentiality protected, and what are the limits of confidentiality? How does the therapeutic process work? What is your primary role as a helper? What is the approximate length of the counseling process? How will termination be handled? What are the main rights and responsibilities of a client? What are some of the main benefits and risks of counseling? Of course, not all these topics can be addressed in one session. Educating clients and obtaining informed consent begins at the first session and continues throughout the duration of the helping process in one way or another. We discuss the topic of informed consent more fully in Chapter 8. For a more completed discussion of informed consent, see Corey, Corey, and Callanan (2011).

Stage 2: Identifying Clients' Problems

During the second stage, the central task is to gather information, conduct an assessment, and identify the client's problems and resources. Typically, people become clients either when they recognize that they need outside help to understand and cope with their problems, or because someone else suggests professional intervention. Clients often need assistance in identifying and clarifying aspects of their lives that are not working for them. The helper's role is to assist clients in identifying problem situations or missed opportunities for full development. This is a time when both the client and helper need to gain insight into the client's strengths, deficiencies, wants, needs, unresolved conflicts, and interpersonal functioning (Welfel & Patterson, 2005).

As soon as possible in the helping process it is crucial to teach clients how to identify and clarify problem areas and how to acquire problem-solving skills they can apply in a variety of difficult situations in everyday living. As a helper, your role is not to identify the nature of clients' problems but to assist them in doing this themselves. In a sense, from the very first meeting you can be most helpful to clients by encouraging them to look within themselves for resources and strengths they can draw on to better manage their lives. Effective helpers also put clients in touch with external resources within the community that they can utilize in meeting the demands of daily living. The confidence your clients have in you will increase if they are convinced that you appreciate the resources both within themselves and in their external world.

By understanding your client's cultural background, you are doing a great deal to build upon the therapeutic working relationship that was begun at the initial session. Although it is not necessary to have an in-depth understanding of your client's culture and worldview, you must have some understanding of your client's basic beliefs and values if you hope to be useful to this person. If you are not aware of the central values that guide your client's behavior and decisions, your client will soon pick up on this and likely not return for further sessions. A more detailed discussion of the importance of understanding clients' cultural values appears in Chapter 7.

Understanding the environmental context. Clients may come to you not to resolve internal conflicts but to better understand and deal with external stressors in their environment. Some people who seek your services may need your assistance in linking them to resources within their community. They may need legal assistance or your help in coping with day-to-day survival issues such as getting a job, arranging for child care, or taking care of a dependent parent. Clients in a crisis situation will require immediate direction in finding external resources to cope effectively with the crisis.

As you listen to your clients, do not assume that they simply need to adjust to problematic situations. They may feel frustration and anger due to societal factors such as being discriminated against in their workplace because of their age, gender, race, religion, or sexual orientation. You will do them a disservice if you encourage them to settle for injustices in an oppressive environment. Instead of merely solving the presenting problems of your clients, you can begin supporting your clients in their efforts to take action within their community to bring about change. Of course, to do this means that you must assume a variety of helping roles: educator, advocate, social change agent, and influencer of policymaking. A more detailed discussion of your role in influencing change within the community is presented in Chapter 13.

Conducting an initial assessment. Assessment consists of evaluating the relevant factors in a client's life to identify themes for further exploration in the counseling process. This assessment does not necessarily have to be completed during the intake interview or even the early phase of helping, nor does it have to be a fixed judgment that the helper makes about the client. To obtain the most accurate results from an assessment, it is first necessary to have established rapport and structured the relationship, which is a task for the first stage. Ideally, assessment is a collaborative effort that is part of the interaction between the client and the helper. Both should be involved in discovering the nature of the person's presenting problem, a process that begins with the initial sessions and continues until the professional relationship ends. Here are a few questions that are helpful to consider during this early assessment phase:

- What appears to be going on in this person's life at this time?
- What are the client's main assets and liabilities?
- Who are the significant people in the client's life? Can they be relied upon for support?
- Is this a crisis situation, or is it a long-standing problem?
- What is the client primarily seeking from the therapeutic relationship, and how can it best be achieved?
- What major internal and external factors are contributing to the client's current problems, and what can be done to alleviate them?
- In what ways can an understanding of the person's cultural background shed light on developing a plan to deal with these problems?
- What significant past events appear to be related to the client's present level of functioning?
- What are the prospects for meaningful change, and how will we determine that change has occurred?

Helpers will develop tentative hypotheses, which they can share with their clients as the process evolves. Additional information is bound to emerge in time, which may call for a modification of the original assessment. This process of assessment does not necessarily have to result in classifying the client under some clinical category. Instead, helpers can describe behavior as they observe it and encourage clients to think about its meaning. In this way assessment becomes a process of thinking about issues with the client rather than the assessment being made solely by the professional. This kind of assessment is vital to the interventions that are selected, and it helps practitioners in conceptualizing a case.

Diagnosis, which is sometimes part of the assessment process, consists of identifying a specific psychological or behavioral problem based on a pattern of symptoms. A **psychological diagnosis** is a general term covering the process of identifying an emotional or behavioral problem and making a statement about the current status of a client. This process also includes identification of possible causes of the person's emotional, psychological, and behavioral difficulties, suggestions for appropriate therapy techniques to deal effectively with the identified problem, and estimates of the chances for a successful resolution. The fourth edition of the American Psychiatric Association's (2000) *Diagnostic and Statistical Manual of Mental Disorders* **(DSM-IV-TR)** is the standard reference for distinguishing one form of psychological disorder from another. The rationale for the traditional diagnostic approach is to allow the therapist to plan treatments tailored to the special needs of the client.

Whether diagnosis should be part of psychotherapeutic practice is a controversial issue. Some mental health professionals see diagnosis as an essential step in any treatment plan, but others oppose a diagnostic model on the assumption that DSM-IV-TR labels stigmatize people. Although you may not yet have had to face the practical question of whether to diagnose a client, you will probably need to come to terms with this issue at some point in your work. More and more agencies now rely on initial assessments and a DSM-IV-TR diagnosis for reimbursement purposes. Because most agency settings require some form of official assessment and diagnosis, being able to carry out these functions competently is likely to be an integral part of your job responsibilities. Herlihy, Watson, and Patureau-Hatchett (2008) state that although there are limitations of the DSM system, it is probably here to stay. They add that the question for practitioners is not *whether* to use the DSM system but *how* to use it in a way that can benefit clients while being culturally sensitive.

In our view, diagnosis does not have to be a matter of categorizing clients; rather, practitioners can think more broadly, describe behavior, and think about its meaning. In this way, diagnosis becomes a process of thinking *about* the client *with* the client. Diagnosis can be viewed as a general descriptive statement identifying a client's style of functioning, but like informed consent, thinking diagnostically is an ongoing process.

Ivey and Ivey (1998) propose reframing the diagnostic model by paying special attention to the interface of multicultural issues, origin of problems, and treatment. Ivey and Ivey suggest that diagnostic systems need more balance and attention to the reality of human experience. In their developmental counseling and therapy model, psychological distress is viewed as the result of biological and developmental factors. Although the stressor may be located within the individual, the broader systemic and cultural contexts must be considered for meaningful assessment. For example, the distress of depression is generally the result of the interaction of the person in the environment. Depression in women or in persons from some cultural groups can result from cultural racism or sexism. Individuals who have been discriminated against may experience depression as a result of environmental factors. It is important for clinicians to understand the various ways that depression is often associated with the racism or sexism that marginalized groups routinely experience in their daily lives (Zalaquett, Fuerth, Stein, Ivey, & Ivey, 2008). From the developmental perspective, the inclusion of culture-related issues such as race, ethnicity, gender, sexual orientation, and spirituality is essential for accurate assessment and diagnosis. Ivey and Ivey (1998) argue that "a diagnosis that is not culture-centered with awareness of multiple contextual issues is incomplete at best and potentially dangerous and misleading" (p. 336). For the first time, the 2005 *ACA Ethics Code* states that counselors may refrain from assigning a DSM diagnosis when it is in the best interest of the client not to do so (Kaplan, 2009).

Even though you may not find diagnosis necessary or useful in your practice, it may behoove you to know enough about diagnosis to refer a client. For example, once you have made a diagnosis of a client who is chronically depressed with possible suicidal tendencies, you are in a position to make an appropriate referral if you do not have the competence to work in this problem area.

Helping clients gain a focus. Some people who come for help feel overwhelmed with a number of problems. By trying to talk about everything that is troubling them in one session, they also may manage to overwhelm the helper. It is necessary to provide a direction for the helping efforts, enabling both the client and the helper to know where to start. To achieve this focus, it is essential to make an assessment of the major concerns of the client. You could say to a client who presents you with a long list of problems: "We won't be able to deal with all your problems in one session. What was going on in your life when you finally decided to call for help?" Here are some other focusing questions: "At this time in your life, what seems most troublesome to you?" "You say that you often wake up in the middle of the night. What do you find yourself thinking about?" "When you don't want to get up in the morning, what is it that you most want to avoid?" "If you could address only one problem today, which one would you pick?"

As a helper, you can be instrumental in encouraging clients to tell their story and to explore their key issues in terms of their experiences, feelings, and behaviors. By focusing on what is salient in the present and by avoiding dwelling on the past, you can assist clients in clarifying their own problems and opportunities for change. A participant in one of our training workshops commented that she was beginning to see the fine line that exists between the therapeutic value of telling one's story versus overwhelming people by getting lost in talking about themselves. She also learned that the purpose of a client disclosing personal information is not to satisfy the helper's curiosity. Client disclosure can provide a sense of the person's struggles, which will aid the helper in identifying a direction for the sessions.

Reflect for a moment on the degree to which you are able to facilitate the process of your clients' being able to tell some aspect of their life story. Do you let clients tell their story, or do you get impatient and want to interrupt them? Do you encourage clients to tell stories in great detail out of curiosity? Do you have a tendency to get lost in the details of their story and miss the essence of their struggle? Are you able to inquire with open-ended questions that help clients flesh out meaningful stories?

Identifying exceptions to one's problems. As the helping relationship deepens and clients present you with information about their life, help them identify and overcome their own distortions. This is a good time to encourage clients to identify exceptions to their problem-saturated lives. Ask them what they can do and have already done to deal with their problems. Ask clients to focus on possible solutions rather than having them define themselves in light of their presenting problem. By reconceptualizing a particular problem, you can assist clients in acquiring a new perspective that will lead to action. You can challenge clients who see very few options to develop a variety of alternatives in coping with a given problem. You can help them distinguish between what they can do and what might be difficult for them to do, and you can invite them to stretch their boundaries. You can also encourage clients to make choices for themselves and to be willing to accept responsibility for their decisions. By providing clients with support and challenge, you facilitate their process of change. For a more detailed treatment of the topic of identifying exceptions to one's problems, see DeJong and Berg (2008).

Stage 3: Helping Clients Create Goals

In the third stage, the helper and the client collaboratively establish goals by determining the specific changes desired. It is the helper's role to assist clients in formulating meaningful goals. Based on these goals, action plans are designed, implemented, and evaluated (Cormier & Hackney, 2005). If clients hope to make actual changes, they have to be willing to go beyond talking and planning; they must translate their plans into action.

Goals refer to desired outcomes of the helping process that are agreed upon by the helper and the client. Thinking in terms of a strengths perspective, the helper pays particular attention to what their clients do well and want to enhance, as well as attending to what problems need to be explored and solved (Murphy & Dillon, 2008). To clarify goals, helpers often ask these questions: What would you like to achieve from our work together? Where would you like to be in your life at this time? What specific feelings, thoughts, and behaviors are you most interested in changing? What would you like to reduce or eliminate from your life? What qualities would you like to acquire that you do not now have? What do you imagine the ideal solution would be to the problems you have presented? How might things be different if you were able to eliminate a key problem from your life? What kind of future do you most want for yourself?

Brian is a young worker who comes to you because he wants help in getting into college. Consider how you might assist Brian in setting his goals. He has put off applying to colleges for several years, and the thought of actually being accepted scares him. However, his job dissatisfaction is so great that it has begun to affect his personal life. Test results show that Brian is performing far below his intellectual abilities. In his work with you, Brian discovers that he has accepted some early messages from his parents that he is ignorant and would never amount to anything, and they attributed his early difficulties in school to laziness. His insight that he unconditionally accepted these early messages has been important. As a helper, you could make a mistake by focusing on his feelings about his parents and endlessly exploring the reasons he feels inadequate. You will better serve this client by helping him define the steps toward his goal. At this stage he is aware of what has stopped him so far in accomplishing his goals. He knows that he must acquire better reading and writing skills before he can successfully compete in college. Now he has clarified a new set of goals, and his task is to identify the specific steps to take in accomplishing them.

Clients need to state their goals in such a manner that both they and the helper will know what changes are desired and both will have a framework to assess the degree to which these goals are being attained. Establishing, refining, and revising goals takes time and continued effort, but doing so will give direction to the helping process. After goals are collaboratively established, it is critical to devise alternative approaches to deal with the identified problems. Guide clients in a brainstorming process to create perspectives that are in line with their values and can lead to action. It is important that these goals be measurable, be realistic in terms of the resources of the client, and be chosen by the client.

Strategies to help clients in crisis. Clients in crisis may feel immobilized and may fail to examine the options available to them. In fact, they may not see any options. Effective helping involves teaching clients to recognize that there are alternatives, some of which are better than others. James (2008) describes three strategies designed to help clients in crisis consider the options open to them: (1) identify **situational supports**, which include people in the client's life from whom they can draw strength during their crisis; (2) discuss **coping mechanisms**, which are the actions, behaviors, or environmental resources that clients can use in getting through a crisis; and (3) emphasize **positive and constructive thinking patterns**, which includes ways of reframing a situation that can lessen stress and anxiety by substantially changing a client's perspective on a problem. Crisis workers are in a position to examine a number of possibilities for action, and they can help their clients develop a different perspective, especially if clients feel that their situation is hopeless and that they are lacking in choices. For a more complete discussion on managing client crises using therapeutic relationship skills, see Cochran and Cochran (2006).

A problem-solving approach. The need of helpers to solve problems for others could easily block them from hearing what clients want to communicate. A common mistake we have observed with trainees is a tendency to short-circuit the exploration of feelings of clients and move too quickly to solving their presenting problem. This problem-solving focus aborts the struggle of clients in expressing and dealing with feelings and thoughts and eventually coming up with alternatives that are best for them.

If you are too intent on providing solutions for every problem, it is possible that you are preoccupied with your own needs for being a competent helper who wants to see results. You may be uncomfortable with the client's struggle, and you may push for resolution without proper exploration. If you were this kind of helper in the case of Brian, you would have spent no time listening and exploring his deep feelings of inadequacy. You would not have assisted him in examining what had kept him time and again from succeeding academically. With your problem-solving orientation, you would have urged him to apply prematurely for college. If Brian had not had an opportunity to express and explore his fears and self-doubts and if he had not acquired any insights into his own part in setting himself up to fail, it is unlikely that he would succeed in college.

Stage 4: Encouraging Client Exploration and Taking Action

The fourth stage of helping deals with exploring alternatives, identifying strategies for action, choosing which combination of strategies will best meet the client's goals, and putting these plans into a realistic action program. A helper's role is to facilitate clients in gaining new perspectives, seeing thing differently, and encouraging them to do things differently (Murphy & Dillon, 2008). One of the tasks of this phase is to facilitate generalization and transfer of learning from the sessions to daily life.

Once the goals of the helper-client relationship have been identified, it becomes necessary to decide on the various avenues by which these goals can be accomplished. Knowing *what* you want to change is the first step, and knowing *how* to bring about this change is the next step. Helpers first assist clients in developing and assessing action strategies for making their vision a reality. To work toward changing a client's thoughts, feelings, and behaviors, it is generally necessary to explore alternatives and confront incongruities. This stage of helping may be the longest, and at times this stage involves a lengthy exploration of an individual's dynamics. The helper's task is to explore possibilities and to assist the client in finding new ways to act more intentionally in the world (Ivey et al., 2010). Confrontation and self-disclosure are both very important aspects that can further client self-exploration, can lead to new insights, and can encourage clients to take action to achieve their personal goals. The crux of this stage also involves collaboratively creating a plan of action that is discussed in the sessions and carried out in daily life. Once an action plan has been formulated, the steps need to be carried out, and then the plan must be evaluated (Egan, 2010).

Confronting (or challenging) clients. Clients typically experience a sense of stagnation. A helper needs to acquire the skills of caring and gentle confrontation of clients' behaviors as a way to enable them to move forward. Confrontation can be viewed as "care-frontation" if it is done out of genuine concern and in a responsible, constructive way. **Confrontation** invites individuals to look at the discrepancies, incongruities, distortions, excuses, defensive behaviors, and evasions that prevent them from taking action to change their lives.

A lack of confrontation often results in stagnation. Without some degree of challenge, clients will persist with self-defeating behavior and develop no new perspectives or skills to make change possible. Helpers cease being effective catalysts to others' growth if all they offer is support. Confrontation is a practice that is often misunderstood, which is our reason for using the term *challenging* as a substitute for confrontation. Confrontation should not be viewed as aggressive or as destructive of a supportive relationship. Unfortunately, there are many misconceptions about the purpose and value of confrontation. Some helpers see it as producing defensiveness and withdrawal in clients. Or they may view it as an adversarial stance between them and their clients, which can lead to premature termination of the helping relationship. Helpers sometimes see confrontation as a negative act with destructive potential and avoid it at all costs, even though it is the very thing they need to provide an impetus for change.

Ask yourself if you are willing to confront others when this may be useful. If you find it difficult to confront others, it is important to understand why. It could be that you want to be liked and approved by your clients. You might fear that they will be angry with you or will not return. Even though challenging others might not be easy for you, it is a skill that you must acquire if you hope to move clients beyond a mere "talking-about" phase of their counseling. It may help to realize that it is not abnormal to feel anxious about challenging others or to be confronted by others. Even though you may be uncomfortable, one of the ways to develop skills in confronting is by doing what is difficult.

Confronting clients effectively entails focusing on their awareness of what they are thinking, feeling, and doing. In other words, you describe what you observe. If this is done effectively, clients are able to see what they are doing and can develop new perspectives on their life situation. They are also influenced to make changes based on this self-understanding. Thus, confronting aims at enabling clients to participate actively and fully in the process of helping themselves. Done with sensitivity, a helper can ultimately enable clients to develop the capacity for self-confrontation that they will need in working through their problems.

Here are some suggestions for making confrontations effective. First of all, earn the right to confront. Know your motivations for confronting. Is it because you want to more deeply understand another, or is it because you want to control the other person? Do you care about your relationships with clients? Confront clients only if you feel an investment in them and if you have the time and effort to continue building the relationship with them. If you have not yet established a working relationship with a client, your confrontation is likely to be received defensively, and rightly so. The degree to which you can confront your clients depends on how much they trust you and how much you trust them (Egan, 2010).

Be willing to be confronted yourself. If you model a nondefensive stance in the counseling relationship, your clients will be much more willing to listen to what you tell them. Before you confront others, imagine being the recipient of what is said. The tone and your general manner of giving your message will have a lot to do with how others hear you. It is also useful to present your confrontations in a tentative manner, as opposed to issuing a dogmatic pronouncement. Confronting is your chance to inspire clients to look at what they most want to change in themselves and what seems to be interfering with this change.

Confrontation is not intended to attack the defenses of clients; rather, it invites them to examine their problematic behaviors and keep moving toward more effective behavior. Confrontations should not be dogmatic statements concerning who or what others are. Here is an example of a confrontation that would be certain to arouse a client's defensiveness and evoke resistance: "I'm impatient with hearing you complain every week about how horrible your life is. I doubt that you will ever change." Here is an intervention that could lead to a more productive exploration of the client's difficulties: "I have noticed that you complain every week about how horrible your life is. But you seem to prevent yourself from taking the first steps leading to change. Are you aware of this, and are you willing to challenge yourself?"

Here is another suggestion for confronting a client who wants his father to change: "You have said several times that most of all you want to be successful, feel good about yourself, and feel proud of your accomplishments. Yet much of what you do and say prevents you from being successful. You've done this for a long time, and you tell me that not feeling good is very familiar. Your father has never given you his approval, and around him you feel insignificant. Are you willing to talk about the possibility that your failures have something to do with your relationship with your father?"

Likewise, in counseling a couple it would be unproductive to tell a husband to "Be quiet and listen to what she has to say!" This confrontation might silence him for the rest of the session, but it would be more helpful to describe what you saw going on between the two of them: "You say you want your wife to tell you how she feels about you, but every time she has tried this in the last 10 minutes, you've interrupted her and told her all the reasons she shouldn't feel the way she does. Are you aware of this? Describe your wife's behavior, rather than labeling it. Would you be willing for the next few minutes to let her talk and not think about what you're going to say in return? When she's finished, I'd like you to tell her how you're affected by what she has said. Focus more on you, and tell her about you." People who are being confronted are less likely to be defensive if they are told what effect they have on others rather than simply being judged and labeled.

Some clients will have numerous reasons for the way they are. You can ask them to accept responsibility for what they are doing rather than relying on excuses for what they are not doing. You can assist clients in redirecting the attention from others to themselves. Other clients may operate on the assumption that they must have approval from everyone. Again, your questioning of their belief system can help them discover the source of their stagnation and whether it is serving them well.

You can also invite clients to consider strengths they possess, but may not be using. Emphasizing strengths is usually more fruitful than dwelling on weaknesses. It helps to be specific: avoid sweeping judgments and focus on concrete behaviors. Remember to describe to clients what you see them doing and how this behavior affects you. It is also useful to encourage a dialogue with clients, and your sensitivity to their responses is a key factor in determining the degree to which they will accept your confrontations.

Here is an example of a helper's challenge to a client who is not making the best use of her strengths: "For several weeks now you've made detailed plans to reach out to a friend. You say that when you do reach out to people they usually like you, and you have no reason to fear that this friend will reject you. Yet you have not made contact with her, and you have many reasons for not doing so. Let's explore what is keeping you from contacting her."

To make the issue of confrontation more concrete, we present examples of other styles of confronting. The first statement illustrates ineffective confrontation; this is followed by an effective confrontation alternative.

• "You're always so cold and aloof, and you make me feel distant from you." This could be changed to: "I am uncomfortable when you talk to me. I'd like to see if we can be different with each other."

• "You're always smiling, and that's not real." An effective confrontation is: "Often when you say you're angry, you're smiling. I have a hard time knowing whether you are angry or happy. Are you aware of this?"

• "If I were your husband, I'd leave you. You're full of hostility, and you'll destroy any relationship." A more effective statement is: "I am scared of your anger. I find it difficult to be open with you. Many of the things you say are hurtful and create distance between us. Is this something you are aware of and something you would like to change?"

In the ineffective statements, the people being confronted are being told how they are, and in some way are being discounted. In the effective statements, the helper doing the confronting is revealing his or her perceptions and feelings about the client and is reporting how the person's behavior is affecting him or her.

If you want to learn more about challenging clients, we recommend Egan's (2010) book, *The Skilled Helper*. He devotes three chapters to the nature of challenging, specific challenging skills, and the wisdom of challenging. We also recommend Ivey et al.'s (2010) chapters that deal with the skills of confrontation. They emphasize supporting while challenging.

Using helper self-disclosure appropriately. Appropriately and timely disclosing aspects of yourself can be a powerful intervention in working with clients and facilitating a process of their self-exploration. It is a mistake to think of self-disclosure in terms of "all" or "none"; it can best be viewed on a continuum. There is a distinction between a helper's self-disclosing statements (disclosing personal information about oneself) and self-involving statements (revealing personal thoughts, feelings, and reactions to the client in the context of here-and-now aspects of the helping relationship). You are bound to have many reactions to your clients in the therapeutic relationship. Strive to let your clients know how you are perceiving and experiencing them.

Letting your clients know how you are affected by what they are saying and doing is frequently more useful to them than revealing aspects of your personal life. If you are having a difficult time listening to a client, for example, it could be useful to let the person know this. You might say: "I've noticed at times that it's difficult for me to stay connected to what you're telling me. I'm able to follow you when you talk about yourself and your own feelings, but I find myself losing interest when you go into great detail about all the things your daughter is doing or not doing." In this statement the client is not being labeled or judged, but the helper is giving his reactions about what he hears when his client tells stories about others. An example of an unhelpful response would be "You're boring me!" This response is a judgment of the client, and the helper assumes no responsibility for his own lack of interest.

It can be therapeutic to talk about yourself if doing so is for a client's benefit, but it is not necessary to reveal detailed stories of your past to form a trusting relationship with others. Inappropriate self-disclosure of your personal problems to your clients can easily distract them from productive self-exploration.

Examine the impact that your disclosures have on others, and be honest with yourself about your own motivations for disclosing. If you often prevent your clients from exploring their issues, this is the time that you could benefit from your own therapy.

Some helpers use self-disclosure inappropriately as a way of unburdening themselves. They take the focus away from the clients and direct it to their own concerns. If your feelings are very much in the foreground and inhibit you from fully attending to a client, it may be helpful for you and your client if you let him know you are distracted and it is your problem, not his. Depending on your relationship with the client, you might share some aspects about your own situation, or you might simply reveal that what the client is struggling with touches you personally, without going into too much detail.

Identifying and assessing action strategies. Insight without action is of little value. Self-understanding and seeing a range of possible alternatives can be significant in the change process, but clients also need to identify specific actions they can take and are willing to carry out in everyday living. Clients often do not accomplish their goals because they devise strategies that are unrealistic. One function of helping at this stage is to assist clients in thinking of many possibilities to achieve their goals. Together, helpers and clients can come up with a range of alternatives for coping with problems, can assess how practical these strategies are, and can decide on the best plans for action. Helpers guide clients to recognize the skills they need to put goals into action. If they don't have certain skills, they can acquire them during the helping sessions or learn about resources that are available to them.

At this stage of helping, the emphasis is on asking clients to come up with specific plans for what they will do today, tomorrow, and the next day to bring about change and to anticipate what might get in the way of their plans. In choosing **action strategies**, clients consider their internal and external resources and limitations and then determine which strategies are best suited to their capabilities. Helpers work with them to ensure that these strategies are specific and realistic, are related to their goals, and are consistent with their value system. This process is especially important in working with clients in crisis situations. Again, it is helpful to work collaboratively with clients so that they will have some degree of responsibility for their plan. Even in crisis intervention, the critical element in developing a plan is that clients do not feel robbed of their power and independence (James, 2008).

The process of creating and carrying out plans enables people to begin to gain effective control over their lives. This is clearly the teaching phase of the helping process, which is best directed toward providing clients with new information and assisting them in the discovery of more effective ways of getting what they want and need. Throughout this planning phase, the helper continually urges clients to assume responsibility for their own choices and actions.

Wubbolding (1988, 2000) writes about the central place of planning and commitment in any change process, emphasizing that when clients make plans and follow through they are taking charge of their lives by redirecting their energy and making action choices. According to Wubbolding, effective plans have the following characteristics:

• The plan should be within the limits of the motivation and capacities of each client. Plans should be realistic and attainable. Helpers do well to caution clients about plans that are too ambitious or unrealistic.

• Good plans are simple and easy to understand. Although plans need to be concrete and measurable, they should be flexible and open to modification as clients gain a deeper understanding of the specific behaviors that they want to change.

• The plan should involve positive action and should be stated in terms of what the client will do.

• It is useful to encourage clients to develop plans that they can carry out independently. Plans that are contingent on what others will do lead clients to sense that they are not steering their own ship but are at the mercy of others.

• Good plans are specific and concrete. Clients can develop specificity when helpers raise questions such as "what?" "where?" "with whom?" "when?" and "how often?"

• Effective plans are repetitive and ideally are performed daily. For people to overcome symptoms of depression, anxiety, negative thinking, or psychosomatic complaints, it is essential for them to replace these symptoms with new patterns of thinking and behaving. Each day, clients might choose a course that will lead to a sense of being in charge of their lives.

• Plans should be done as soon as possible. Helpers can ask questions such as "What are you willing to do today to begin to change your life?" "You say you'd like to stop depressing yourself. What are you going to do now to attain this goal?"

• Effective planning involves process-centered activities. For example, clients may state that they will do any of the following: apply for a job, write a letter to a friend, take a yoga class, substitute nutritious food for unhealthy food, devote 2 hours a week to volunteer work, or take a vacation they have been wanting.

• Before clients carry out their plan, it is a good idea for them to evaluate it to determine if it is realistic, attainable, and reflective of what they need and want. After the plan has been carried out in real life, it is useful to evaluate it again. Helpers can raise the question with the client, "Is your plan helpful?" If the plan does not work, it can be reevaluated and alternatives can be considered.

• For clients to commit themselves to their plan, it is useful for them to firm it up in writing.

• Part of developing a plan for action involves a discussion of the main costs and benefits of each strategy as well as a discussion of the possible risks involved and the chances for success. It is the helper's task to work with clients in constructively dealing with any hesitations they might have to formulating plans or carrying them out.

Resolutions and plans are meaningless unless there is a decision to carry them out. It is crucial that clients commit themselves to a definite plan that they can realistically accomplish. The ultimate responsibility for making plans and following through on them rests with the client. It is up to each client to determine ways of carrying these plans outside the helping relationship and into the everyday world. Effective helping can be the catalyst that leads to self-directed, satisfying, and responsible living.

Carrying out an action program. Clients are encouraged to see the value in actively trying new behavior rather than being passive and leaving action to chance. One way of fostering an active stance by clients is to formulate clear contracts. In this way clients are continually confronted with what they want and what they are willing to do. Contracts are also a useful frame of reference for evaluating the outcomes of helping. Discussion can be centered on how well the contract is being met and what modifications of it might be in order.

If certain plans do not work out well, this is a topic for exploration in a subsequent session. For example, if a mother does not follow through with her plan to deal with her son who is getting in trouble in school, the counselor can explore with her what stopped her from carrying it out. Contingency plans are also developed. The counselor might role-play different ways the mother could deal with setbacks or with her son's lack of cooperation. In this way clients learn how to deal with reverses and how to predict possible obstacles to their progress.

Stage 5: Termination

Termination, the fifth stage, assists clients in maximizing the benefits from the helping relationship and deciding how they can continue the change process. During this stage, clients consolidate their learning and make long-range plans. A helper's role at this time is to prepare clients for termination, to encourage them to express any feelings or thoughts about ending the relationship, to discuss what they have accomplished, to talk about what may have been missed, and to talk about future plans (Moursund & Erskine, 2004).

Just as the initial session sets the tone for the helping relationship, the ending phase enables clients to maximize the benefits from the relationship and decide how they can continue the change process. As a helper, your goal is to work with clients in such a way that they can terminate the professional relationship with you as soon as possible and continue to make changes on their own. As mentioned earlier, in settings where brief therapy is the standard, it is especially important that termination and issues pertaining to restrictions on time be addressed at the initial session. If an agency policy specifies that clients can be seen for only six sessions, for example, clients have a right to know this from the outset.

Working in a short-term context, the final phase of the helping process should always be in the background. With brief interventions, the goal is to teach clients, as quickly and efficiently as possible, the coping skills they need to live in self-directed ways. Your overriding goal is to increase the chances that your client will not continue to need you. It is critical to remember that if you are an effective helper you will eventually "put yourself out of business"—at least with your current clients. Remember that your role is to get clients working effectively on their own, not to keep them dependent on you for help. If you can teach your clients ways of finding their own solutions to problems, they can use what they learn in dealing not only with present concerns but also with any future problems that occur.

Preparing clients for termination. In cases of structured, time-limited counseling, both you and your client know from the beginning the approximate number of sessions available. Brief therapy traditionally involves 12 to 25 sessions, depending on client circumstances (Miller & Marini, 2009). However, in many settings clients may be limited to fewer sessions, perhaps as few as 6. Although clients may know cognitively that they have only a limited number of sessions, they may emotionally deny this restriction of their counseling experience. Termination should be discussed at the first session and be explored as necessary throughout the course of the helping relationship. In this way, termination does not come as a surprise to the client.

The limitation of time can help both you and your clients establish short-term, realistic goals of helping. Toward the end of each session, you can ask clients the degree to which they see themselves reaching the goals they have established. By reviewing the course of treatment, clients are in a position to identify what is and is not working for them in the helping process. Each session can be assessed in light of having a specific number of sessions devoted to accomplishing preset goals.

Ideally, termination is the result of a mutual decision by the client and the helper that the goals of the helping process have been accomplished. Effective termination provides clients with closure to their experience and with the incentive to continue applying what they learned in the helping relationship to the challenges that lie ahead of them (Welfel & Patterson, 2005).

Terminating when clients are not benefiting. Ethical standards state that it is improper to continue a professional relationship if it is clear that a client is not benefiting. The problem is to assess whether the client is really being helped. Consider this example: You have been seeing a client for some time who typically reports that she has nothing to talk about in the sessions. You have talked to her about her unwillingness to disclose much of herself in the counseling sessions. The client agrees yet continues her behavior. Finally, you suggest termination because, in your opinion, she is not benefiting from the counseling relationship. The client is reluctant to terminate despite her lack of involvement in the sessions. What you would do if you were confronted with this situation?

When a client who is not making progress does not wish to terminate, Younggren and Gottlieb (2008) suggest an open, collaborative stance on the part of the therapist. When a client does not seem to be benefiting from treatment, it is critical that the therapist explore with the client the reasons for the lack of progress. However, ultimately it is the therapist's responsibility to determine whether further progress is likely to occur and if termination is in order. Younggren and Gottlieb caution helpers about the risk of malpractice in such situations: "We contend that it is a significant error to continue to treat someone when no progress is being made simply because the patient values the relationship. Rather, termination must be executed in a sensitive and careful manner for the benefit of both the patient and the practitioner and may include timely and appropriate referral. We fear that to do otherwise increases the risk of legal/regulatory action against the psychotherapist" (p. 502).

Taking steps to avoid fostering dependency. Helpers can foster clients' dependent attitudes and behaviors in many subtle ways. Sometimes helpers actually prevent clients from ending a professional relationship. Instead of helping clients find their own direction, helpers may do too much for them, which results in clients assuming too little responsibility for action and change. While your clients may temporarily become dependent on you, clinical and ethical issues arise if you foster their dependency and actually prevent their progress. Ask yourself these questions as a way of determining the degree to which you encourage either dependent or independent behavior:

- Do I have a hard time terminating a case? Do I have trouble "losing" a client? Am I concerned about a reduction in my income?
- Do I encourage clients to think about termination of the professional relationship, and do I assist them in preparing for termination?
- Might I need some clients more than they need me? Do I have a need to be needed? Am I flattered when clients express dependency on me?
- Do I challenge clients to do for themselves what they are able to do? How do I respond to clients when they press me for answers?
- To what degree do I encourage clients to look within themselves for potential resources to find their own answers?

Some helpers may foster dependence in their clients as a way of feeling important. They convince themselves that they are exceptional and that they can direct their clients' life. When clients become passive and ask for answers, these helpers respond all too quickly with problem-solving solutions. Such actions may not be helpful in the long run, for clients are being reinforced to depend on you. Your main task as a helper is to encourage clients to rely on their own resources rather than on yours. By reinforcing the dependency of your clients, you are telling them that you do not trust that they can help themselves or that they can function independently of you.

Skills for ending the helping relationship. Basically, the interventions for endings pertain to assisting clients in consolidating their learning and determining how they can proceed once they stop coming in for treatment. Here are some considerations for effectively accomplishing these tasks:

• Remind clients of the approaching ending of the sessions with you. This should be done a couple of sessions before the final one. You might ask clients to think about any unfinished business they have and what they would most like to talk about in the final two meetings with you. You could even ask at a session prior to the last one, "If this were our last meeting, what would you want to talk about?"

• If you are not limited to a specified number of sessions, and both you and your client determine when termination is appropriate, one option is to space out the final few sessions. Instead of meeting weekly, your client might come in every 3 weeks. This schedule allows more opportunity to practice and to prepare for termination.

• Review the course of treatment. What lessons did clients learn, how did they learn them, and what do they intend to do with what they have learned? What did they find most helpful in the sessions with you? What did they think about their own participation in this process?

• Encourage clients to talk about their feelings of separation. Just as they may have had fears about seeking help, they may have different fears about ending the work with you.

• Be clear about your own feelings about endings. Helpers are often ambivalent about letting go of clients. It is possible to hold back clients because of your own reluctance to terminate with a client, for whatever reason. It is essential that you reflect on the degree to which you may need your clients more than they need you.

• It is a good idea to have an open-door policy, meaning that clients might be encouraged to return at a later time should they feel a need for further learning. Although professional helping is best viewed as a terminal process, at a later period of development clients may be ready to deal with a new set of problems or concerns in ways they were not willing to do when they initially began counseling. Clients may need only a few sessions to get refocused.

• Assisting clients to translate their learning into action programs is one of the most important functions during the action phase and the ending phase of helping. If clients have been successful, the ending stage is a *commencement;* they now have some new directions to follow in dealing with problems as they arise. Furthermore, clients acquire some needed tools and resources for continuing the process of personal growth. For this reason, discussing available programs and making referrals are especially timely toward the end of your work with clients. In this way the end leads to new beginnings.

For a useful discussion of guidelines for ending therapeutic relationships, see Cochran and Cochran (2006).

By Way of Review

• Skills and knowledge are important in becoming an effective professional, but your personal qualities are equally important in determining your success as a helper.

• Your view of the helping process is largely a function of your beliefs about human nature and about how people change. It is essential that you clarify your beliefs about what brings about change.

• Effective helpers hold positive beliefs about people; have a healthy self-concept; ground their interventions in values; and possess empathy, congruence, warmth, compassion, genuineness, and unconditional positive regard.

• Generalizations that helpers make about clients tend to foster a self-fulfilling prophecy within clients. If helpers view clients as being highly dependent and unable to find their own way, they will most likely live up to this expectation.

• Examine your assumptions to determine whether they are helpful for clients. Challenge your beliefs and make them your own through this process of self-examination.

• There are five stages in the helping process. Stage 1 is the time for creating rapport and structure in the relationship. Stage 2 consists of helping clients identify and clarify their problems. In Stage 3 the client and the helper collaboratively create goals. Stage 4 involves encouraging clients to engage in self-exploration and develop an action plan aimed at change. This is a time to take action and to assist clients in translating what they have learned in counseling to everyday life situations. Stage 5 deals with termination and the consolidation of learning. Specific helper strategies are required at each of these stages. Developing these skills takes time and supervised practice. Your own life experiences play a vital role in your ability to be present and to be effective in working with clients.

What Will You Do Now?

1. Identify a few of your key beliefs and assumptions that stand out after you have read this chapter. To examine how you acquired these beliefs and assumptions, talk with someone you know who tends to hold similar beliefs.

Then seek out somebody with a different perspective. With both of these people, discuss how you developed your beliefs.

2. Consider the skills needed for effective helping, and select what you consider to be your one major asset and your one major limitation, and write them down. How do you see your main asset enabling you to be an effective helper? How might your main limitation get in the way of working successfully with others? What can you do to work on the area that limits you? You might ask people you know well to review your statements about yourself. Do they see you as you see yourself?

3. Write a one-page essay that describes your personal view of what helping is about. You might imagine that a supervisor had asked you to describe your views about counseling or that in a job interview you had been instructed to "Tell us briefly how you see the helping process." You could also imagine that someone who is not sophisticated in your field had said to you: "Oh, you're a counselor. What do you do?"

4. After reflecting on your beliefs about people and about the helping process, write some key ideas in your journal pertaining to the role that your beliefs play in the manner in which you might intervene in the lives of clients. How do your beliefs influence the suggestions you make to clients? How are your beliefs the groundwork for the strategies from which you will draw in dealing with client populations?

5. As you review the stages of the helping process, ask yourself what you consider to be your most important tasks at each of the different stages. Write in your journal about some of the challenges you expect to face when working with people at each of these stages. For example, might termination be a difficult process for you? Would you have difficulty appropriately sharing your life experiences with your clients? Might you have difficulty confronting clients? What can you do to develop the personal characteristics and skills you will need to effectively intervene at each of the stages of helping?

6. For the full bibliographic entry for each of these sources, consult the References at the back of the book. For comprehensive overviews of stages in the helping process, descriptions of systematic skill development, and intervention strategies, see Cochran and Cochran (2006), Cormier and Hackney (2005), DeJong and Berg (2008), Egan (2010), Ivey, Ivey, and Zalaquett (2010), James (2008), Moursund and Erskine (2004), Murphy and Dillon (2008), Okun and Kantrowitz (2008), Shulman (2009), Teyber (2006), and Welfel and Patterson (2005). Consult James (2008) for an excellent survey text on crisis intervention strategies and Kanel (2007) for a practical guide to crisis-counseling techniques.

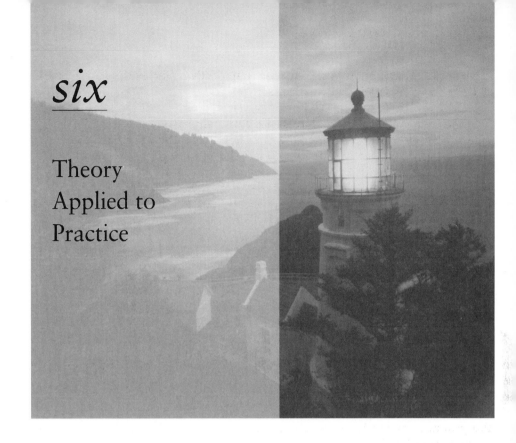

six

Theory
Applied to
Practice

Focus Questions

1. Why is theory relevant to practice?

2. The psychodynamic approaches emphasize understanding how childhood experiences influence the person you are today. Do you value understanding the past as a key to the present? How might you work with a client from the perspective of the past? the present? the future?

3. The experiential approaches stress the value of a client's direct experience rather than being taught by the counselor. How much do you trust a client's ability to lead the way in a helping relationship?

4. In the experiential approaches, the client–counselor relationship is the most important determinant for therapeutic outcomes. What specific things can a helper do to form a collaborative working relationship with a client?

5. The cognitive-behavioral approaches give primary attention to how thinking influences the way we feel and act. Do you see value in focusing on a client's thinking processes?

6. The postmodern approaches de-emphasize the therapist as expert and view the client as the expert. What do you think of this position?

7. Family systems approaches consider the whole family rather than a single individual. What unique value do you see of working with a client's issues based on his or her family of origin? Would you like to learn more about working with a family?

8. What are the advantages and disadvantages of brief models of therapy? How do brief, solution-focused intervention strategies fit the requirements of managed care programs?

9. How do you determine whether an intervention you are planning to use is suitable for you or for the client?

10. What do you understand by developing your own integrative perspective on the helping process? What do you think it would take to effectively be able to integrate some basic concepts and techniques from various theoretical orientations?

Aim of the Chapter

The purpose of this chapter is to provide you with a brief overview of some of the major theories of counseling that have applicability to a variety of helping relationships. We consider the role of theory as a guiding factor for practicing effectively. You will be introduced to the following five general theoretical orientations: psychodynamic models, experiential and relationship-oriented approaches, cognitive-behavioral therapies, the postmodern approaches, and the family systems perspective. We also present our own integrative approach, emphasizing the role of thinking, feeling, and acting in human behavior, which is based on selected ideas from most of the theories presented in this chapter.

Your theoretical orientation provides a map for making interventions, and developing this perspective takes considerable time and experience. A theory provides a structure for organizing information you get about a client, designing appropriate interventions, and evaluating the outcomes. We stress the importance of developing a personal stance toward counseling that fits the person you are and is flexible enough to meet the unique needs of the client population with which you work. The purpose of this chapter is to stimulate your thinking about how to design a framework for practice.

Theory as a Roadmap

There are many different theoretical approaches to understanding what makes the helping process work. Different practitioners might work in a variety of ways with the same client, largely based on their theory of choice. Their theory will provide them with a framework for making sense of the multitude of interactions that occur within the therapeutic relationship. Some helpers focus on feelings, believing that what clients need most is to identify and express feelings that have been repressed. Other helpers emphasize gaining insight and explore the reasons for actions and interpret clients' behavior. Some are not much concerned about having clients develop insight or express their feelings. Their focus is on behavior and assisting clients to develop specific action plans to change what they are doing. Other practitioners encourage clients to focus on examining their beliefs about themselves and about their world; they believe change will result if clients can eliminate faulty thinking and replace it with constructive thoughts and self-talk.

Helpers may focus on the past, the present, or the future. It is important to consider whether you see the past, present, or future as being most productive. This is more than just a theoretical notion. If you believe your clients' past is a crucial aspect to explore, many of your interventions are likely to be designed to assist them in understanding their past. If you think your clients' goals and strivings are important, your interventions are likely to focus on the future. If you are oriented toward the present, many of your interventions will emphasize what your clients are thinking, feeling, and doing in the moment.

Each of these choices represents a particular theoretical orientation. Attempting to practice without having an explicit theoretical rationale is like flying a plane without a flight plan. If you operate in a theoretical vacuum and are unable to draw on theory to support your interventions, you may flounder in your attempts to help people change.

Theory is not a rigid set of structures that prescribes, step by step, what and how you should function as a helper. Rather, we see theory as a general framework that enables you to make sense of the many facets of the helping process, providing you with a map that gives direction to what you do and say. Ultimately, the most meaningful perspective is one that is an extension of your values and personality. Your theory needs to be appropriate for your client population, setting, and the type of counseling you provide. A theory is not something divorced from you as a person. At best, a theory becomes an integral part of the person you are and an expression of your uniqueness.

Our Theoretical Orientation

Neither of us subscribes to any single theory in its totality. Rather, we function within an integrative framework that we continue to develop and modify as we practice. We draw on concepts and techniques from most of the contemporary counseling models and adapt them to our own unique personalities. Our conceptual framework takes into account the *thinking*, *feeling*, and *behaving* dimensions of human experience. Thus, our theoretical orientations and styles of practice are primarily a function of the individuals we are.

We value those approaches that emphasize the *thinking* dimension. We typically challenge clients to think about the decisions they have made about themselves. Some of these decisions may have been necessary for their psychological survival as children but now may not be functional. We want clients to be able to make necessary revisions that allow them to be more fully themselves. One way we do this is by asking clients to pay attention to their "self-talk." Here are some questions we encourage clients to ask themselves: "How are my problems actually caused by the assumptions I make about myself, about others, and about life? How do I create problems by the thoughts and beliefs I hold? How can I begin to free myself by critically evaluating the sentences I repeat to myself?" Many of the techniques we use are designed to tap clients' thinking processes, to help them think about events in their lives and how they have interpreted these events, and to work on a cognitive level to change certain belief systems.

Thinking is only one dimension that we pay attention to in our work with clients. The *feeling* dimension is also extremely important. We emphasize this facet of human experience by encouraging clients to identify and express their feelings. Clients are often emotionally frozen due to unexpressed and unresolved emotional concerns. If they allow themselves to experience the range of their feelings and talk about how certain events have affected them, their healing process is facilitated. If individuals feel listened to and understood, they are more likely to express more of the feelings that they have kept to themselves.

Thinking and feeling are vital components in the helping process, but eventually clients must express themselves in the *behaving* or *doing* dimension. Clients can spend many hours gaining insights and expressing pent-up feelings, but at some point they need to get involved in an action-oriented program of change. Their feelings and thoughts can then be applied to real-life situations. Examining current behavior is the heart of the helping process. We tend to ask questions such as these:"What are you doing? What do you see for yourself now and in the future? Does your present behavior have a reasonable chance of getting you what you want, and will it take you in the direction you want to go?" If the emphasis of the helping process is on what people are doing, there is a greater chance that they will also be able to change their thinking and feeling.

In addition to highlighting the thinking, feeling, and behaving dimensions, we help clients consolidate what they are learning and apply these new behaviors to situations they encounter every day. Some strategies we use are contracts, homework assignments, action programs, self-monitoring techniques, support systems, and self-directed programs of change. These approaches all stress the role of commitment on the clients' part to practice new behaviors, to follow through with a realistic plan for change, and to develop practical methods of carrying out this plan in everyday life.

Underlying our integrated focus on thinking, feeling, and behaving is our philosophical leaning toward the existential approach, which places primary emphasis on the role of choice and responsibility in the process of change. We invite people to look at the choices they *do* have, however limited they may be, and to accept responsibility for choosing for themselves. We help clients discover their inner resources and learn how to use them in resolving their difficulties. We do not provide answers for clients, but we facilitate a process that will lead clients to greater awareness of the knowledge and skills they can draw on to solve both their present and future problems.

Most of what we do in our therapeutic work is based on the assumption that people can exercise their freedom to change situations, even though the range of this freedom may be restricted by external factors. It is important for helpers to do more than assume that clients are capable of changing their internal world. Helpers also have a role to play in bringing about change in the external environment when societal or community conditions are directly contributing to a client's problems.

Individuals cannot be understood without considering the various systems that affect them—family, social groups, community, church, and other cultural forces. For the helping process to be effective, it is critical to understand how individuals influence and are influenced by their social world. Effective helpers need to acquire a holistic approach that encompasses all facets of human experience.

As we work with an individual, we are not consciously thinking about what theory we are using. We adapt the techniques we use to fit the needs of the individual rather than attempting to fit the client to our techniques. In deciding on techniques to introduce, we take into account an array of factors about the client population. We consider the client's readiness to confront an issue, the client's cultural background, the client's value system, and the client's trust in us as helpers. A general goal that guides our practice is helping clients identify and experience whatever they are feeling, identifying ways in which their assumptions influence how they feel and behave, and experimenting with alternative modes of behaving. We have a rationale for using the techniques we employ, and our interventions generally flow from some aspects of the theories that we describe in the remainder of this chapter.

One way to understand how the various major theoretical orientations apply to the counseling process is to consider five categories under which most contemporary systems fall. These are (1) the *psychodynamic approaches,* which stress insight in therapy (psychoanalytic and Adlerian therapy); (2) the *experiential* and *relationship-oriented approaches,* which stress feelings and subjective experiencing (existential, person-centered, and Gestalt therapy); (3) the *cognitive-behavioral approaches,* which stress the role of thinking and doing and tend to be action-oriented (behavior therapy, rational emotive behavior therapy, cognitive therapy, and reality therapy); (4) the *postmodern approaches,* which stress a collaborative and consultative stance on the therapist's part (solution-focused brief therapy and narrative therapy); and (5) *family systems approaches,* which stress understanding the individual within the entire system of which he or she is a part.

Although we have separated the theories into five general groups, this categorization is somewhat arbitrary. Overlapping concepts and themes make it difficult to neatly compartmentalize these theoretical orientations. What follows is a brief overview of the basic assumptions, key concepts, therapeutic goals, therapeutic relationship, techniques, multicultural applications, and contributions underlying each of these approaches to the helping process.

Psychodynamic Approaches

Psychodynamic approaches provide the foundation from which many diverse theoretical orientations have sprung. Although most helpers will not have the training to practice psychoanalytically, this point of view is useful in gaining an understanding of client dynamics and how therapy can assist clients in working through some deeply engrained personality problems. Psychoanalytic therapy has progressed far beyond Freud; many contemporary forms of relational psychoanalysis can be adapted to brief therapeutic approaches.

Along with Freud, Alfred Adler was a major contributor to the development of the psychodynamic approach to therapy. Although influenced by many of Freud's ideas, Adler developed a very different approach to therapy. Adlerians put the focus on reeducating individuals and reshaping society. Adler was the forerunner of a subjective approach to psychology that focuses on internal determinants of behavior such as values, beliefs, attitudes, goals, interests, and the individual perception of reality. He was a pioneer of an approach that is holistic, social, goal oriented, systemic, and humanistic. As you will see, many of Adler's key concepts are found in other theories that emerged later in time.

Psychoanalytic Approach

Overview and basic assumptions. The **psychoanalytic approach** rests on the assumption that normal personality development is based on dealing effectively with successive psychosexual and psychosocial stages of development. Faulty personality development is the result of inadequately resolving a specific developmental conflict. Practitioners with a psychoanalytic orientation are interested in the client's early history as a way of understanding how past situations contribute to a client's present problems.

Key concepts. The psychoanalytic approach is an in-depth and generally longer-term exploration of personality. Some of the key concepts that form this theory include the structure of personality, consciousness and unconsciousness, dealing with anxiety, the functioning of ego-defense mechanisms, and the developmental stages throughout the life span.

Therapeutic goals. A primary goal is to make the unconscious conscious. Restructuring personality rather than solving immediate problems is the main goal. Childhood experiences are reconstructed in therapy, and these experiences are explored, interpreted, and analyzed. Successful outcomes of psychoanalytic therapy result in significant modification of an individual's personality and character structure.

Therapeutic relationship. Psychoanalytically oriented therapists try to relate objectively with warm detachment. Both transference and countertransference are central aspects in the relationship. The focus is on resistances that occur in the therapeutic process, on interpretation of these resistances, and on working through transference feelings. Through this process, clients explore the parallels between their past and present experience and gain new understanding that can be the basis for personality change.

Techniques. All techniques are designed to help the client gain insight and bring repressed material to the surface so that it can be dealt with in a conscious way. Major techniques include maintaining the analytic framework, free association, interpretation, dream analysis, analysis of resistance, and analysis of transference. These techniques are geared to increasing awareness, acquiring insight, and beginning a working-through process that will lead to a reorganization of the personality.

Multicultural applications. The psychosocial approach that emphasizes turning points at various stages of life has relevance for understanding diverse client populations. Therapists can assist clients in identifying and dealing with the influence of environmental situations on their personality development. The goals of brief psychodynamic therapy can provide a new understanding for current problems. With this briefer form of psychoanalytically oriented therapy, clients can relinquish old patterns and establish new patterns in their present behavior.

Contributions. The theory provides a comprehensive and detailed system of personality. It emphasizes the legitimate place of the unconscious as a determinant of behavior, highlights the significant effect of early childhood development, and provides techniques for tapping the unconscious. Several factors can be applied by practitioners who are not psychoanalytically oriented, such as understanding how resistance is manifested and can be therapeutically explored, how early trauma can be worked through successfully, and understanding of the manifestations of transference and countertransference in the therapy relationship. Many other theoretical models have developed as reactions against the psychoanalytic approach.

The Adlerian Approach

Overview and basic assumptions. According to the **Adlerian approach,** people are primarily social beings, influenced and motivated by societal forces. Human nature is viewed as creative, active, and decisional. The approach focuses on the unity of the person and on understanding the individual's subjective perspective. The subjective decisions each person makes regarding the specific direction of this striving form the basis of the individual's lifestyle (or personality style). The **lifestyle** consists of our beliefs and assumptions about others, the world, and ourselves; these views lead to distinctive behaviors that we adopt in pursuit of our life goals. We can shape our own future by taking risks and making decisions in the face of unknown consequences. Clients are not viewed as being "sick" or suffering from some disorder that needs to be "cured." Rather, they are seen as being discouraged and functioning on the basis of self-defeating and self-limiting assumptions, which generate problem-maintaining, ego-protective behaviors. Thus, clients are seen as being in need of encouragement to correct mistaken perceptions of self and others and to learn to initiate new behavioral interaction patterns.

Key concepts. Consciousness, not the unconscious, is the center of personality. The Adlerian approach, based on a growth model, stresses the individual's positive capacities to live fully in society. It is characterized by seeing unity in the personality, understanding a person's world from a subjective vantage point, and stressing life goals that give direction to behavior. **Social interest,** the heart of this theory, involves a sense of identification with humanity, a feeling of belonging, and a concern with bettering society. **Inferiority feelings** often serve as the wellspring of creativity, motivating people to strive for mastery, superiority, and perfection. People attempt to compensate for both imagined and real inferiorities, which helps them overcome handicaps.

Therapeutic goals. Counseling is not simply a matter of an expert therapist making prescriptions for change. It is a collaborative effort, with the client and therapist working on mutually accepted goals. Change is aimed at both the cognitive and behavioral levels. Adlerians are mainly concerned with confronting clients' mistaken notions and faulty assumptions. Working cooperatively with clients, therapists try to provide encouragement so that clients can develop socially useful goals. Some specific goals include fostering social interest, helping clients overcome feelings of discouragement, changing faulty motivation, restructuring mistaken assumptions, and assisting clients to feel a sense of equality with others.

Therapeutic relationship. The client–therapist relationship is based on mutual respect, and both client and counselor are active. Clients are active parties in a relationship between equals. Through this collaborative partnership, clients recognize that they are responsible for their behavior. The emphasis is on examining the client's lifestyle, which is expressed in everything the client does. Therapists frequently interpret this lifestyle by demonstrating connections between the past, the present, and the client's future strivings.

In the therapeutic process, the client's relative levels of functioning in all the basic **life tasks** are explored—social, love-intimacy, occupational, and spiritual—so as to more fully understand the social context of the client's life situation. The Adlerian therapist seeks to work with the client in developing a deeper and more complete understanding of his or her basic personality structure. This involves placing emphasis on the individual's lifestyle—or the cognitive framework or schema from which the individual attempts to understand life and to make behavior choices. More specifically, the therapist seeks to ascertain the faulty, self-defeating perceptions and assumptions about self, others, and life that maintain the problematic behavioral patterns the client brings to therapy.

Techniques. Adlerians have developed a variety of cognitive, behavioral, and experiential techniques that can be applied to a diverse range of clients in a variety of settings and formats. They are not bound to follow a specific set of procedures; rather, they can tap their creativity by applying those techniques that they think are most appropriate for each client. Some specific techniques they often employ are attending, encouragement, confrontation, summarizing, interpreting experiences within the family, early recollections, suggestion, and homework assignments.

Multicultural applications. The interpersonal emphasis of the Adlerian approach is most appropriate for counseling people from diverse backgrounds. The approach offers a range of cognitive and action-oriented techniques to help people explore their concerns in a cultural context. Adlerian practitioners are flexible in adapting their interventions to each client's unique life situation. Adlerian therapy has a psychoeducational focus, a present and future orientation, and is a brief, time-limited approach. All of these characteristics make the Adlerian approach suitable for working with a wide range of client problems.

Contributions. Adler founded one of the major humanistic approaches to psychology. Perhaps the greatest contribution of the Adlerian perspective is the degree to which its basic concepts have been integrated into other therapeutic approaches. There are significant linkages between Adlerian theory and most of the present-day theories.

Experiential and Relationship-Oriented Approaches

Therapy is often viewed as a journey taken by counselor and client, a journey that delves deeply into the world as perceived and experienced by the client. This journey is influenced by the quality of the person-to-person encounter in the therapeutic situation. The value of the therapeutic relationship is a common denominator among all therapeutic orientations, yet some approaches place more emphasis than others do on the role of the relationship as a healing factor. This is especially true of the existential, person-centered, and Gestalt approaches. These **relationship-oriented approaches** (sometimes known as experiential approaches) are all based on the premise that the quality of the client–counselor relationship is primary, with techniques being secondary. The **experiential approaches** are grounded on the premise that the therapeutic relationship fosters a creative spirit of inventing techniques aimed at increasing awareness, which enables clients to change some of their patterns of thinking, feeling, and behaving.

Some of the key concepts common to all experiential approaches that are assumed to be related to effective therapeutic outcomes include the following:

- The quality of the person-to-person encounter in the therapeutic situation is the catalyst for positive change.
- The counselor's main role is to be present with clients during the therapeutic hour. This implies that the counselor has good contact with the client and is centered.
- Clients can best be invited to grow by a counselor modeling authentic behavior.
- A therapist's attitudes and values are at least as critical as his or her knowledge, theory, or techniques.
- Counselors who are not sensitively tuned in to their own reactions to a client run the risk of becoming technicians rather than artists.
- The I-Thou relationship enables clients to experience the safety necessary for risk-taking behavior.
- Awareness emerges within the context of a genuine meeting between the counselor and the client, or within the context of I-Thou relating.
- The basic work of therapy is done by the client. The counselor's job is to create a climate in which the client is likely to try out new ways of being.

These somewhat overlapping notions give a sense of the paramount importance of the therapeutic relationship. Counselors who operate in the framework of the relationship-oriented therapies will be much less anxious about using the "right technique." Their techniques are most likely designed to enhance some aspect of the client's experiencing rather than being used to stimulate clients to think, feel, or act in a certain manner.

The Existential Approach

Overview and basic assumptions. The **existential perspective** holds that we define ourselves by our choices. Although outside factors restrict the range of our choices, we are ultimately the authors of our lives. We are thrust into a meaningless world, yet we are challenged to accept our aloneness and create a meaningful existence. Because we have the capacity for awareness, we are basically free. Along with our freedom, however, comes responsibility for the choices we make. People who seek therapy often lead a **restricted existence**, or function with a limited degree of self-awareness; they see few alternatives for dealing with life situations and may feel trapped. The therapist's job is to confront these clients with the restricted life they have chosen and to help them become aware of their own part in creating this condition. As an outgrowth of the therapeutic venture, clients are able to recognize outmoded patterns of living, and they begin to accept responsibility for changing their future.

Key concepts. There are six key propositions of existential therapy: (1) We have the capacity for self-awareness. (2) Because we are basically free beings, we must accept the responsibility that accompanies our freedom. (3) We have a concern to preserve our uniqueness and identity; we come to know ourselves in relation to knowing and interacting with others. (4) The significance of our existence and the meaning of our life are never fixed once and for all; instead, we re-create ourselves through our projects. (5) Anxiety is part of the human condition. (6) Death is also a basic human condition, and awareness of it gives significance to living.

Therapeutic goals. The principal goal is to challenge clients to recognize and accept the freedom they have to become the authors of their own lives. Therapists confront clients on ways in which they are avoiding their freedom and the responsibility that accompanies it. The existential approach places primary emphasis on understanding clients' current experience, not on using therapeutic techniques.

Therapeutic relationship. The client–therapist relationship is of paramount importance, for the quality of the I-Thou encounter offers a context for change. Instead of prizing therapeutic objectivity and professional distance, existential therapists value being fully present, and they strive to create caring relationships with clients. Therapy is a collaborative relationship in which both client and therapist are involved in a journey into self-discovery.

Techniques. Existential therapy reacts against the tendency to view therapy as a system of well-defined techniques; it affirms looking at those unique characteristics that make us human and building therapy on them. The approach places primary emphasis on understanding the client's current experience. Existential therapists are free to adapt their interventions to their own personality and style, as well as paying attention to what each client requires. Therapists are not bound by any prescribed procedures and can use techniques from other therapeutic models. Interventions are used in the service of broadening the ways in which clients live in their world. Techniques are tools to help clients become aware of their choices and their potential for action.

Multicultural applications. Because the existential approach is based on universal human themes, and because it does not dictate a particular way of viewing reality, it is highly applicable when working in a multicultural context. In working with cultural diversity, it is essential to recognize the commonalities and similarities among clients. Themes such as relationships, finding meaning, anxiety, suffering, and death are concerns that transcend the boundaries that separate cultures. Clients in existential therapy are encouraged to examine the ways their present existence is being influenced by social and cultural factors.

Contributions. The person-to-person therapeutic relationship lessens the chances of dehumanizing therapy. The approach has something to offer counselors regardless of their theoretical orientation. The basic ideas of this approach can be incorporated into practice regardless of the counselor's particular theory. It provides a perspective for understanding the value of anxiety and guilt, the role and meaning of death, and the creative aspects of being alone and choosing for oneself. As applied to *brief therapy,* the existential approach focuses on encouraging clients to examine issues such as assuming personal responsibility, expanding their awareness of their current situation, and making a commitment to deciding and acting. A time-limited framework can serve as a catalyst for clients to become maximally involved in their therapy sessions.

The Person-Centered Approach

Overview and basic assumptions. Person-centered therapy was originally developed by Carl Rogers in the 1940s as a reaction against psychoanalytic therapy. Based on a subjective view of human experience, the **person-centered approach** emphasizes the client's resources for becoming self-aware and for resolving blocks to personal growth. It puts the client, not the therapist, at the center of the therapeutic process. It is the client who primarily brings about change. Rogers did not present his approach as being a final model, but expected the theory and practice to evolve over time. By participating in the therapeutic relationship, clients actualize their potential for growth, wholeness, spontaneity, and inner-directedness.

Key concepts. A key concept is that clients have the capacity for resolving life's problems effectively without interpretation and direction from an expert therapist. Clients are able to change without a high degree of structure and direction from the therapist. This approach emphasizes fully experiencing the present moment, learning to accept oneself, and deciding on ways to change.

Therapeutic goals. A major goal is to provide a climate of safety and trust in the therapeutic setting so that the client, by using the therapeutic relationship for self-exploration, can become aware of obstacles to growth. The client tends to move toward more openness, greater self-trust, and more willingness to evolve as opposed to being a static entity. The client learns to live by internal standards as opposed to taking external cues for what he or she should become. The aim of therapy is not merely to solve problems but to assist a client's growth process to enable him or her to better cope with present and future problems.

Therapeutic relationship. The person-centered approach emphasizes the attitudes and personal characteristics of the therapist and the quality of the client–therapist relationship as the prime determinants of the outcomes of therapy. The qualities of the therapist that determine the relationship include genuineness, nonpossessive warmth, accurate empathy, unconditional acceptance of and respect for the client, permissiveness, caring, and the ability to communicate those attitudes to the client. Effective therapy is based on the quality of the relationship between therapist and client. The client is able to translate his or her learning in therapy to outside relationships with others.

Techniques. Because this approach stresses the client–therapist relationship as a necessary and sufficient condition leading to change, it specifies few techniques. Techniques are always secondary to the therapist's attitudes. The approach minimizes directive techniques, interpretation, questioning, probing, diagnosis, and collecting history. It maximizes active listening and hearing, expressing empathy, reflection of feelings, and clarification.

Multicultural applications. The emphasis on universal, core conditions provides the person-centered approach with a framework for understanding diverse worldviews. Empathy, being present, and respecting the values of clients are essential attitudes and skills in counseling culturally diverse clients. Person-centered counselors convey a deep respect for all forms of diversity and value understanding the client's subjective world in an accepting and open way.

Contributions. One of the first therapeutic orientations to break from traditional psychoanalysis, the person-centered approach stresses the active role and responsibility of the client. It is a positive and optimistic view and calls attention to the need to account for a person's inner and subjective experiences. Emphasizing the crucial role of the therapist's attitude, this approach makes the therapeutic process relationship-centered rather than technique-centered.

Gestalt Therapy

Overview and basic assumptions. Gestalt therapy is an experiential and existential approach based on the assumption that individuals and their behavior must be understood in the context of their present environment. The therapist's task is to facilitate clients' exploration of their present experience. Clients carry on their own therapy as much as possible by doing experiments designed to heighten awareness and to engage in contact. Change occurs naturally as awareness of "what is" increases. Heightened awareness can also lead to a more thorough integration of parts of the client that were fragmented or unknown.

Key concepts. This approach focuses on the here and now, direct experiencing, awareness, bringing unfinished business from the past into the present, and dealing with unfinished business. Other concepts include energy and blocks to energy, contact and resistance to contact, and paying attention to nonverbal cues. Clients identify their own unfinished business from the past that is interfering with their present functioning by reexperiencing past situations as though they were happening in the present moment.

Therapeutic goals. The goal is attaining awareness and greater choice. Awareness includes knowing the environment and knowing oneself, accepting oneself, and being able to make contact. Clients are helped to note their own awareness process so that they can be responsible and can selectively and discriminatingly make choices. With awareness the client is able to recognize denied aspects of the self and proceed toward reintegration of all its parts.

Therapeutic relationship. This approach stresses the I-Thou relationship. The focus is not on the techniques employed by the therapist but on who the therapist is as a person and the quality of the relationship. Factors that are emphasized include the therapist's presence, authentic dialogue, gentleness, direct self-expression, and a greater trust in the client's experiencing. The counselor assists clients in experiencing all feelings more fully and lets them make their own interpretations. Technical expertise is important, but the therapeutic engagement is paramount. Rather than interpreting the meaning of experience for clients, the therapist focuses on the "what" and "how" of their behavior.

Techniques. Although the therapist functions as a guide and a catalyst, presents experiments, and shares observations, the basic work of therapy is done by the client. Therapists do not force change on clients; rather, they create experiments within a context of the I-Thou dialogue in a here-and-now framework. These experiments are the cornerstone of experiential learning. Although the therapist suggests the experiments, this is a collaborative process with full participation by the client. **Gestalt experiments** take many forms: setting up a symbolic dialogue between a client and a significant person in his or her life; assuming the identity of a key figure through role playing; reliving a painful event; exaggerating a gesture, posture, or some nonverbal mannerism; or carrying on a dialogue between two conflicting aspects within an individual.

Multicultural applications. Gestalt therapy can be used creatively and sensitively with culturally diverse populations if interventions are used flexibly and in a timely manner. Gestalt practitioners focus on understanding the person and not on the use of techniques. Experiments are done with the collaboration of the client and with the attempt to understand the background of the client's culture.

Contributions. Gestalt therapy recognizes the value of working with the past from the perspective of the here and now. This orientation emphasizes doing and experiencing as opposed to merely talking about problems in a detached way. Gestalt therapy gives attention to nonverbal and body messages, which broaden the field of material to be explored in a helping relationship. It provides a perspective on growth and enhancement, not merely a treatment of disorders. The method of working with dreams is a creative pathway to increased awareness of key existential messages in life.

Cognitive-Behavioral Approaches

This section describes some of the main **cognitive-behavioral approaches,** which include behavior therapy, rational emotive behavior therapy, cognitive therapy, and reality therapy. Although the cognitive-behavioral approaches are quite diverse, they do share these attributes: (1) a collaborative relationship between client and therapist, (2) the premise that psychological distress is largely a function of disturbances in cognitive processes, (3) an emphasis on changing cognitions to produce desired changes in affect and behavior, and (4) a time-limited and educational treatment focusing on specific target problems. The cognitive-behavioral approaches are based on a structured, psychoeducational model, and they tend to emphasize the role of homework, place responsibility on the client to assume an active role both during and outside of therapy sessions, and draw from a variety of cognitive and behavioral techniques to facilitate change. Of all the therapeutic models, the cognitive-behavioral therapies have gained most in popularity and are increasingly being used as the basis for practice with a wide variety of client populations, with a multitude of problems, and in many different settings.

Behavior Therapy

Overview and basic assumptions. Behavioral approaches assume that people are basically shaped by both learning and the sociocultural environment. Due to the diversity of views and strategies, it is more accurate to think of behavioral therapies rather than a unified approach. The central characteristics that unite the diversity of views of the field of behavior therapy are a focus on observable behavior, current determinants of behavior, learning experiences to promote change, and rigorous assessment and evaluation.

Key concepts. Behavior therapy emphasizes current behavior as opposed to historical antecedents, precise treatment goals, diverse therapeutic strategies tailored to these goals, and objective evaluation of therapeutic outcomes. Therapy focuses on behavior change in the present and on action programs. Concepts and procedures are stated explicitly, tested empirically, and revised continually. There is an emphasis on measuring a specific behavior before and after an intervention to determine if, and to what degree, behaviors change as a result of a procedure.

Therapeutic goals. A hallmark of behavior therapy is the identification of specific goals at the outset of the therapeutic process. The general goals are to increase personal choice and to create new conditions for learning. An aim is to eliminate maladaptive behaviors and to replace them with more constructive patterns. Generally, client and therapist collaboratively specify treatment goals in concrete, measurable, and objective terms.

Therapeutic relationship. Although the approach does not place primary emphasis on the client–therapist relationship, a good working relationship is an essential precondition for effective therapy. The skilled therapist can conceptualize problems behaviorally and make use of the therapeutic relationship in bringing about change. The assumption is that clients make progress primarily because of the specific behavioral techniques used rather than by the relationship with the therapist. The therapist's role is to teach concrete skills through the provision of instructions, modeling, and performance feedback. Therapists tend to be active and directive and to function as consultants and problem solvers. Clients must also be actively involved in the therapeutic process from beginning to end, and they are expected to cooperate in carrying out therapeutic activities, both in the sessions and outside of therapy.

Techniques. Assessment and diagnosis are done at the outset to determine a treatment plan. Behavioral treatment interventions are individually tailored to specific problems experienced by different clients. Any technique that can be demonstrated to change behavior may be incorporated in a treatment plan. A strength of the approach lies in the many and varied techniques aimed at producing behavior change, a few of which are relaxation methods, systematic desensitization, in vivo desensitization, flooding, assertion training, and self-management programs.

Multicultural applications. Behavioral approaches can be appropriately integrated into counseling with culturally diverse client populations when culture-specific procedures are developed. The approach emphasizes teaching clients about the therapeutic process and stresses changing specific behaviors. By developing their problem-solving skills, clients learn concrete methods for dealing with practical problems within their cultural framework.

Contributions. Behavior therapy is a short-term approach that has wide applicability. It emphasizes research into and assessment of the techniques used, thus providing accountability. Specific problems are identified and explored, and clients are kept informed about the therapeutic process and about what gains are being made. The approach has demonstrated effectiveness in many areas of human functioning. The concepts and procedures are easily grasped. The therapist is an explicit reinforcer, consultant, model, teacher, and expert in behavioral change.

Rational Emotive Behavior Therapy (REBT)

Overview and basic assumptions. Albert Ellis is considered the father of rational emotive behavior therapy and the grandfather of cognitive-behavior therapy. **Rational emotive behavior therapy** rests on the premise that thinking, evaluating, analyzing, questioning, doing, practicing, and redeciding are the basics of behavior change. REBT assumes that individuals are born with the potential for rational thinking but that they also uncritically accept irrational beliefs. The cognitive-behavioral approaches are based on the assumption that a reorganization of one's self-statements will result in a corresponding reorganization of one's behavior.

Key concepts. REBT holds that although emotional disturbance is rooted in childhood, people keep repeating irrational and illogical beliefs. Emotional problems are the result of one's beliefs, not events, and these beliefs need to be challenged. Clients are taught that the events of life themselves do not disturb us; rather, our interpretation of events is what is critical.

Therapeutic goals. The goal of REBT is to eliminate a self-defeating outlook on life, to reduce unhealthy emotional responses, and to acquire a more rational and tolerant philosophy. Two main goals of REBT are to assist clients in the process of achieving unconditional self-acceptance and unconditional acceptance of others. To accomplish these goals, REBT offers clients practical ways to identify their underlying faulty beliefs, to critically evaluate these beliefs, and to replace them with constructive beliefs. Clients learn how to substitute preferences for demands.

Therapeutic relationship. In REBT, a warm relationship between the client and the therapist is not essential. However, the client needs to feel unconditional positive regard from the therapist. Therapy is a process of reeducation, and the therapist functions largely as a teacher in active and directive ways. As clients begin to understand how they continue to contribute to their problems, they need to actively practice changing their self-defeating behavior and converting it to rational behavior.

Techniques. REBT utilizes a wide range of cognitive, emotive, and behavioral methods with most clients. This approach blends techniques to change clients' patterns of thinking, feeling, and acting. Techniques are designed to induce clients to critically examine their present beliefs and behavior. REBT focuses on specific techniques for changing a client's self-defeating thoughts in concrete situations. In addition to modifying beliefs, REBT helps clients see how their beliefs influence what they feel and what they do.

From a cognitive perspective, REBT demonstrates to clients that their beliefs and self-talk keep them disturbed. A few of the *cognitive techniques* that are frequently used by REBT practitioners include teaching the A-B-C's of REBT, active disputation of faulty beliefs, teaching coping self-statements, psychoeducational methods, and cognitive homework.

Emotive techniques include unconditional acceptance, rational emotive imagery, the use of humor, shame-attacking exercises, and rational emotive role playing. Although this approach does not give priority to feelings, as clients explore what they are thinking and how they are acting, feelings often surface. When feelings do emerge, they can be addressed.

Behavioral techniques include self-management strategies, modeling, use of reinforcements and penalties, carrying out homework in daily life, and practicing a wide range of coping skills as a way to deal with challenges. Behavioral techniques tend to work best when they are used in combination with emotive and cognitive methods.

Multicultural applications. Some factors that make REBT effective in working with diverse client populations include tailoring treatment to each individual, addressing the role of the external environment, the active and directive role of the therapist, the emphasis on education, relying on empirical evidence, the focus on present behavior, and the brevity of the approach. REBT practitioners function as teachers; clients acquire a wide range of skills they can use in dealing with the problems of living. This educational focus appeals to many clients who are interested in learning practical and effective methods of bringing about change.

Contributions. REBT is a comprehensive, integrative approach to therapy aimed at changing disturbances in thinking, feeling, and behaving. REBT has taught us how people can change their emotions by changing the content of their thinking. Counseling is brief and places value on active practice in experimenting with new behavior so that insight is carried into doing.

Cognitive Therapy (CT)

Overview and basic assumptions. Aaron Beck is a pioneer of cognitive therapy who made important contributions in understanding and treating disorders such as depression and anxiety. **Cognitive therapy** rests on the premise that cognitions are the major determinants of how we feel and act. CT assumes that the internal dialogue of clients plays a major role in their behavior. The ways in which individuals monitor and instruct themselves and interpret events shed light on the dynamics of disorders such as depression and anxiety.

Key concepts. According to CT, psychological problems stem from commonplace processes such as faulty thinking, making incorrect inferences on the basis of inadequate or incorrect information, and failing to distinguish between fantasy and reality. Cognitive therapy consists of changing dysfunctional emotions and behaviors by modifying inaccurate and dysfunctional thinking.

Therapeutic goals. The goal of cognitive therapy is to change the way clients think by using their automatic thoughts to reach the core schemata and begin to introduce the idea of schema restructuring. Changes in beliefs and thought processes tend to result in changes in the way people feel and how they behave. Clients in CT are encouraged to gather and weigh the evidence in support of their beliefs. Through the collaborative therapeutic effort, they learn to discriminate between their own thoughts and the events that occur in reality.

Therapeutic relationship. Cognitive therapy emphasizes a collaborative effort by both therapist and client to frame the client's conclusions in the form of a testable hypothesis. Cognitive therapists are continuously active and deliberately interactive with the client; they also strive to engage the client's active participation and collaboration throughout all phases of therapy.

Techniques. Cognitive therapy emphasizes a Socratic dialogue to help clients discover their misconceptions for themselves. Through a process of guided discovery, the therapist functions as a catalyst and guide who helps clients understand the connection between their thinking and the ways they feel and act. Cognitive therapists teach clients how to be their own therapist. This includes educating clients about the nature and course of their problems, about how cognitive therapy works, and how their thinking influences their emotions and behaviors. Techniques in CT are designed to identify and test the client's misconceptions and faulty assumptions. Homework is often used, which is tailored to the client's specific problems and arises out of the collaborative therapeutic relationship. Homework is generally presented as an experiment, and clients are encouraged to create their own self-help assignments as a way to keep working on issues addressed in their therapy sessions.

Multicultural applications. Cognitive therapy tends to be culturally sensitive because it uses the individual's belief system, or worldview, as part of the method of self-change. The collaborative nature of CT offers clients the structure many clients want, yet the therapist still strives to enlist clients' active participation in the therapeutic process. Because of the way CT is practiced, with emphasis on enlisting the full participation of clients, it is ideally suited to working with clients from diverse backgrounds.

Contributions. Cognitive therapy has been demonstrated to be effective in the treatment of anxiety, phobias, and depression. This approach has received a great deal of attention by clinical researchers. Many specific cognitive techniques have been supported by empirical evidence as being useful in teaching clients ways to change their belief systems.

Reality Therapy

Overview and basic assumptions. Founded and developed by William Glasser in the 1960s, reality therapy posits that people are responsible for what they do. Based on existential principles, reality therapy holds that we choose our own destiny. **Choice theory** rests on the assumption that humans are internally motivated and behave to control the world around them according to some purpose within them. Choice theory, which is the underlying philosophy of the practice of reality therapy, provides a framework that explains the why and how of human behavior. **Reality therapy** is based on the assumption that human beings are motivated to change (1) when they determine that their current behavior is not getting them what they want and (2) when they believe they can choose other behaviors that will get them closer to what they want. Clients are expected to make an assessment of their current behavior to determine specific ways they may want to change.

Key concepts. The core concept of this approach is that behavior is our best attempt to control our perceptions of the external world so they fit our internal world. **Total behavior** includes four inseparable but distinct components of acting, thinking, feeling, and the physiology that accompany our actions. A key concept of reality therapy and choice theory is that no matter how dire our circumstances may be, we always have a choice. An emphasis of reality therapy is on assuming personal responsibility and on dealing with the present.

Therapeutic goals. The overall goal of this approach is to help people find better ways to meet their needs for survival, love and belonging, power, freedom, and fun. Changes in behavior should result in the satisfaction of basic needs. Clients are expected to make a self-evaluation of what they are doing, thinking, and feeling to assess whether this is getting them what they want and to assist them in finding a better way to function.

Therapeutic relationship. The therapist initiates the therapeutic process by becoming involved with the client and creating a supportive and challenging relationship. Practitioners teach clients how to make significant connections with others. Throughout therapy the counselor avoids criticism, refuses to accept clients' excuses for not following through with agreed-on plans, and does not easily give up on clients. Instead, counselors continue to ask clients to evaluate the effectiveness of what they are choosing to determine if better choices may be possible.

Techniques. The practice of reality therapy can best be conceptualized as the cycle of counseling, which consists of two major components: (1) the counseling environment and (2) specific procedures that lead to change in behavior. Reality therapy is active, directive, and didactic. Skillful questioning and various behavioral techniques are employed to help clients make a comprehensive self-evaluation.

Some of the specific procedures in the practice of reality therapy have been developed by Wubbolding (2000). These procedures are summarized in the **WDEP model**, which refers to the following clusters of strategies:

W = wants: exploring wants, needs, and perceptions
D = direction and doing: focusing on what clients are doing and the direction that this is taking them
E = evaluation: challenging clients to make an evaluation of their total behavior
P = planning and commitment: assisting clients in formulating realistic plans and making a commitment to carry them out

For a more detailed summary of the procedures that lead to change, see Wubbolding (2000).

Multicultural applications. Reality therapists demonstrate their respect for the cultural values of their clients by helping them explore how satisfying their current behavior is both to themselves and to others. After clients make this self-assessment, they identify those areas of living that are not working for them. Clients are then in a position to formulate specific and realistic plans that are consistent with their cultural values.

Contributions. As a short-term approach, reality therapy can be applied to a wide range of clients. Reality therapy consists of simple, clear concepts that are easily understood by many in the human services field, and the principles can be used by parents, teachers, and clergy. As a positive and action-oriented approach, it appeals to a variety of clients who are typically viewed as difficult to treat. This approach teaches clients to focus on what they are able and willing to do in the present to change their behavior.

Postmodern Approaches

This section describes two of the main **postmodern approaches,** solution-focused brief therapy and narrative therapy. In these approaches the therapist disavows the role of expert, preferring a more collaborative and consultative stance. Both solution-focused brief therapy and narrative therapy are based on the optimistic assumption that people are healthy, competent, resourceful, and possess the ability to construct solutions and alternative stories that can enhance their lives.

Solution-Focused Brief Therapy (SFBT)

Overview and basic assumptions. Solution-focused brief therapy is based on the assumption that the therapist is not the expert on a client's life; rather, the client is the expert on his or her own life. Complex problems do not necessarily require complex solutions, and the therapist helps clients recognize the competencies they already possess. Change is constant and inevitable, and small changes pave the way for bigger changes. Attention is given to what clients are doing that is working and to helping them build on their potential, strengths, and resources.

Key concepts. A central concept of SFBT includes a movement from talking about problems to talking about and creating solutions. Therapy is kept simple and brief. There are exceptions to every problem, and by talking about these exceptions, clients are able to conquer what seem to be major problems in a brief period of time.

Therapeutic goals. The solution-focused model emphasizes the role of clients in establishing their own goals and preferences. This is done when a climate of mutual respect, dialogue, inquiry, and affirmation are a part of the therapeutic process. Working together in a collaborative relationship, both therapist and client develop useful and meaningful treatment goals, and ultimately, clients construct meaningful goals that will lead to a better future.

Therapeutic relationship. SFBT is a collaborative venture; the therapist strives to carry out therapy *with* an individual, rather than doing therapy *on* an individual. Therapists recognize that clients are the primary interpreters of their own experiences. Solution-focused therapists adopt a "not knowing" position, or a nonexpert stance, as a way to put clients in the position of being the experts about their own lives. The therapist-as-expert is replaced by the client-as-expert. Together the client and the therapist establish clear, specific, realistic, and personally meaningful goals that will guide the therapy process. This spirit of collaboration opens up a range of possibilities for present and future change.

Techniques. Solution-focused therapists use a range of techniques. Some therapists ask the client to externalize the problem and focus on strengths or unused resources. Others challenge clients to discover solutions that might work. Techniques focus on the future and how best to solve problems rather than on understanding the cause of problems. Solution-focused brief therapy techniques that are frequently used include pre-therapy change, exception questions, the miracle question, scaling questions, homework, and summary feedback.

Solution-focused brief therapists often ask clients at the first session, "What have you done since you called for an appointment that has made a difference in your problem?" Asking about **pre-therapy change** tends to encourage clients to rely less on the therapist and more on their own resources to reach their goals.

Exception questions direct clients to those times in their lives when their problems did not exist. Exploring exceptions offers clients opportunities for discovering resources, engaging strengths, and creating possible solutions.

The **miracle question** allows clients to describe life without the problem. This question involves a future focus that encourages clients to consider a different kind of life than one dominated by a particular problem. The miracle question focuses clients on searching for solutions. Examples are "How will you know when things are better?" and "What will be some of the things you will notice when life is better?"

Scaling questions require clients to specify improvement on a particular dimension on a scale of zero to 10. This technique enables clients to see progress being made in specific steps and degrees.

Therapists may provide summary feedback in the form of genuine affirmations or pointing out particular strengths that clients have demonstrated.

Multicultural applications. Solution-focused therapists learn from their clients about their experiential world rather than approaching clients with a preconceived notion about their worldview. The nonpathologizing stance taken by solution-focused practitioners moves away from dwelling on what is wrong with a person to emphasizing creative possibilities. Instead of aiming to make change happen, the SFBT practitioner attempts to create an atmosphere of understanding and acceptance that allows a diverse range of individuals to utilize their resources for making constructive changes.

Contributions. A key contribution of SFBT is the optimistic orientation that views people as being competent and able to create better solutions. Problems are viewed as ordinary difficulties and challenges of life. A strength of solution-focused brief therapy is the use of questioning, especially future-oriented questions that challenge clients to think about how they might solve potential problems in the future.

Narrative Therapy

Overview and basic assumptions. Narrative therapy is based partly on examining the stories that people tell and understanding the meaning of the story. Each of these stories is true for the individual who is telling the story; there is no absolute reality. Narrative therapists strive to avoid making assumptions about people out of respect for each client's unique story and cultural heritage.

Key concepts. Some key concepts of **narrative therapy** include a discussion of how a problem has been disrupting, dominating, or discouraging the person. The therapist attempts to separate clients from their problems so that they do not adopt a fixed view of their identity. Clients are invited to view their stories from different perspectives and eventually to co-create an alternative life story. Clients are asked to find evidence to support a new view of themselves as being competent enough to escape the dominance of a problem and are encouraged to consider what kind of future they could expect if they were competent.

Therapeutic goals. Narrative therapists invite clients to describe their experience in fresh language, which tends to open new vistas of what is possible. The heart of the therapeutic process from the perspective of narrative therapy involves identifying how societal standards and expectations are internalized by people in ways that constrain and narrow the kind of life they are capable of living. Narrative therapists collaborate with clients to help them experience a heightened sense of agency or ability to act in the world.

Therapeutic relationship. Narrative therapists do not assume that they have special knowledge about the lives of clients. Clients are the primary interpreters of their own experiences. In the narrative approach, the therapist seeks to understand clients' lived experience and avoids efforts to predict, interpret, or pathologize. Through a systematic process of careful listening, coupled with curious, persistent, and respectful questioning, the therapist works collaboratively with clients to explore the impact of the problem and what they are doing to reduce its effects. Through this process, client and therapist co-construct enlivening alternative stories.

Techniques. Narrative therapy emphasizes the quality of the therapeutic relationship and the creative use of techniques within this relationship. Narrative therapy's most distinctive feature is captured by the statement, "The person is not the problem, but the problem is the problem." Narrative therapists engage clients in *externalizing conversations* that are aimed at separating the problem from the person's identity. The assumption is that clients can develop alternative and more constructive stories once they have separated themselves from their problems.

Multicultural applications. With the emphasis on multiple realities and the assumption that what is perceived to be true is the product of social construction, narrative therapy is a good fit with diverse worldviews. Narrative therapists operate on the premise that problems are identified within social, cultural, political, and relational contexts rather than existing within individuals.

Contributions. As narrative therapists listen to clients' stories, they pay attention to details that give evidence of clients' competence in taking a stand against an oppressive problem. Problems are not viewed as pathological manifestations but as ordinary difficulties and challenges of life. In the practice of narrative therapy, there is no recipe, no set agenda, and no formula to follow that will ensure a desired outcome. This therapeutic approach encourages practitioners to use creativity when working with clients.

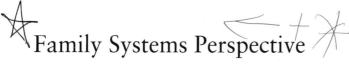

Family Systems Perspective

Family therapy involves a conceptual shift from individual dynamics to interaction within the system. A **family systems perspective** views the family as a functioning unit and as an entity unto itself that adds up to more than the sum of its members. By focusing on the internal dynamics of an individual without adequately considering interpersonal dynamics, only an incomplete picture of that individual is revealed. Family therapists subscribe to the basic notion that families are systems and that a treatment approach that comprehensively addresses the other family members as well as the "identified" client is required. Goldenberg and Goldenberg (2008) point to the need for therapists to view all behavior, including the symptoms expressed by the individual, within the context of the family and society. The Goldenbergs add that a systems orientation does not preclude dealing with the dynamics within the individual but that this approach broadens the traditional emphasis. It is not possible to accurately assess an individual's concerns without observing the interaction of the other family members as well as the broader context in the community and in society.

Family therapy is more than an approach to working with a family; it is a perspective that sheds light on the individual's and the family's development over time. It also provides a lens through which to view connections in the world. It takes into consideration the influence of an individual's neighborhood, community, church, work environment, school, and other systems. Indeed, the family systems perspective holds that significant change within an individual is not likely to be made or maintained unless the client's network of intimate relationships is taken into account. Even if an individual makes changes, those changes are not likely to be maintained if there is little support for, or if there is opposition to, the changes from the individual's family and other social relationships.

Family Systems Therapy

Overview and basic assumptions. Family systems approaches rest on the assumption that individuals are best understood through assessing the interactions of the entire family. It is also grounded on the assumptions that a client's problematic behavior may (1) serve a function or purpose for the family; (2) be a function of the family's inability to operate productively, especially during developmental transitions; or (3) be a symptom of dysfunctional patterns handed down across generations. All these assumptions challenge traditional individual therapy frameworks for conceptualizing human problems and their formation.

One of the systemic principles is that symptoms are an expression of a dysfunction within the family system—not the individual—and dysfunctions are often passed across several generations. The family provides the context for understanding how individuals behave. Actions by any individual family member will influence all the other members, and their reactions will have a reciprocal effect on the individual.

Another systemic principle is that each family member is part of a whole pie, even though it is easy for the members to think of themselves as separate pieces of the pie without an integral connection. The system assumes its own personality. You cannot pluck yourself out of your family system, for you are dynamically related to it. If you restrict yourself exclusively to your internal dynamics, without considering your interpersonal dynamics, you are not getting a full picture of yourself.

From a systems perspective, being a healthy person involves both a sense of belonging to your family system and a sense of separateness and individuality. An individual's level of functioning can be seen as a manifestation of the way the family is functioning.

Key concepts. Family therapy is a diverse field with respect to concepts, techniques, and approaches. The key concepts presented here address some of the themes that unite the many different systemic approaches.

Family therapy tends to be brief because families who seek professional help typically want resolution of some problematic symptom. In addition to being short-term, solution-focused, and action-oriented, family therapy tends to deal with present interactions. One way in which it differs from many individual therapies is its emphasis on how current family relationships contribute to the development and maintenance of symptoms.

Almost all of the family therapies are concerned with here-and-now interactions in the family system. By dealing with interactions in the here and now, patterns that have existed over time can be changed. The family therapy perspective emphasizes verbal and nonverbal communication. Family therapists have a keen interest in the process of family interaction and in teaching patterns of communication. Some approaches to family therapy assume that the central aim of communication is attaining power in interpersonal relationships.

Therapeutic goals. Family or relationship therapy is aimed at helping the members change the patterns of relationships that are not working well and helping the family create new ways of interacting. The general goal is to bring about a change within a system, predicated on the assumption that if a system changes so will the individuals within the system. The specific goals are determined by the practitioner's specific orientation or by a collaborative process between the family and the therapist.

An integrative approach to the practice of family therapy must include guiding principles that help organize goals, interactions, observations, and ways to promote change. Some theories focus on perceptual and cognitive change, others deal mainly with changing feelings, and others emphasize behavioral change.

Therapeutic relationship. Family therapists function as models, teachers, and coaches. Although the skills of the therapist are crucial, the therapist's ability to establish rapport and create a working relationship with all family members is what counts. What most approaches have in common is their commitment to helping family members learn new and more effective ways of interacting.

Key to the family systems approach is that neither the individual nor the family is blamed for a particular dysfunction. The family is empowered through the process of identifying and exploring interaction patterns. If change is to come about in a family or between individual members of a family, the family must be aware of the systems that influence them.

For Bitter (2009), the relationship a practitioner creates with a family is far more important than the techniques he or she employs. Bitter identifies the following personal characteristics and orientations of effective family practitioners: presence; acceptance, interest, and caring; assertiveness and confidence; courage and risk-taking; openness to change; paying attention to goals and purposes of a family; working in patterns; appreciating the influence of diversity; being sincerely interested in the welfare of others; tending to the spirit of the family and its members; and involvement, engagement, and satisfaction in working with families. These personal characteristics influence the manner in which techniques are delivered.

Techniques. Diverse techniques are available to family therapists, but the intervention strategies they employ are best considered in conjunction with their own personal characteristics. It is essential that therapists use skills and techniques that fit their personality and that are appropriate for the goals of therapy. Bitter (2009), Goldenberg and Goldenberg (2008), and Nichols (2008) emphasize that techniques are tools for achieving therapeutic goals, yet these intervention strategies do not make a family therapist.

Faced with the demands of clinical practice, practitioners need to be flexible in selecting intervention strategies that will meet specific therapeutic objectives and contribute to specific outcomes. Many therapy procedures can be borrowed from various models, depending on what is likely to work best with a given family. The central consideration is what is in the best interests of the family.

Today, family therapists explore both the individual culture of the family and the larger culture to which the family belongs. They look for ways in which culture can inform their work with a family. Therapeutic interventions are no longer applied universally, regardless of the culture involved, but rather are designed to complement the family system within the larger community of which it is a part.

Multicultural applications. Many cultures value interdependence over independence, and this is a key strength of the family systems approach. When working with clients who especially value grandparents, parents, and aunts and uncles in some form of cooperative family unit, it is easy to see that family approaches have a distinct advantage over individual therapy. By understanding and appreciating the diversity of family systems, the therapist can contextualize family experiences in relation to the larger culture of which they are now a part.

Contributions. One of the key contributions of the family systems approach is that neither the individual nor the family is blamed for a particular dysfunction. Rather than blaming either the "identified patient" or a family, the entire family has an opportunity to examine the multiple perspectives and interactional patterns that characterize the unit and to participate in finding solutions. The family is empowered through the process of identifying and exploring internal, developmental, and purposeful interaction patterns. At the same time, a systems perspective recognizes that individuals and families are affected by external forces and systems. If change is to occur in families or within individuals, therapists must be aware of as many systems of influence as possible.

An Integrative Approach to the Helping Process

An **integrative model** refers to a perspective based on concepts and techniques drawn from various theoretical approaches. One reason for the current trend toward an integrative approach to the helping process is the recognition that no single theory is comprehensive enough to account for the complexities of human behavior when the full range of client types and their specific problems are taken into consideration. According to Dattilio and Norcross (2006), most clinicians now acknowledge the limitations of basing their practice on a single theoretical system and are open to the value of integrating various therapeutic approaches. Those clinicians who are open to an integrative perspective may find that several theories play crucial roles in their personal approach. Each theory has its unique contributions and its own domain of expertise. By accepting that each theory has strengths and weaknesses and is, by definition, different from the others, practitioners have some basis to begin developing a counseling model that fits them. Dattilio and Norcross contend that the ultimate goal of an integrative approach is to enhance the efficacy, efficiency, and applicability of psychotherapy.

We encourage you to remain open to the value inherent in each of the theories of counseling. All the theories we described have some unique contributions as well as some limitations. Study all the contemporary theories to determine which concepts and techniques you can incorporate into your approach to practice. You will need to have a basic knowledge of various theoretical systems and counseling techniques to work effectively with diverse client populations in various settings. Functioning exclusively within the parameters of one theory may not provide you with the therapeutic flexibility that you need to deal creatively with the complexities associated with diverse client populations.

Each theory represents a different vantage point from which to look at human behavior, but no one theory has the total truth. Because there is no "correct" theoretical approach, it is well for you to search for an approach that fits who you are and to think in terms of working toward an integrated approach that addresses thinking, feeling, and behaving. To develop this kind of integration, you need to be thoroughly grounded in a number of theories, be open to the idea that these theories can be unified in some ways, and be willing to continually test your hypotheses to determine how well they are working.

If you are currently a student in training, it is unrealistic to expect that you will already have an integrated and well-defined theoretical model. An integrative perspective is the product of a great deal of reading, study, clinical practice, research, and theorizing. With time and reflective study, the goal is to develop a consistent conceptual framework that you can use as a basis for selecting from the multiple techniques that you will eventually be exposed to. Developing your personalized approach that guides your practice is a lifelong endeavor that is refined with experience.

Of necessity, this discussion of the various theoretical orientations has been brief. Eventually you will likely take a course on theories of counseling that will enable you to see the broader picture of how theory can be translated into action in the helping relationship. For a more elaborate discussion of the different theoretical approaches described in this chapter, see *The Art of Integrative Counseling* (Corey, 2009a) and *Theory and Practice of Counseling and Psychotherapy* (Corey, 2009c). Three other useful books that contain chapters on each of the theories described are *Current Psychotherapies* (Corsini & Wedding, 2008), *Systems of Psychotherapy: A Transtheoretical Analysis* (Prochaska & Norcross, 2010), and *Theories of Psychotherapy and Counseling* (Sharf, 2008).

By Way of Review

- A theoretical orientation that integrates thinking, feeling, and behaving provides the basis for developing interventions that can be used flexibly with clients at various stages of the helping process.

- A theory can be very practical in the sense that it can guide interventions.

- Because there is no one "right" theoretical approach, you would do well to consider adopting an approach that is congruent with your personality and values.

- Before you can integrate the theories, you need to first study and master the various theories. It is not possible to integrate that which you do not know.

- Psychodynamic theories provide a foundation upon which many of the contemporary theories have been designed.

- Experiential therapies are based on the therapist developing a quality relationship with clients. In many respects, the relationship-oriented therapies are grounded on the assumption that clients can be the experts of their own lives. The therapist functions as a facilitator to help clients tap their internal resources.

- Cognitive-behavioral therapies place emphasis on how thinking influences emotions and behavior. These approaches stress the value of taking action if change is desired.

- The postmodern approaches are based on the optimistic assumption that people are healthy, competent, resourceful, and possess the ability to construct solutions and alternative stories that can enhance their lives. Individuals, not therapists, are seen as the experts on their lives.

- An assumption of the systems approach is that change in any one part of the system affects all parts of that system.

• A family systems perspective provides a lens through which to view connections in the world by taking into consideration the influence of an individual's family, neighborhood, community, church, school, and work environment.

What Will You Do Now?

1. In small groups explore how you might answer this question if it were posed to you in a job interview: "What is your theoretical orientation, and how do you think this will influence the way you work with diverse client populations?"

2. Review the different theories described and reflect on what concepts of the various theories you could apply to your personal life. How can you use some of these approaches to better understand yourself?

3. As a small group exercise, discuss some the following aspects of the various theories presented:

• The role of the helper
• Key concepts you would most want to borrow from each theory
• Techniques that you find useful from each theory
• View of the client–counselor relationship
• Multicultural applications of each theory
• Major contributions of each theory

4. In small groups, take some time to discuss what you need to know and specific skills you need to have to be able to effectively work with families. If you were asked by your supervisor in your fieldwork placement to join him or her in conducting family sessions in the agency, what would be your response?

5. For the full bibliographic entry for each of these sources, consult the References at the back of the book. For an introduction to the contemporary theories of counseling, see Corey (2009c), Corsini and Wedding (2008), Prochaska and Norcross (2010), and Sharf (2008). For a discussion of integrative counseling, see Corey (2009a). For an overview of the major theories of family therapy, see Bitter (2009), Goldenberg and Goldenberg (2008), Hanna (2007), and Nichols (2008). Thomlison (2002) is a good source as a family assessment workbook.

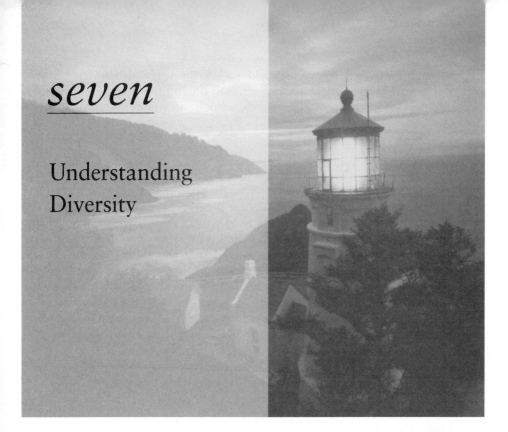

seven

Understanding Diversity

Focus Questions

1. How much thought have you given to your own cultural background, and how has it influenced you?

2. How prepared are you to work with client populations that differ from you significantly in a number of ways (age, gender, culture, ethnicity, sexual orientation, socioeconomic status, and educational background)? What life experiences can you draw from to bridge differences between you and your clients?

3. What values do you hold that could make it difficult for you to work with clients who have a different worldview? For example, if you value self-determination and this is not a central value in your client's culture, could this pose a problem for you?

4. What would you do if a client wondered if you would be able to help him because of differences in worldview or culture?

5. How much involvement have you had with people with disabilities? How do you generally feel in their presence? What personal characteristics or experience do you have that could facilitate your work with this special population?

6. What are some societal stereotypes pertaining to people with disabilities? How could you work to change these beliefs in your community?

7. In your college program, how much attention is given to developing awareness of your cultural assumptions, knowledge about diverse cultural groups, and skills for working in a pluralistic society?

8. What can you do to increase your ability to make contact with clients who are different from you? What does it take for you to become a culturally skilled helper?

9. Are you aware of how others perceive you? Have you explored your own identity or multiple identities?

10. What are you willing to do to expand your current attitudes and worldview?

Aim of the Chapter

In most places where you might work, it will be necessary for you to relate effectively to a wide variety of clients. At this point in your development as a helper, it is essential that you be open to learning how to establish contact with clients who differ from you in age, gender, ethnicity, race, culture, ability, socio-economic status, sexual orientation, life circumstances, or basic values. You do not need to be of the same point of view or the same background as your client, nor is it necessary for you to experience the same life circumstances to form an effective therapeutic alliance. However, it is necessary for you to have a range of experiences upon which to draw in understanding the human condition. Universal human themes link people in spite of their differences. Your open-ness to learn from the lessons that life has presented to you, your respect for contrasting perspectives, your interest in understanding the diverse world-views of the clients you will meet, and your capacity for examining narrow views of reality are critical skills. Even if you have grown up in a monocultural world, you can learn about people with a worldview different from your own. Through concerted efforts on your part, it is possible to expand your current attitudes and views.

To function effectively as a helper, you must familiarize yourself with your clients' cultural attributes and realize how cultural values operate in the helping process. It is important to know about specific differences in various aspects of life and to realize how these differences can affect your work. (See Chapter 2 for a discussion of how your values may affect your interventions as a helper.) All helpers must seriously consider these issues, regardless of their racial, ethnic, or cultural background.

This chapter offers a perspective on how to work with diversity in the help-ing relationship. By understanding how your own cultural background has con-tributed to who you are, you have a basis for understanding other viewpoints. You will probably take a course in cultural diversity, which is likely to cover gender concerns, ageism, racism, multicultural issues, physical disabilities, and issues pertaining to sexual orientation. This can be enlightening and can help broaden your vision of the world. By honoring cultural diversity, you can formu-late alternative perspectives and develop appropriate tools for working with diverse client populations.

A Multicultural Perspective on Helping

We look at **multicultural helping** from a broad perspective and do not limit our consideration of this topic to race and ethnicity. Pedersen (2000) defines cultural groups by *ethnographic* variables (nationality, ethnicity, language, and religion), *demographic* variables (age, gender, and place of residence), *status* variables (edu-cational and socioeconomic background), and formal and informal *affiliations.* According to Pedersen, the multicultural perspective provides a conceptual framework that both recognizes the complex diversity of a pluralistic society and suggests bridges of shared concern that link all people, regardless of their differences. This perspective looks at both the unique dimensions of a person and the common themes we share with those who are different.

Arredondo and her colleagues (1996) make a distinction between multiculturalism and diversity. **Multiculturalism** puts the focus on ethnicity, race, and culture. In the context of training helpers, the term **multicultural** refers to five major cultural groups in the United States and its territories: African/Black, Asian, European/White, Hispanic/Latino, and Native American. **Diversity** refers to other individual differences and characteristics by which persons may self-define. This includes but is not limited to an individual's age, gender, sexual orientation, religion or spiritual identification, physical ability/disability, social and economic class background, and residential location.

Due to the changing demographics of American society, Lee and Ramsey (2006) believe it is imperative that multicultural counseling address differences in gender, social class, language, sexual orientation, disability, and race and ethnicity between the helper and client. They write:

> Broadly conceptualized, multicultural counseling considers the personality dynamics and cultural backgrounds of both counselor and client in creating a therapeutic environment in which these two individuals can purposefully interact. Multicultural counseling, therefore, takes into consideration the cultural background and individual experiences of diverse clients and how their psychosocial needs might be identified and met through counseling. (p. 5)

When you become a helper, you will encounter many individuals from cultures different from your own. In many instances, your first step toward helping people involves understanding their cultural values.

The Need for a Multicultural Emphasis

In the past two decades we have seen an increased awareness on the part of the helping professions to address the special issues involved in working with people of various cultures. Lee and Ramsey (2006) contend that because of the changing demographics in American society, a new paradigm is needed for the helping professions. They state that these changing demographics are not limited to racial and ethnic aspects but encompass other areas of diversity including sexual orientation, disability, and socioeconomic status. Because of these changes in demographics, it is important for human service professionals to embrace a broad multicultural perspective if they hope to understand the behavior of culturally diverse client populations.

Pedersen (2008) believes that effective counselors cannot afford to ignore their own culture or the culture of their clients through encapsulation. He claims that whether we are aware of it or not, culture controls our lives and defines reality for each of us. Cultural factors are an integral part of the helping process, and culture influences the interventions we make with our clients. Adopting a multicultural perspective enables us to think about diversity without polarizing issues into "right" or "wrong." According to Pedersen, when two people argue from culturally different assumptions, they can disagree without one being right and the other being wrong. Depending on the cultural perspective from which a problem is considered, there can be several appropriate solutions. In some cases, a similar problem may have very different solutions depending on one's culture. For example, helpers may encourage some clients to express feelings of hurt to parents but respect other clients' practice of restraint in self-expression so as not to offend their elders.

A multicultural perspective respects the needs and strengths of diverse client populations, and it recognizes the experiences of these clients. However, it would be a mistake to perceive individuals as simply belonging to a group. The differences between individuals within the same group are often greater than the differences between groups. Pedersen (2000) indicates that individuals who share the same ethnic and cultural background are likely to have sharp differences. Not all Native Americans have the same experiences, nor do all African Americans, all Asian Americans, all Euro-Americans, all women, all old people, or all people who are physically challenged. Helpers, regardless of their cultural background, must be prepared to deal with the complex differences among individuals from a variety of groups. They need to be prepared to deal with diversity in areas such as race, culture, ethnicity, sexual orientation, disability status, religion, socioeconomic status, gender, and age (Lee & Ramsey, 2006).

Pedersen (2000) believes that multicultural awareness can make your job easier and more fun; it can also increase rather than decrease the quality of your life. Adopting a perspective that cultural differences are positive attributes that add to relationships will expand your ability to work with diverse client groups. We hope you will view the tapestry of culture woven into the fabric of all helping relationships not as a barrier to break through but as a garment that provides comfort in your clients' search for meaning.

Ethical Dimensions in Multicultural Practice

Becoming an ethical and effective helper in a multicultural society is a continuing process, not a one-time destination. Effective **multicultural counseling** evolves from three primary practices. First, helpers must be aware of their own assumptions, biases, and values about human behavior, and of their own worldview as well. Second, helpers need to become increasingly aware of the cultural values, biases, and assumptions of diverse groups in our society, and come to an understanding of the worldview of culturally different clients in nonjudgmental ways. Third, with this knowledge helpers will begin to develop culturally appropriate, relevant, and sensitive strategies for intervening with individuals and with systems (Hansen, Pepitone-Arreola-Rockwell, & Greene, 2000; Lee, 2006a; Sue & Sue, 2008).

Lee (2006a) maintains that counselors must address diversity in a way that is both culturally responsive and ethically responsible. Counselors who are culturally responsive have a greater chance of working ethically and effectively with diverse cultural groups. Those counselors who are unaware of cultural dynamics and their impact on client behavior are at risk of practicing unethically.

Dolgoff, Loewenberg, and Harrington (2009) assert that discrimination in providing services is often linked to racial and cultural factors, socioeconomic class, and gender. They claim that discrimination and misdiagnosis can be due to biased attitudes on the part of practitioners. For example, people in lower socioeconomic classes consistently receive more severe diagnoses than do individuals in higher socioeconomic classes. Diller (2007) claims that discrimination involves more than simply refusing to offer services to certain client groups. Discrimination by helpers can take any one of these forms:

- Being unaware of one's own biases and how they can inadvertently be communicated to clients.
- Being unaware that some of the theories studied during a training program may be culture bound.
- Being unaware of differences in cultural definitions of health and illness.
- Being unaware of the need to match treatment modalities to clients' cultural backgrounds.

Recognizing diversity in our society and embracing a multicultural approach in the helping relationship have become fundamental tenets of professional codes of ethics, and the ethics codes specify that discrimination by helping professionals is unethical. Most ethics codes mention the practitioner's responsibility to recognize the special needs of diverse client populations. Watson, Herlihy, and Pierce (2006) maintain that counselors have been slow to recognize a connection between multicultural competence and ethical behavior. They further state that reliance on ethics codes alone does not guarantee multicultural competence. Respecting diversity implies a commitment to acquiring the knowledge, skills, and personal awareness that are essential to working effectively with a wide variety of client groups. The ACA (2005) ethics code explains this requirement:

> Counselors encourage client growth and development in ways that foster the interest and welfare of clients and promote formation of healthy relationships. Counselors actively attempt to understand the diverse cultural backgrounds of the clients they serve. Counselors also explore their own cultural identities and how these affect their values and beliefs about the counseling process. (A: Introduction)

The *Ethical Standards of Human Service Professionals* (NOHS, 2000) contain six principles aimed at the human service professional's responsibility to the community and society, with a specific emphasis on ethics and human diversity. Human service professionals must adhere to these standards:

- Advocate for the rights of all members of society, particularly those who are members of minorities and groups at which discriminatory practices have been directed.
- Provide services without discrimination or preference based on age, ethnicity, culture, race, disability, gender, religion, sexual orientation, or socioeconomic status.
- Become knowledgeable about the cultures and communities within which they practice.

- Become aware of their own cultural backgrounds, beliefs, and values, recognizing the potential impact these values may have on their relationships with others.
- Become aware of sociopolitical issues that differently affect clients from diverse backgrounds.
- Seek the training, education, experience, and supervision necessary to ensure their effectiveness in working with culturally diverse client populations.

To practice ethically, helpers must pay attention to the issues involved in working with culturally diverse populations. Dolgoff and colleagues (2009) remind us that people often belong to several groups and have multiple identities. Even if an individual is primarily identified with a single culture, his or her identify can be based on a number of factors. Dogoff and colleagues caution helpers to avoid stereotyping persons by a primary group identity. It is important to understand the concept of a plurality of identities.

Helpers may misunderstand clients of a different gender, race, age, religion, social class, educational level, or sexual orientation. If practitioners fail to integrate these diversity factors into their practice, they are infringing on the client's cultural autonomy and basic human rights, which will reduce the chance of establishing an effective helping relationship. For some clients religious values may be important. Other clients may focus on gender or age discrimination. By paying attention to what a client is saying, helpers can discover which aspects of a client's identity are most salient for this person at this time.

Overcoming Cultural Tunnel Vision

Our work with students in a human services training program has shown us that students struggle with **cultural tunnel vision.** Many students are unaware of the difficulty of dealing with clients who have a cultural background different from their own. They have limited cultural experiences, and in some cases they see it as their role to transmit their values to their clients. Some students have made inappropriate generalizations about a particular group of clients. For example, some students in training may assert that certain groups of people are unresponsive to psychological intervention because of a lack of motivation to change.

In a sense, all helping relationships are multicultural. Both those providing help and those receiving help bring to their relationship attitudes, values, and behaviors that can vary widely. One mistake is to deny the importance of these cultural variables; another mistake is to overemphasize such cultural differences to the extent that helpers lose their spontaneity and thus fail to be present for their clients. You need to understand and accept clients who have a different set of assumptions about life, and you need to be alert to the likelihood of imposing your own worldview. In working with clients with different cultural experiences, it is important that you resist making value judgments for them.

The **culturally encapsulated counselor,** a concept introduced by Wrenn (1962, 1985), exhibits the characteristics common to cultural tunnel vision. Think about how broad your own vision is as you consider these traits of culturally encapsulated counselors:

- Define reality according to one set of cultural assumptions
- Show insensitivity to cultural variations among individuals
- Accept unreasoned assumptions without proof or ignore proof because that might disconfirm their assumptions
- Fail to evaluate other viewpoints and make little attempt to accommodate the behavior of others
- Remain trapped in one way of thinking, resist adaptation, and reject alternatives

Encapsulation is a potential trap that all helpers are vulnerable to falling into. If you accept the idea that certain cultural values are supreme, you limit yourself by refusing to consider alternatives. If you possess cultural tunnel vision, you are likely to misinterpret patterns of behavior displayed by clients who are culturally different from you. Unless you understand the values of other cultures, you are likely to misunderstand these clients. Because of this lack of understanding, you may label certain client behaviors as resistant, you may make an inaccurate diagnosis of a particular behavior as maladaptive, and you may impose your own value system on the client. For example, some Latinas might resist changing what you view as dependency on their husband. If you work with Latina clients, you need to appreciate that they might possess the value of remaining with their husband, even if he is unfaithful. Latino tradition tells these women that no matter what, it is not appropriate to leave one's husband. If you are unaware of this traditional value, you could make the mistake of pushing such women to take an action that will violate their belief system.

It is important that helpers respect the cultural heritage of their clients and that they avoid encouraging clients to give up this culture so that they can assimilate into the dominant culture. Certainly, clients need to consider the consequences of not accepting certain values of the society in which they live, but they should not be pressured to accept wholesale a set of values that may be unacceptable to them. Although clients who inhabit more than one culture are likely to struggle with finding ways to integrate what is best for them from both cultures, the synthesis can be rich with possibilities.

Helpers from all cultural groups need to examine their expectations, attitudes, biases, and assumptions about the helping process and also about persons from diverse groups. Realize that there is no sanctuary from cultural bias. We tend to carry our bias around with us, yet we often do not recognize this fact. It takes a concerted effort and vigilance to monitor our biases and value systems so that they do not interfere with establishing and maintaining successful helping relationships.

Western and Eastern Values

The theories and practices of the helping process that you have learned are grounded in Western assumptions, yet most of the world differs from mainstream U.S. culture. Hogan (2007) points out that the mainstream culture in the

United States derives from the Anglo-Saxon culture of the English who colonized America. She summarizes the underlying value orientations of the mainstream culture as characterized by an emphasis on a patriarchal nuclear family; "getting things done" and keeping busy; measurable and visible accomplishments; individual choice, responsibility, and achievement; self-reliance and self-motivation; the pragmatic notion of "If an idea works, use it"; change and novel ideas; and equality, informality, and fair play. The degree to which these values fit culturally diverse client groups needs to be carefully considered by human service practitioners.

Some writers in the multicultural field are critical of the strong individualistic bias of contemporary theories and the lack of emphasis on broader social contexts such as families, groups, and communities (Duran, Firehammer, & Gonzalez, 2008; Ivey, D'Andrea, Ivey, & Simik-Morgan, 2007; Pedersen, 2003; Sue, Ivey, & Pedersen, 1996). Pack-Brown, Thomas, and Seymour (2008) write that "the cultural encapsulation of the counseling field helps to perpetuate various cultural biases that are antithetical to the worldview, values, and psychological well-being of many persons from diverse cultural groups and backgrounds" (p. 297). According to Duran, Firehammer, and Gonzales (2008), oppression has resulted in "soul wounding" for persons in diverse groups. Intervention strategies based on Western assumptions may not be congruent with the values of some clients and may perpetuate forms of injustice and institutional racism. Duran and colleagues claim that Western counseling interventions have at times been used to promote social control and conformity rather than the psychological well-being of minority culture clients.

The Western model of helping does have certain limitations when applied to cultural groups such as Asian Americans, Latinos, Native Americans, and African Americans. Seeking professional help is not typical for many people from diverse backgrounds. In most non-Western cultures, in fact, informal groups of friends and relatives provide a supportive network. Many of the clients with whom you will work have a cultural heritage associated with non-Western values. Some of the interventions you have learned will be of questionable value if you do not modify your techniques.

Eastern and Western are not just geographic terms but also represent philosophical, social, political, and cultural orientations. It is typical to examine individualism and collectivism through comparisons between the cultures of the West, which reflect individualism, and those of the East, which reflect collectivism (Sampson, 2000). Ho (1985) states that a comparison of Western and Eastern systems shows some striking differences in value orientations. **Western culture** places a prime value on choice, the uniqueness of the individual, self-assertion, and strengthening the ego. By contrast, the **Eastern view** stresses interdependence, downplays individuality, and emphasizes losing oneself in the totality of the cosmos. From the Western perspective, the primary values are the primacy of the individual, youth, independence, nonconformity, competition, conflict, and freedom. The guiding principles for action (**individualism**) are found in the fulfillment of individual needs and individual responsibility. From the Eastern perspective, the primary values are the primacy of relationships, maturity, compliance, conformity, cooperation, harmony, and security. The guiding principles for action (collectivism) are found in the achievement of collective goals and collective responsibility.

Behavioral orientations also differ. The Western view encourages expression of feelings, striving for self-actualization, and individual success, whereas the Eastern view encourages control of feelings, striving for collective actualization, and group achievements. Western approaches emphasize outcomes such as improving the environment, changing one's coping behavior, learning to manage stress, and changing objective reality in other ways to improve one's way of life. Eastern approaches emphasize acceptance of one's environment and inner enlightenment.

Sampson (2000) maintains that individualism and collectivism have become increasingly important cultural variables that have significant effects on an individual's experiences and behavior. He contends that it is not necessary to pit individualism against collectivism. Recognizing both individualism *and* collectivism, independence *and* interdependence, as aspects of a total process can encourage clients to move toward a synthesis of these characteristics.

Some time ago we presented a series of workshops in Hong Kong for human service professionals. This gave us the opportunity to rethink the relevance of applying Western approaches to working with non-Western clients. Almost all the participants in these workshops were Chinese, but some of them had obtained their graduate training in social work or counseling in the United States. These professionals experienced struggles in retaining the values that were basic to their Chinese heritage while also integrating a Western counseling viewpoint that appealed to them.

In talking with these practitioners, we learned that their focus is on the individual in the context of the social system. In their interventions they pay more attention to the family than to individuals' interests. They are learning how to balance a stress on personal development with what is in the best interest of the family and society. They are able to respect the values of their clients, who are also mostly Chinese, yet at the same time challenge them to think of some ways they may want to change. Many of the helping professionals in Hong Kong told us that they had to demonstrate patience and understanding with their clients. They saw it as essential to form a trusting relationship before engaging in confrontation. Although this necessity applies to counseling in general, it seems especially important for non-Western clients.

Case example: Considering cultural differences.* A counselor, Doug, receives a telephone request from the oldest male in a traditional extended family that had recently migrated from a northern state in India. Kishore is requesting counseling concerning his younger sister, who is having difficulty adjusting to their new country and has recently tried to run away from her family. He states that there is disagreement between his sister, Savita, and the

* We thank Tim Bond, University of Bristol, UK, and Lina Kashyap, Tata Institute of Social Sciences, Mumbai, India, for contributing this case study.

rest of her family about whom she should marry. Doug's usual practice would be to respond positively to the inquiry but to insist on the potential client speaking directly to him to arrange an appointment.

Doug wonders what he should do in these circumstances, particularly in view of the cultural differences. It becomes clear that the brother intends to attend the counseling sessions with his younger sister, Savita. This is contrary to Doug's usual practice of seeing client's alone. He hesitates before deciding whether to accept these arrangements.

Your stance. If you were the counselor in this situation, how would you respond to this phone call? Consider these issues in forming your opinion:

- What are the indications of cultural differences between the counselor and the prospective clients?
- Who is the client?
- How far should the counselor go in adapting his usual practices to respond to these cultural differences?
- In what ways will counseling be ethically compromised if the counselor proceeds as requested?
- How far does the available ethical guidance from your applicable professional counseling organization help or hinder responding to these circumstances?

Discussion. This case study directs attention to potential tensions between cultural competence and meeting other ethical requirements. The ethical guidance issued by most professional associations requires cultural sensitivity and competence and warns against prejudice. However, the ethics codes seldom offer more precise instructions on how to achieve these requirements, nor do they provide advice on how to resolve conflicts between any adaptations made in response to cultural differences and other ethical requirements.

The culturally most significant feature of this case is that Kishore is reaching out beyond the family for help. Typically, within his culture problems are resolved or contained within the family, and there is great reluctance to communicate the private business of the family to outsiders. If the problem is of such significance that it justifies breaking the family's privacy, the counselor should recognize the seriousness of this request and the family's sense of concern and vulnerability in requesting help in this way. They are taking a major step outside their cultural norms. One of the first challenges for the counselor is to recognize the scale of risk that the family is taking and the significance of responding in a culturally appropriate way in order to offer a sense of reassurance and safety.

The second culturally significant feature is that the request for counseling is from the oldest male, who has responsibility for the well-being of all family members. This creates new challenges for the counselor who will need to balance being respectful of the oldest male's responsibility whilst working with other members of the family who will also be expected to defer to the oldest male. Kishore's desire to be present in the counseling sessions may be interpreted as his way of communicating his care and concern for his sister or as a way of exercising control. It is unlikely that this will become clear in an initial phone call, and it may take several sessions before the balance between care and control and the nature of the relationship between brother and sister becomes apparent.

As the counselor, Doug is faced with a critical decision about whether to start his work on the basis suggested by the brother or to attempt to ensure that Savita both wants counseling and is seen on her own to ascertain her wishes. The first might be more culturally appropriate for his client, and the second more respectful of a Western sense of individual autonomy and women's rights. As Doug has little information about Savita's views about her situation, he may decide to offer an initial meeting with both of them to discuss their situation and to agree on how he will work with them. A single meeting may not be sufficient to enable Savita to speak freely; her cultural background may encourage reticence over speaking freely, or even at all, in the presence of men. A tradition of modesty may discourage her from making eye contact with a stranger who is male. Doug will have to be sensitive and patient to win her trust sufficiently for her to communicate her views. He may want to keep an open mind as to whether a female counselor would be more appropriate if Savita is to become the primary client.

Doug's multicultural competence may be tested in other ways. Actions can be as important as words in providing a sense of security across cultural differences. One of the ways in which he might open the meeting would be to offer a cup of tea or water as a culturally appropriate way of demonstrating a respectful welcome, even if offering refreshments is not his normal practice with clients.

At some point Doug will need to decide who constitutes the "client." This is both an ethically and professionally significant decision that cannot be made without taking cultural values into account. Professional ethical guidance for counselors tends to be based on assumptions about nuclear families and the rights of all family members to be autonomous. The basic unit of ethical concern is the individual. These are culturally specific assumptions characteristic of North America and some areas of Europe, including Britain. In extended family systems, the basic unit of ethical concern may be the family as a whole rather than any individual within it. From this perspective, it could be a mistake to understand the request for help in personal terms relating to the two named individuals. Instead, it may be better understood as a request on behalf of the whole family, including other significant unnamed people such as the mother or an older sister.

Deciding how to interpret the request and its implications for establishing how to deliver the counseling is likely to be one of the primary tasks of the initial assessment. It is also ethically significant. Should the counselor work with the autonomy of the family as whole, even if this is at the expense of individual autonomy, or prioritize individual autonomy at the expense of family identity? How the counselor should position himself with respect to existing family structures and gender relationships is another challenging issue that will require careful consideration throughout the counseling relationship. When a counselor is working with people from an unfamiliar cultural background, there is a strong case for obtaining appropriate cultural mentoring in addition to any external therapeutic support or supervision. Some professional bodies strongly recommend or require this additional cultural mentoring.

The decision about who is the client will determine how the counselor approaches issues of informed consent, whose consent ought to be sought, and the management of confidentiality between family members. The emphasis on consent that is characteristic of most professional ethics codes may fail to convey the level of respect that is the intended ethical purpose of this practice. Many counselors would consider it to be good practice to discuss these issues with the prospective clients to determine their wishes before making a final decision about how to proceed. The extent to which such discussions are possible and desirable will depend on the degree of urgency and purpose for which counseling is being sought.

Many of the helping professions express doubts about how far an ethical principle founded on respect for individual autonomy can adequately address the needs of people from a collectivist culture. Could a professional ethic that emphasizes the principle of respect for individual autonomy in itself be culturally insensitive and exclude people who hold other cultural values?

Examining Your Cultural Assumptions

Pedersen (2003) contends that it is critical for practitioners to consider behaviors in a cultural context to achieve accurate assessment, meaningful understanding, and appropriate intervention. For Pedersen, anything less is culturally biased. Without being aware of their cultural assumptions and biases, helpers could cause harm to those they serve. A central task helpers face in becoming culturally competent involves acknowledging that they bring their cultural biases, prejudices, and stereotypes to their work with clients (Pack-Brown et al., 2008).

Culturally learned basic assumptions, whether we are aware of them or not, significantly influence the ways in which we perceive and think about reality and how we act. A willingness to examine such assumptions opens doors to seeing others from their vantage point rather than from a preconceived perspective. Helpers often unwittingly make cultural assumptions on a variety of topics. Reflect on how your understanding of these issues is likely to influence your work with clients.

Assumptions about self-disclosure. Self-disclosure is highly valued in counseling, and most helpers assume that no effective helping can occur unless clients reveal themselves in the helping relationship. One way to facilitate meaningful disclosure on the part of clients is for helpers to model appropriate self-disclosure. Ivey, Ivey, and Zalaquett (2010) comment that helper self-disclosure can increase client self-disclosure, create trust between counselor and client, and establish a more equal relationship in the interview. However, some writers have reservations about the value of helper self-disclosure, contending that the helping process can work quite well without this kind of sharing.

Ivey and colleagues (2010) make some points worth your consideration. Unless clients work through the obstacles to some level of disclosure, they are not likely to be able to participate in the helping relationship. However, you can recognize and appreciate that some of your clients will struggle in letting you know the nature of their problems. This struggle in itself is a useful focus for exploration. Rather than expecting such clients to disclose freely, you can demonstrate respect for their values and at the same time ask them what they want from you. With your support and encouragement, clients can sort through their values and socialization pertaining to self-disclosure and decide the degree to which they want to change.

Some forms of helping place less stress on verbal disclosure, such as music therapy, occupational and recreational therapy, and other forms of activity therapy. Helpers can also assume an advocacy role for the client in the system, can help clients build on their natural sources of support, or can teach clients to use the resources within the community. As you will see in Chapter 13, a number of community-based interventions may be more appropriate for some clients than traditional approaches to helping.

Assumptions about family values. D. Sue (1997) has written about some traditional Chinese family values. Filial piety is a significant value in Chinese American families, emphasizing obedience to parents and respect and honor for them. They value family bonds and unity more than self-determination and independence. Family communication patterns are based on cultural tradition and emphasize appropriate roles and status. Academic achievement is prized. Helpers who fail to understand and appreciate these values are likely to err by pushing Chinese American clients to change in directions that are not consistent with their values.

In one of his multicultural workshops, Paul Pedersen related that many Asian students with whom he worked reflected values from their family when they were confronted with a problem. They first tended to reflect inward for some answer. If they did not find an answer within themselves, they tended to go to someone in the family. If neither of these routes worked, they were likely to seek guidance from a teacher, a friend, or someone they considered wise. If none of these avenues resulted in a satisfactory solution, they might then consult a professional helper.

Assumptions about nonverbal behavior. Clients can disclose themselves in many nonverbal ways, but cultural expressions are prone to misinterpretation. Personal space requirements, eye contact, handshaking, dress, formality of greeting, perspective on time, and so forth all vary among cultural groups. Mainstream Americans often feel uncomfortable with silence and tend to fill in quiet gaps with words. In some cultures, in contrast, silence indicates a sign of respect and politeness. You could misinterpret a quiet client's behavior if you did not realize that the client might be waiting for you to ask questions. It is good to keep in mind that there are no universal meanings of nonverbal behaviors.

You may have been systematically trained in a range of microskills: attending, open communication, observation, hearing clients accurately, noting and reflecting feelings, and selecting and structuring, to mention a few (Ivey et al., 2010). Although these behaviors are aimed at creating a positive therapeutic relationship, individuals from certain ethnic groups may have difficulty responding positively or understanding the intent of the counselor's attitudes and behavior. The helper whose confrontational style involves direct eye contact, physical gestures, and probing personal questions may be seen as offensively intrusive by clients from other cultures.

In American middle-class culture, direct eye contact is usually considered a sign of interest and presence, and a lack thereof is interpreted as evasiveness. It is common for individuals to maintain more eye contact while listening and less while talking. Some research indicates that African Americans may reverse this pattern by looking more when talking and slightly less when listening. Among some Native American and Latino groups, eye contact by the young is a sign of disrespect. Some cultural groups generally avoid eye contact when talking about serious subjects (Ivey et al., 2010). Clearly, helpers who pathologize a client's lack of eye contact may not be understanding or respecting important cultural differences. Helpers need to acquire sensitivity to a wide range of cultural differences to reduce the probability of miscommunication, misdiagnosis, and misinterpretation of nonverbal behaviors.

Assumptions about trusting relationships. Many, but not all, mainstream Americans tend to form quick relationships and to talk easily about their personal life. This characteristic is often reflected in their helping style. Thus, the helper expects that the client will approach their relationship in an open and trusting manner. Doing this is very difficult for some clients, however, especially given that they are expected to talk about themselves in personal ways to a stranger. It may take a long time to develop a meaningful working relationship with a client who is culturally different from you.

Assumptions about self-actualization. Helping professionals commonly assume that it is important for the individual to become self-actualized. But some clients are more concerned about how their problems or changes are likely to affect others in their life. You will recall that in the Eastern orientation one of the guiding principles is achievement of collective goals. Likewise, Native Americans judge their worth primarily in relation to how their behavior contributes to the harmonious functioning of their tribe. Native Americans have a value system that is fundamentally different from that of the dominant culture, determining their self-worth in reference to the betterment of the tribe rather than their own gain (Anderson & Ellis, 1988).

Assumptions about directness and assertiveness. Although the Western orientation prizes directness, some cultures see it as a sign of rudeness and as something to be avoided. If you are not aware of this cultural difference, you could make the mistake of interpreting a lack of directness as a sign of being unassertive rather than as a sign of respect. Getting to the point immediately is valued in Western culture, but clients from other cultures may prefer to delay dealing with their problems or to cope with them in indirect ways. It is easy to put the responsibility on the client when the therapy interventions do not work. However, if therapists cannot connect to clients using the techniques in which they were trained, it is their responsibility to find other ways to work with their clients.

A helper may judge certain clients as being "nonassertive," with the implication that this is negative and something that needs to be changed. If you are operating from a Western orientation, you are likely to assume that your clients are better off if they can behave in assertive ways, such as telling people what they think, feel, and want. It is critical to recognize that being direct and assertive is just one way of being; counselors should avoid assuming that assertive behavior is the norm and is desirable for everyone. Certain clients might be offended if it were automatically assumed that they would be better off if they were more assertive. For example, assume that you are working with a woman who rarely asks for what she wants, allows others to decide her priorities, and almost never denies a request or demand from anyone in her family. If you worked hard at helping her become an assertive woman, it could very well create conflicts within her family system. If she changed her role, she might no longer fit in her family or in her culture. Therefore, it is crucial that both you and your clients consider the consequences of examining and modifying their cultural values.

One way to respect your clients is to listen to what they say they value. Ask your clients what behaviors are and are not working in their lives. If clients tell you that being indirect or unassertive is problematic for them, then this should be explored. However, if such behaviors are not posing difficulty for them, you need to monitor how your biases may be operating when you attempt to change clients in directions that they are not interested in pursuing. Asking your clients what they want from you is a way of decreasing the chances that you will impose your cultural values on them. On this point, consider the following case.

Case example: Is listening to your client enough?   Mac, a successful psychologist, has concerns about much of the multicultural movement. He sees it as more trendy than useful. "I do not impose my values. I do not tell clients what to do. I listen, and if I need to know something, I ask. How am I to know whether a Japanese American client is more American than Japanese or vice versa unless I ask him? My belief is that the client will tell you all you need to know."

Your stance. What is your reaction to Mac's attitude? How would you determine the level of acculturation of a client of yours? What is your reaction to Mac expecting his client to educate him on culture issues?

Discussion. We react not so much to what Mac says as to what is implied by what is said. Certainly, it is important for clients to tell counselors what they need to know. However, Mac seems to downplay the necessity for ongoing education and sensitivity to cultural issues, which might enable him to ask more effective questions. It is not the responsibility of Mac's clients to educate him. Listening to our clients is not enough; we also need to be formally and informally educated.

Review the basic cultural assumptions that influence you and determine where you might be imposing your views. What forces have shaped your basic assumptions? Are you open to considering the relevance of such assumptions in working with clients who are different from you?

Challenging Your Stereotypical Beliefs

Although you may assume you are without bias, stereotypical beliefs could well affect your practice. **Stereotyping** involves assuming that the behavior of an individual will reflect or be typical of that of most members of his or her cultural group. This assumption leads to statements such as these: "Asian American clients are emotionally repressed." "African American clients are suspicious and will not trust professional helpers." "White people are arrogant." "Native Americans have very low motivation."

Sue (2005) contends that **modern racism** is often subtle, indirect, and unintentional, which allows people to remain oblivious to its existence. According to Sue, racism frequently operates outside the level of conscious awareness. Helpers who view themselves as being without any stereotypes, biases, and prejudices are most likely underestimating the impact of their socialization. Such helpers can be even more dangerous than those who are more open about their biases and prejudices. According to Pedersen (2000), this form of racism emerges unintentionally from well-meaning and caring professionals who are no more nor less culturally biased than segments of the general public. He believes that unintentional racists must be challenged either to become intentional racists or to modify their attitudes and behaviors. The key to changing the unintentional racist lies in examining basic underlying assumptions, such as those we described earlier.

In addition to cultural stereotypes, some stereotypes are associated with special populations, such as people with disabilities, older people, and people who are homeless. Statements that lump together individuals within a group reflect a myth of uniformity. In your professional work you need to realize that there are variations within cultural groups and that such differences may be at least as important as those among different groups. In your attempt to be culturally sensitive, be careful to avoid further stereotyping of certain groups.

Although cultural differences both among and within groups may be obvious, it is important not to go to the extreme of focusing exclusively on the differences that can separate us. In working with mental health professionals in foreign countries, we have become even more convinced that there are some basic similarities among the peoples of the world. Universal experiences can bind people together. Although personal circumstances differ, most people experience the pain of making decisions and attempting to live with integrity in the world. It is essential to be respectful of the real cultural differences that exist, and it is equally important that we not forget the common denominators of all people.

Understanding People With Disabilities*

Part of understanding diversity involves understanding how ability and disability are relevant factors in the delivery of human services. In ways similar to people of color, people with disabilities have to face prejudice, hostility, lack of

* We want to acknowledge Dr. Mark Stebnicki, Professor and Director of the Graduate Program in Rehabilitation Counseling at East Carolina University, for his consultation with us and helpful input in revising this section on understanding people with disabilities.

understanding, and discrimination on the basis of their physical, emotional, or mental abilities. DePoy and Gilson (2004) point out that diversity categories such as race, ethnicity, and gender fall under a similar analytic lens. Individuals without disabilities frequently view people with disabilities through the same distorted spectacles with which they see others who differ from them. The clarity of a helper's vision can be impaired by myths, misconceptions, prejudices, and stereotypes about people with disabilities.

It is important to recognize the potential of people with disabilities. Helpers' attitudes are a key factor in successfully intervening in the lives of people with disabilities. Dispelling myths and misconceptions when helping people with disabilities achieve their goals can be just as necessary as when working with persons who have addiction issues, intense marital conflicts, or are survivors of extraordinary stressful and traumatic events.

Examining Stereotypes Pertaining to Physical Disabilities

People with physical disabilities do not want to be labeled with language such as "crippled," afflicted," "special," or "handicapped." Many advocates believe that the environment itself and others' negative attitudes toward persons with disabilities are the real handicapping conditions (Smart, 2009). Historically, much of the language used to refer to "the disability experience," as portrayed in the print and electronic media, has communicated a condescending attitude toward persons with disabilities. For example, some with spinal cord injuries are concerned that others may perceive them as being "physically or mentally deficient" in some way. Marini (2007) notes that spinal cord injury has profound implications for socialization, employment outlook, self-esteem, and basic independent functioning. Overall, persons with disabilities remain the most disenfranchised group in almost every society, regardless of their ethnicity. Minorities with disabilities are the least educated and have the highest unemployment rate in the United States, with some unemployment estimates ranging from 66 to 70% (Roessler & Rubin, 1998; Szymanski & Parker, 2003). Persons with disabilities are often unemployed and underemployed, and many live below the poverty line (Olkin, 2009). Olkin states that people with disabilities generally report psychosocial issues more than physical barriers as major impediments in living with a disability.

Individuals without disabilities often try to hide their feelings of awkwardness in the presence of a person with a disability through exaggerated attention and kindness. Helpers may have learned a variety of negative messages about disability, and they may experience some initial discomfort. It is essential for helpers to demonstrate a willingness to examine their own attitudes when they are working with people who have any kind of disability. A critical aspect of self-awareness is to recognize, understand, and manage one's countertransference in working with clients with disabilities (Olkin, 2009). Although people with disabilities share some common concerns, it is a mistake to think of them as all being the same. There is considerable diversity among people within a particular ethnic group, and the same can be said about people with physical disabilities.

As with any special population with which you work, it is important that you identify your assumptions. For example, you could assume that certain careers might be out of reach for a client with a disability. But to make this assumption without checking it out with your client is tantamount to limiting his or her options. Inaccurate assumptions may result in faulty case conceptualizations and problem formulation (Smart, 2009). Smart notes that many of our assumptions about individuals who have disabilities are inaccurate and may impede the helping process and further disable the client. This would be a good time for you to reflect on any stereotypes that you may have toward people with disabilities and to scrutinize your assumptions about why they are seeking counseling.

A major role of practitioners who work with people with disabilities is to help these individuals to understand the prejudice and discrimination that surrounds disability. According to Palombi (in Cornish, Gorgens, Monson, Olkin, Palombi, & Abels, 2008), persons with disabilities often experience many of the same prejudices and kinds of discrimination as other underrepresented groups. For practitioners to effectively work with persons with disabilities, it is essential that helpers recognize their own biases and address them. If practitioners fail to do this, the result may be a perpetuation of attitudinal barriers based on ignorance, false beliefs, and prejudice (Cornish et al., 2008). Helpers need to be able to assist their clients who have a disability develop an understanding of the impact that societal stereotypes have on their view of themselves. Mackelprang and Salsgiver (1999) put this matter cogently:

> Stereotypical attitudes are pervasive in society, and human service professionals are as susceptible to them as anyone. Close monitoring of personal reactions to people with disabilities can help professionals identify and deal with their personal attitudes based on stereotypical beliefs. (p. 9)

Pushing Through Perceived Limitations

If you work with people with disabilities, you must develop attitudes and intervention skills that will enable your clients to recognize the strengths and resources they possess. As a helper, you may encounter clients who have been disabled from birth, adolescents recently disabled due to traumatic injury (perhaps a sports injury or an automobile accident), adults who have had a stroke or heart disease, those with rapid onset disabilities that may or may not be permanent, or adults who have been diagnosed with a chronic degenerative condition such as Parkinson's disease, multiple sclerosis, or type I (insulin dependent) diabetes.

The kinds of help persons with disabilities need may encompass a broad range of services. Primarily, these individuals could benefit from psychosocial adjustment services with the intention of optimizing their level of independent functioning, developing positive coping skills, cultivating resiliency strategies, and achieving optimal levels of wellness. Some clients may need help finding community resources to enable them to participate fully in the workforce. Others may need counseling to overcome the anxiety and depression that is often present when it looks like all of life has been turned on its head in a single moment. The rehabilitation plan should be highly individualized and presented in such a way that each person can reach his or her optimal level of medical, physical, psychological, emotional, vocational, and social functioning. Persons with disabilities often have complex issues; it is best not to judge these clients or their needs based on your first meetings with them. You should not assume that people with disabilities are seeking counseling only because of their disability.

To provide ethical and effective services to individuals with disabilities, Smart (2009) believes helpers must seek further training about the experience of disability: "Certainly, information about each client's identity and feelings about his or her disability must come from that individual, but obtaining a broad knowledge of the disability experience is essential" (p. 643). Palombi (in Cornish et al., 2008) contends that many practitioners are unaware of the unique needs and struggles of persons with disabilities, and thus, they may not be able to provide ethical and competent care.

Cornish and her colleagues state that professionals are not being adequately trained to provide services to clients with disabilities despite the likelihood that they will work with this population. Practitioners must engage in self-reflection to accurately determine whether they are competent to provide services to persons with disabilities. If not, appropriate referral skills are necessary. Cornish and her colleagues (2008) contend that "it is essential to provide ethical treatment to persons with disabilities, minimize barriers to care, and train future psychologists in these endeavors" (p. 489).

Olkin (2009) describes disability-affirmative therapy as being designed "to help counselors incorporate disability knowledge and culture into the treatment, making for a powerful combination to achieve desired results" (p. 369). A premise of disability-affirmative therapy is that "incorporating information about disability will inform the case formulation such that it neither overinflates nor underestimates the role of disability" (p. 355).

Mackelprang and Salsgiver (1999) provide these guidelines for practice with persons with disabilities:

- Operate on the assumption that people are capable or potentially capable.
- Critically evaluate the assumption that the problem with disability lies with the person and that individuals with disabilities must be changed before they can function adequately in society.
- Recognize that people with disabilities often face discrimination and oppression, as do other minority groups. Realize that your interventions might well involve political advocacy and actions on your part to eliminate policy barriers that prevent individuals from accessing society's benefits.
- Empower persons with disabilities with interventions based on the assumption that these individuals have the right to control their own lives.

Reflect on these basic assumptions and principles as you strive to formulate your own guidelines for effective practice with people with disabilities.

Case example: Challenging our perceptions. I (Marianne) gave a talk to people with disabilities at a residential facility. The kinds of questions they raised were not any different from those of other groups that I have addressed, and many of the residents emphasized that they were no different from people without disabilities. Later, I asked a staff member at this institution to ask a few residents this question: "What would you like to tell helpers in training about yourself to assist them in better dealing with special populations?" Some of the residents gave these responses:

- "I would like them to know that I want to be treated as a normal person even though I am in a wheelchair. Look at the person, not at the wheelchair. Don't be afraid of us."
- "I'm a very good person. I'm a very smart person. I have a disability, but I also have intelligence."
- "I can think and feel just like a normal person."

The staff member said a great deal in very few words in a letter to me about her perceptions of the people she helps:

> They have lived in institutions for most of their adult lives. They say they are no different from people without disabilities, but I think that they have enormous hearts. The people I have known have no prejudice and are very loving and giving. They also have a greater appreciation for the very simple things in life that most of us take for granted each day. They are unique individuals and I feel fortunate to have worked with them.

Your stance. Consider your own attitudes and assumptions about people you meet who have disabilities. Do you go out of your way to "help" these individuals? Do you conveniently "avoid" getting too close to them? How might your own reactions affect your work as a helper with this population?

Discussion. Societal attitudes are slowly changing as well-known individuals demonstrate a basic truth—having a disability does not mean that the person is disabled. One example is Erik Weihenmayer, who was born with a degenerative eye disorder that resulted in losing his sight by age 13. In *Touch the Top of the World,* Weihenmayer (2001) chronicles a life of determination that led to him accomplishing incredible physical feats. He is a world-class athlete, acrobatic skydiver, long-distance biker, marathon runner, skier, mountaineer, ice climber, and rock climber. He was the first man with blindness to gain the summit of Mt. McKinley and to scale the 3,300-foot rock wall of El Capitan. In the spring of 2001 he earned the distinction of being the first person who was blind to climb above 29,000 feet to reach the summit of Mount Everest. So far he has climbed five of the seven highest mountains in the world, and his goal is to reach all seven summits on each of the seven continents. Weihenmayer is living proof that sensory disabilities do not necessarily limit a person's ability to reach his dreams. His story and the stories of others, though less dramatic, demonstrate that misconceptions regarding disabilities can be challenged. Weihenmayer's accomplishments give new meaning to the term "physically challenged."

Most of us are familiar with the Special Olympics, in which people with physical disabilities participate at the highest levels. Indeed, many people who are not so well known are challenging themselves to reach phenomenal goals in their daily lives. Such individuals continue to teach us about ourselves and the capacity of the human spirit to overcome any obstacle. And what about clients who have a disability but who lack hope and want to give up? If helpers accept their hopelessness and despair, they will be of little therapeutic value to their clients. Human service professionals need to discover their clients' strengths and work toward empowerment.

Multicultural Counseling Competencies

Increasingly, helpers will come into contact with culturally diverse client populations who may not share their worldview of what constitutes normality and abnormality. Because the helping professions seem to continue to emphasize a monocultural approach to training and practice, many helpers are ill prepared to deal effectively with cultural diversity (Sue & Sue, 2008). Although referral is sometimes an appropriate course of action, it should not be viewed as a solution to the problem of inadequately trained practitioners. With the increasing number of culturally diverse clients seeking professional help, and with the decreasing number of resources to meet these needs, helpers may not always be able to make a referral, even in those cases where they deem this necessary. Given this reality, we recommend that students in the human service professions, regardless of their racial or ethnic background, receive training in multicultural helping.

Working with culturally diverse client populations requires that helpers possess the awareness, knowledge, and skills to effectively deal with the concerns of the people with whom they work. Although it is unrealistic to expect you to have an in-depth knowledge of all cultural backgrounds, it is feasible to have a comprehensive grasp of general principles for working successfully with cultural diversity. If you are open to the values inherent in a diversity perspective, you will find ways to avoid getting trapped in provincialism, and you will be able to challenge the degree to which you may be culturally encapsulated (see Wrenn, 1985).

Sue and his colleagues (1982, 1992) developed a conceptual framework for **multicultural counseling competencies** and standards in three areas. The first area deals with the helper's beliefs and attitudes about race, culture, gender, and sexual orientation. The second dimension involves knowledge and understanding of the worldview of the helper and specific knowledge of the diverse groups with whom he or she works. The third area deals with skills and intervention strategies needed to serve diverse client groups. Sue and Sue (2008) have summarized these competencies as they apply to practice. Arredondo and her colleagues (1996) updated and operationalized these competencies, and Sue and his colleagues (1998) extended multicultural counseling competencies to individual and organizational development. Hansen and colleagues (2000) have identified and described some minimal multicultural competencies for practice, and Egan (2006) has developed list of multicultural competencies he has adapted from various sources. These multicultural competencies have been endorsed by the Association for Multicultural Counseling and Development (AMCD), by the Association for Counselor Education and Supervision (ACES), and by the

American Psychological Association (APA, 2003). For an updated and expanded version of these competencies, see *Multicultural Counseling Competencies 2003: Association for Multicultural Counseling and Development* (Roysircar et al., 2003). Refer also to the APA's (2003) *Guidelines on Multicultural Education, Training, Research, Practice, and Organizational Change for Psychologists.*

The essential attributes of **culturally skilled helpers,** compiled from these sources, are presented next. You can use this checklist to identify areas of *multicultural competence* you now possess as well as areas in which you need to acquire additional knowledge and skills.

Beliefs and Attitudes of Culturally Skilled Helpers

Put a check mark in the box before each of the beliefs and attitudes in this section that you think you already hold or each area of awareness that you already possess.

With respect to beliefs and attitudes, culturally skilled helpers . . .

☐ become aware of their own personal culture and how they might come across to those who differ from them in a multitude of ways.

☐ are aware of how their own cultural heritage, gender, class, ethnic identity, sexual orientation, disability, and age shape their values, assumptions, and biases related to identified groups.

☐ gain awareness of their personal and culture biases toward individuals or groups other than their own.

☐ do not allow their personal biases, values, or problems to interfere with their ability to work with clients who are different from them.

☐ believe that cultural self-awareness and sensitivity to one's own cultural heritage are essential for any form of helping.

☐ are aware of their negative and positive emotional reactions toward others that may prove detrimental to establishing collaborative helping relationships.

☐ have moved from being culturally unaware to knowing their cultural heritage.

☐ learn about the ways in which they are both alike and different from the person they are helping.

☐ seek to examine and understand the world from the vantage point of their clients.

☐ become aware of how any aspect of diversity (age, disability, race) can become a target of negative behaviors.

☐ are able to recognize the limits of their multicultural competence and expertise.

☐ respect clients' religious and spiritual beliefs and values.

☐ recognize their sources of discomfort with differences that exist between themselves and others.

☐ welcome diverse value orientations and diverse assumptions about human behavior and, thus, have a basis for sharing the worldview of their clients as opposed to being culturally encapsulated.

☐ rather than maintaining that their cultural heritage is superior, are able to accept and value the many forms of diversity.

☐ are able to identify and understand the central cultural constructs of their clients and to avoid applying their own cultural constructs inappropriately to people with whom they work.

☐ respect indigenous helping practices and respect help-giving networks within the community.

☐ monitor their functioning through consultation, supervision, and further training or education.

☐ understand that mainstream Western helping strategies might not fit all people or all problems and realize how they may need to adapt their interventions to the needs of their clients.

Knowledge of Culturally Skilled Helpers

Put a check mark in the box before each type of knowledge in this section that you think you already possess.

With respect to knowledge areas, culturally skilled helpers . . .

☐ possess knowledge about their own racial and cultural heritage and how it affects them personally and in their work.

☐ possess knowledge and understanding about how oppression, racism, prejudice, discrimination, and stereotyping affect them personally and professionally.

☐ do not impose their values and expectations on clients from differing cultural backgrounds and avoid stereotyping clients.

☐ strive to understand the worldviews, values, and beliefs of those with whom they work.

☐ understand the basic values underlying the helping process and know how these values may clash with the cultural values of diverse groups of people.

☐ are aware of the institutional barriers that prevent some individuals from utilizing the mental health services available in their communities.

☐ have knowledge of the potential bias in assessment instruments and use procedures and interpret findings keeping in mind the cultural and linguistic characteristics of clients.

☐ possess specific knowledge and information about the particular individuals with whom they are working.

☐ are knowledgeable about communication style differences and how their style may clash with or foster the helping process with persons from different cultural groups.

☐ are knowledgeable about the community characteristics and the resources in the community as well as those in the family.

☐ learn about the basics of family structure and gender roles of groups with whom they work.

☐ understand how people in various cultures feel about asking for professional help.

☐ have knowledge about sociopolitical influences that impinge upon the lives of ethnic and racial minorities, including immigration issues, poverty, racism, stereotyping, stigmatization, and powerlessness.

☐ view diversity in a positive light, which enables them to meet and resolve the challenges that arise in their work with a wide range of client populations.

☐ know how to help clients make use of indigenous support systems. In areas where they are lacking in knowledge, they seek resources to assist them.

Skills and Intervention Strategies of Culturally Skilled Helpers

Put a check mark in the box before each of the skill areas in this section that you think you already possess.

With respect to specific skills, culturally skilled helpers . . .

☐ take responsibility for educating their clients to the way the helping process works, including matters such as goals, expectations, legal rights, and the helper's orientation.

☐ familiarize themselves with relevant research and the latest findings regarding mental health and mental disorders that affect diverse client populations.

☐ are willing to seek out educational, consultative, and training experiences to enhance their ability to work with culturally diverse client populations.

☐ assess their level of cross-cultural and personal-cultural competence and do what they can to become a culturally competent helper.

☐ are open to seeking consultation with traditional healers or religious and spiritual leaders to better serve culturally different clients, when appropriate.

☐ use methods and strategies and define goals consistent with the life experiences and cultural values of their clients and modify and adapt their interventions to accommodate cultural differences.

☐ establish rapport with and convey empathy to clients in culturally sensitive ways.

☐ have the ability to design and implement nonbiased and effective interventions for clients from identified groups.

☐ are able to initiate and explore issues of difference between themselves and their clients, when it is appropriate.

☐ are not limited to only one approach in helping but recognize that helping strategies may be culture bound.

☐ are able to send and receive both verbal and nonverbal messages accurately and appropriately.

☐ are able to exercise institutional intervention skills on behalf of their clients.

☐ become actively involved with individuals outside of the office (community events, celebrations, and neighborhood groups) to the extent possible.

☐ are committed to understanding themselves as racial and cultural beings and are actively seeking a nonracist identity.

☐ actively pursue and engage in professional and personal-growth activities to address their limitations.

☐ consult regularly with other professionals regarding issues of culture to determine whether or where referral may be necessary.

Reflection questions. Now that you have completed the checklist, summarize and think about the implications of your current level of awareness, knowledge, and skills. As a way to assess your present level of multicultural competence, reflect on the following questions:

- Are you familiar with how your own culture has a present influence on the way you think, feel, and act? What steps could you take to broaden your base of understanding, both of your own culture and of other cultures?
- Are you able to identify your basic assumptions, especially as they apply to diversity in culture, ethnicity, race, gender, class, religion, and sexual orientation? To what degree are you clear about how your assumptions are likely to affect your practice as a helper?
- How open are you to being flexible in applying the techniques you use with clients?
- How prepared are you to understand and work with clients of different cultural backgrounds?
- To what degree are you now able to differentiate your own cultural perspective from that of a person from another culture?
- Is your academic program preparing you to gain the awareness, knowledge, and skills you will need to work with diverse client populations?
- What kinds of life experiences have you had that will better enable you to understand and counsel people who have a different worldview?
- Can you identify any areas of your personal-cultural biases that could inhibit your ability to work effectively with people who are different from you? If so, what steps might you take to challenge your biases?

Social Justice Competencies

Becoming increasingly aware of the ways that oppression and discrimination operate in the lives of our clients is a fundamental part of ethical practice, and we must translate this awareness into various forms of social action. Multiculturalism and social justice are ultimately intertwined (Crethar, Torres Rivera, & Nash, 2008). The **social justice perspective** is based on the premise that oppression, privilege, and social inequities do exist and have a negative impact on the lives of many persons from diverse cultural groups. For us to be able to effectively work with a range of persons from diverse backgrounds, it is critical that we acquire competencies in the social justice perspective, and it is essential that we incorporate these competencies into our practice. We can play a significant role in making society a better place by challenging systemic inequities. Crethar and Ratts (2008) address the question of why social justice is a concern in the counseling field:

> Social justice in counseling represents a multifaceted approach in which counselors strive to simultaneously promote human development and the common good through addressing challenges related to both individual and distributive justice. This approach includes empowerment of individuals and groups as well as active confrontation of injustice and inequality in society, both as they impact clientele and in their systemic contexts. (p. 24)

From a social justice perspective, the goal of helping is to promote the empowerment of people who are marginalized and oppressed in our society (Herlihy & Watson, 2007). This perspective reflects a valuing of fairness and equal treatment for marginalized and devalued individuals and groups of people who do not share equally in society; it also includes the right to participate in making decisions on matters that affects their lives (Constantine, Hage, Kindaichi, & Bryant, 2007; Crethar & Ratts, 2008; Crethar et al., 2008).

In their clinical and research work in the areas of multicultural competence and social justice, Constantine and colleagues (2007) identify nine social justice competencies essential to effectively delivering services to diverse client populations:

- Become knowledgeable about the ways that oppression and social inequities can operate on individual, societal, and cultural levels.
- Engage in self-reflection on issues of race, ethnicity, oppression, power, and privilege in your own life.
- Develop an ongoing awareness of how your position of power or privilege could replicate experiences of injustice in your interactions with clients or community organizations.
- Question therapeutic practices that appear inappropriate for individuals from certain groups.
- Learn about indigenous models of health and healing and be willing to collaborate with such resources, when appropriate, as a way to implement culturally relevant interventions.
- Consider the various types of social injustices that can occur within an international context, which may have global implications.
- Strive to implement comprehensive prevention and remedial mental health intervention programs designed to meet the needs of marginalized groups of people.
- Collaborate with community organizations in partnerships to promote trust, minimize power differentials, and provide culturally relevant services.
- Acquire advocacy skills and develop system intervention skills necessary to bring about social change within institutions, neighborhood, and communities.

These social justice competencies, like the multicultural competencies, are not achieved once and for all. It is best to think of these competencies as a part of a lifelong journey in developing attitudes and behaviors that will equip you to best serve a wide range of client groups.

Recognizing Your Own Limitations

As a culturally skilled helper, you have the ability to recognize the limits of your multicultural competency and expertise. When necessary, you will refer clients to more qualified individuals or resources. It is not realistic to expect that you will know everything about the cultural background of people with whom you will work. There is much to be said for letting your clients teach you about relevant aspects of their culture. Ask clients to provide you with the information you will need to work effectively with them. In working with culturally diverse individuals, it helps to assess the degree of acculturation and identity development that has taken place. This is especially true for individuals who have had the experience of living in another culture. They often have allegiance to their own home culture but find certain characteristics of their new culture attractive. They may experience conflicts when integrating the values from the two cultures in which they live. These core struggles can be productively explored in the context of a collaborative helping relationship.

We encourage you to accept your limitations and to be patient with yourself as you expand your vision of how your culture continues to influence the person you are today. It is not helpful to overwhelm yourself with all that you do not know or to feel guilty over your limitations or parochial views. You will not become a more effective and culturally skilled helper by expecting to be completely knowledgeable about the cultural backgrounds of all your clients, by thinking that you should have a complete repertoire of skills, or by demanding perfection. Instead, recognize and appreciate your efforts toward becoming a more diversity-competent helper.

The first step is to become more willing to accept diversity as a value and to take actions to increase your ability to work with a range of clients. You can also recognize when referral is in the best interest of your client. It is important to commit to lifelong learning and to take the steps necessary to continually upgrade your knowledge and skills to better serve diverse client populations (NOHS, 2000). This kind of continuing education extends throughout your professional career.

Multicultural Training

To enable helpers to utilize a multicultural perspective in their work, we support specialized training through formal courses and supervised field experiences with diverse client populations. We believe that a self-exploratory class should be required for helpers so that they can better identify their cultural and ethnic blind spots. In addition to enabling students to learn about cultures other than their own, such a course could offer opportunities for trainees to learn more about their own race, ethnicity, and culture.

A good program should include at least one course dealing exclusively with multicultural issues and persons from diverse backgrounds. However, reliance on a single-course offering designed to address the interface of professional ethics, multicultural counseling competence, and social justice counseling issues is not adequate for assisting counselors to deal successfully with the demands they will face (Bemak & Chung, 2007). In addition to a separate course, a broad range of ethical decision-making skills related to multicultural counseling should be integrated throughout the curriculum and infused in all aspects of the training program (Pack-Brown et al., 2008). For example, a fieldwork or internship seminar can introduce ways that helping strategies can be adapted to the special needs of diverse client populations and show how some techniques may be quite inappropriate for culturally different clients. The integration of multiculturalism and gender awareness can certainly be a thread running through relevant formal courses. In addition, there could be at least one required field placement or internship in which trainees have multicultural experiences. Ideally, the supervisor at this agency will be well versed in the cultural variables of that particular setting and also be skilled in cross-cultural understanding. Further, trainees should have access to both individual and group supervision on campus from a faculty member.

Supervised experience, along with opportunities for trainees to discuss what they are learning, is the core of a good program. We encourage you to select supervised field placements and internships that will challenge you to work on gender issues, cultural concerns, developmental issues, and lifestyle differences. You will not learn to deal effectively with diversity by working exclusively with clients with whom you are comfortable and whose culture is familiar to you. You can learn a great deal by going out into the community and interacting with diverse groups of people who face myriad problems. Through well-selected internship experiences, you will not only expand your own consciousness but increase your knowledge of diverse groups. This will provide a basis for acquiring intervention skills.

Pedersen (2000) has identified an effective multicultural training program as including the components of awareness, knowledge, skill development, and experiential interaction, all of which are integrated in actual practice. As you have seen, awareness of personal attitudes and of attitudes toward diverse client populations is integral to becoming an effective helper. From a knowledge perspective, helpers need to understand what makes a diverse population special. They need to know what behavior is acceptable within the diverse population and how this behavior differs from that of other groups.

Hansen and her colleagues (2000) point out that both awareness and knowledge competencies are essential prerequisites to developing effective multicultural skills. The skills they identify as being crucial include being able to (a) conduct culturally sensitive interviews and assessments; (b) form accurate and nonbiased conceptualizations; (c) design and implement effective treatment plans; and (d) accurately evaluate the adequacy of their skills and to take corrective actions when needed. Skill development is a necessary but not sufficient component of learning to work with diverse populations. The skills themselves are not unique, but the ways in which these skills are applied to particular clients should be the focus of training. Effective training will pay sufficient attention to each of these domains. If any of them are neglected, helpers are at a disadvantage.

Training programs have come a long way in the past decade, but they still have some way to go if they are to meet the goal of equipping helpers with the knowledge and skills required to meet the needs of diverse clients. As a student, you can take some small, yet significant, steps toward recognizing and examining the impact of your own cultural background and learning about cultures different from your own. Deciding to act upon even a few of the suggestions listed here is one way to move in the direction of becoming a culturally skilled helper.

By Way of Review

• Multiculturalism can be considered as the fourth force in the helping professions. This perspective recognizes and values diversity in helping relationships and calls on helpers to develop strategies that are culturally appropriate.

• A multicultural perspective on the helping process takes into consideration specific values, beliefs, and actions related to race, ethnicity, gender, age, ability, religion, language, socioeconomic status, sexual orientation, political views, and geographic region. Multicultural counseling, broadly conceptualized, considers the personality dynamics and cultural backgrounds of both helper and client in establishing a context where these people can interact meaningfully.

• To function effectively with clients of various cultures, you need to know and respect specific cultural differences and realize how cultural values operate in the helping process.

• Be aware of any tendencies toward cultural tunnel vision. If you have limited cultural experiences, you may have difficulties relating to clients who have a different view of the world. You are likely to misinterpret many patterns of behavior displayed by such clients.

• It is important to pay attention to ways in which you can express unintentional racism through your attitudes and behaviors. One way to change this form of racism is by making your assumptions explicit.

• There are some striking differences in value orientations between Western and Eastern cultures. A main difference is the Western emphasis on individualism and the Eastern emphasis on collectivism. Individualism and collectivism are not necessarily oppositional concepts, for they are both elements of a total system. These value orientations have important implications for the process of helping.

• In working with people from other cultures, avoid stereotyping and critically evaluate your assumptions about the use of self-disclosure, nonverbal behavior, trusting relationships, self-actualization, and directness and assertiveness.

• Rather than thinking of cultural differences as barriers to effective helping relationships, learn to welcome diversity as something positive. Recognize that consciously dealing with cultural variables in helping can make your job easier, not more difficult.

• As a helper it is essential that you demonstrate a willingness to examine your own attitudes when you are working with people who have any kind of disability.

• Many individuals with disabilities achieve extraordinary success; keep your focus on clients' potential rather than their perceived limitations.

• Effective multicultural helpers have been identified in terms of the specific knowledge, beliefs and attitudes, and skills they possess.

• Social justice addresses issues of oppression, privilege, and social inequities. Helping professionals need to take an active stance in addressing social justice issues that are manifested in society by acquiring social justice competencies.

• Acquiring and refining multicultural and social justice competencies should be thought of as a lifelong developmental process that requires ongoing reflection, training, and continuing education.

• Helpers who view differences as positive attributes will be most likely to meet and resolve the challenges that arise in multicultural helping situations.

What Will You Do Now?

1. If your program does not require a course on cultural diversity, consider taking such a course as an elective. You might also ask if you can sit in on some class sessions in various courses that deal with special populations. For example, in one university these are a few of the courses offered: The Black Family, The Chicano Family, American Indian Women, The African Experience, The Chicano and Contemporary Issues, Afro-American Music Appreciation, The White Ethnic in America, Women and American Society, The Chicano Child, and Barrio Studies.

2. On your campus you will probably find a number of student organizations for particular cultural groups. Approach some members of one of these organizations for information about the group. See if you can attend one of their functions to get a better perspective on their culture.

3. Think of ways to broaden your cultural horizons. Go to a restaurant, social event, church service, concert, play, or movie with a person from a cultural background that is different from your own. Ask this person to teach you about salient aspects of his or her culture.

4. If your grandparents originally came from another country, interview them about their experiences growing up in their culture. If they are bicultural, ask them about any experiences with combining both cultures. What have been their experiences in assimilation? Do they retain their original cultural identity? What do they most value in both cultures? Do what you can to discover the ways in which your cultural roots have some influence on your thinking and behavior today. In Chapter 3 you were introduced to the importance of discovering how your family of origin continues to influence you. This exercise can help you develop a richer appreciation of your cultural heritage.

5. Helpers are likely to encounter clients with a variety of disabilities. Some broad types of disabilities include mobility disabilities, visual disabilities, deafness, developmental disabilities, psychiatric disabilities, and cognitive disabilities. In groups of three or four, select a broad category and research the kinds of help available in your community for persons with this disability. What additional services would benefit this special population? Present your findings in class.

6. For the full bibliographic entry for each of the sources listed here, consult the References at the back of the book. For a state-of-the-art book on multicultural perspectives on supervision and training, practice, and research and on models of racial and ethnic identity development, see Ponterotto, Casas, Suzuki, and Alexander (1995). For a good overview of counseling strategies and issues for various ethnic and racial groups, consult Atkinson (2004). Pedersen (2000) deals extensively with the topic of developing multicultural awareness, knowledge, and skills. For a discussion of unintentional racism in counseling, see Ridley (2005). Sue, Ivey, and Pedersen (1996) deal in a comprehensive manner with multicultural counseling from the perspectives of theory, practice, and research. See Lee (2006c) for a useful treatment of multicultural issues in counseling. Sue and Sue (2008) have written a comprehensive text on helping diverse client populations. For a framework for developing cultural competency in the areas of cultural awareness, knowledge acquisition, and skill development, see Lum (2007); and for a useful treatment of culturally diverse social work practice, see Lum (2004).

Ethics in Action *CD-ROM Exercises*

7. Review role-play segment 12 in Part Three on the CD-ROM. How would you respond if your client presented you with a gift and told you that in his culture this was a way to express appreciation? How might the cultural context make a difference in deciding to accept or not accept a gift?

8. Put yourself into role-play segment 3, Culture Clash, in Part Two on the CD-ROM. You are the counselor, and your client directly questions you about your background, wondering if you are able to understand her life experience and thus help her. When you consider the range of differences between you and a given client, what specific differences concern you the most? Role-play a situation where a clash between you and a client might develop (such as a difference in age, race, sexual orientation, or culture).

9. Refer to the CD-ROM section entitled "Becoming an Effective Multicultural Practitioner," which is found in Part Two immediately following role-play segment 3. Complete the self-examination of multicultural counseling competencies. Bring your answers to class and explore in small discussion groups what you need to learn to become competent as a counselor of clients whose cultural backgrounds differ from your own.

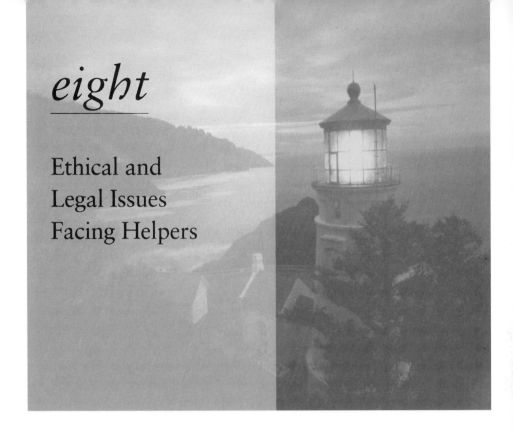

eight

Ethical and Legal Issues Facing Helpers

Focus Questions

1. What ethical issues most concern you at this stage in your professional development?

2. When you are faced with an ethical dilemma, how do you go about resolving the conflicts involved, and how do you make an ethical decision? What specific steps would you take?

3. What are the main purposes of the codes of ethics for helping professionals?

4. There are limits to confidentiality in any helping relationship. What would you want your clients to know about the purposes and limitations of confidentiality?

5. In what ways can the use of technology violate a client's privacy?

6. What do you consider to be the most essential components of informed consent?

7. How are you likely to secure informed consent from your clients?

8. In keeping records on your clients, what do you think is most important to document?

9. What are some of the key ethical issues that need to be considered in a managed care context?

10. What steps can you take to lessen the chances of a malpractice suit?

Aim of the Chapter

Regardless of what helping profession you decide on, you will face ethical dilemmas. Part of becoming a competent practitioner involves being able to apply the ethics code of your professional organization to practical situations in your work. In this chapter we introduce you to an array of ethical and legal concerns you may encounter.

There has been an increased interest in ethics in the mental health professions during the past two decades. Articles pertaining to ethical and legal issues in the helping field are common in professional journals, and many books have been written in the field of professional ethics. Most undergraduate and graduate programs include a discussion of these topics in various courses, with separate courses in ethical and legal issues now required in most graduate programs. We encourage you to take an ethics course or, at the very least, to read a book on professional ethics, and to attend professional conferences and workshops dealing with ethics and the law.

Inventory of Ethical Issues

What are some of your major concerns about ethical practice? Perhaps at this point you have not even raised this question. For each statement in this inventory, indicate the response that most closely identifies your beliefs and attitudes. Use the following code:

   5 = I *strongly agree* with this statement.
   4 = I *agree* with this statement.
   3 = I am *undecided* about this statement.
   2 = I *disagree* with this statement.
   1 = I *strongly disagree* with this statement.

____ 1. When an ethical concern arises, the best way to deal with it is to refer to the code of ethics.

____ 2. If I were faced with an ethical dilemma in one of my cases, I would take the initiative in seeking guidance from one of my professors or supervisors.

____ 3. It would be hard for me to refer a client to another professional, even if I felt this was in the client's best interest.

____ 4. I do not have enough time to keep clinical records on my clients and document everything that goes on in the helping process.

____ 5. It would be difficult for me to decide when I had to break confidentiality.

____ 6. If I were uncertain about keeping a client's confidence, I would want to discuss this with my client.

____ 7. It is my responsibility to resolve any ethical dilemmas that arise, and I would not involve my client in this decision-making process.

____ 8. I am uncertain about how to resolve ethical dilemmas.

____ 9. I often doubt whether I know enough or possess the skills needed to effectively help others.

____ 10. I am not at all certain that I know what to do if a client poses a danger to self or to others.

____ 11. I am likely to be too ready to offer advice and too quick to find solutions to my clients' problems.

____ 12. I am uncertain what "appropriate action" includes under my obligation to warn and protect others.

____ 13. What constitutes ethical practice is very much a concern of mine.

____ 14. I know the steps I am likely to take if I become aware of unethical behavior on the part of my colleagues.

____ 15. I am concerned about the possibility of becoming involved in a malpractice suit as a result of something I do or don't do as a helper.

Once you have finished this inventory, spend a few minutes reflecting on the specific areas you are most concerned about. This reflection can help you read the chapter more actively and formulate ethical questions. Identify a few of the areas in which you are uncertain about your position, and discuss these ambiguities in class.

Ethical Decision Making

Ethical practice involves far more than merely knowing and following a professional code of ethics. In dealing with ethical dilemmas, you will rarely find clear-cut answers. Most of the problems are complex and defy simple solutions. Making ethical decisions involves acquiring a tolerance for dealing with gray areas and for coping with ambiguity. Although knowing the ethical standards of your profession is essential, this knowledge alone is not sufficient. Ethics codes are not dogmatic; however, they do provide guidance in assisting you in making the best possible decisions for the benefit of your clients and yourself. Standards vary among agencies. It is necessary for you to become aware of the specific policies and practices of the agency in which you are working.

In our teaching we find that students often begin an ethics course with the expectation that they will get definitive answers to some of the questions raised in their fieldwork. They typically do not think they will have to engage in personal and professional self-exploration to find the best course of action. At times, readers of our book, *Issues and Ethics in the Helping Professions* (G. Corey, Corey, & Callanan, 2011), comment that it raises many more questions than it answers. We tell them that the book's purpose is to assist them in developing the resources to deal intelligently with ethical dilemmas.

Consider the example of Gerlinde, who became aware of unethical practices in a community agency where she was an intern. She and other interns were expected to take on some difficult clients. She realized that doing so would mean that she was clearly practicing beyond the boundaries of her competence. To make the situation worse, supervision at the agency was not always available.

Her superior was overextended and not able to provide regular supervision. In her fieldwork seminar on campus, she learned that supervisors are ethically and legally responsible for what interns do. Gerlinde had some trouble deciding what to do. She did not want to change placements in the middle of the semester, yet she was struggling with the appropriateness of confronting her supervisor about the situation. Unclear about how to proceed, she made an appointment with her fieldwork professor on campus to discuss her concerns.

In consultation with her professor, Gerlinde explored a number of alternatives. She might approach her agency supervisor herself and be more assertive in getting an appointment. Another option could be a meeting with her agency supervisor and her professor to explore the situation. It might be decided that this particular agency was inappropriate for students. What was important was that Gerlinde knew she could get help in dealing with her problem. Sometimes students who are in similar predicaments arrive too quickly at the conclusion that they will merely tolerate things as they are rather than deal with an uncomfortable situation.

At the beginning of the course, Gerlinde thought that clear answers were available for the variety of situations that would surface. By the end of the semester, she was learning to appreciate that ethics codes are not laws; they are standards that provide guidance in dealing with a range of ethical dilemmas. She had also learned the value of initiating the consultation process in ethical decision making.

Another example involves interpreting the ethical standard that the client's welfare should be the primary consideration in the therapeutic relationship. Consider the case of a client who is talking about her struggles in an alcoholic family. As the therapist listens, he is reminded painfully of the alcohol addiction of his own parents. He wonders whether he should tell this to his client. Why would he want to make this disclosure? Will his disclosure meet his own needs or the needs of the client? How will he know whether the disclosure will help or hinder the client?

Ethical issues in the helping field are often complex and multifaceted, and they defy simplistic solutions. There are gray areas that require decision-making skills. Thinking about ethical issues and learning to make wise decisions is an ongoing process that requires an open mind.

Law and Ethics

Laws and ethics codes provide guidelines for acceptable professional practice, yet neither offers clear-cut answers to most situational problems. Law defines the minimum standards society will tolerate; these standards are enforced by government agencies. All of the codes of ethics state that practitioners must act in accordance with relevant federal and state statutes and government regulations. Sometimes practitioners are not sure if they have a legal problem, nor know what to do once a legal issue has been identified (Remley & Herlihy, 2010). It is essential that practitioners be able to identify legal problems as they arise in their work; many of the situations helpers encounter that involve ethical and professional judgment will also have legal implications. Unlike law,

ethics represents aspirational goals, or the maximum or ideal standards set by the profession. Ethical standards are enforced largely by professional associations. Codes of ethics are conceptually broad in nature and generally are subject to interpretation by practitioners.

Knowledge of the ethics codes and legal guidelines applicable to a helper's practice are essential for practicing ethically and for minimizing legal liability. Hermann (2006b) points out that ethical and legal issues are distinct concepts but that they overlap significantly. As a helper, not only must you follow the ethics codes of your profession but you must also know your state's laws and your legal responsibilities. However, merely becoming familiar with local and state laws that govern your profession is not enough to enable you to make sound decisions. Your professional judgment will play a key role in resolving cases, from both an ethical and a legal perspective. Moreover, the law is not "fact specific"; rules of law must be considered in light of the particular facts of a given situation.

You may encounter a situation in which there is a conflict between the law and ethical practice. In such cases, fulfilling both ethical and legal obligations can demand a great deal of reflection on your part as well as consultation with other professionals. Knapp, Gottlieb, Berman, and Handelsman (2007) offer some recommendations. Practitioners first need to verify what the law requires and determine the nature of their ethical obligations. Sometimes practitioners do not understand their legal requirements and may assume there is a conflict between the law and ethics when none exists. When laws and ethics collide and conflict cannot be avoided, practitioners "should either obey the law in a manner that minimizes harm to their ethical values or adhere to their ethical values in a manner that minimizes the violation of the law" (p. 55). Many times apparent conflicts between the law and ethics can be avoided if clinicians anticipate problems and take proactive measures.

Helpers who work with minors and certain involuntary populations are especially advised to know the laws and ethical standards restricting their practices. At times ethical standards may conflict with legal standards and requirements for working with minors. For example, counselors may want to honor a minor's ethical right to confidentiality, yet may also encounter a parent's demand for information that a particular state law allows (Wheeler & Bertram, 2008). Some areas that may be governed by law include confidentiality, parental consent, informed consent, protection of client welfare, and civil rights of institutionalized persons. Because most helpers do not possess detailed legal knowledge, it is a good idea for helpers to obtain legal consultation about the procedures they use in their practice. Awareness of legal rights and responsibilities as they pertain to helping relationships protects clients and shields practitioners from needless lawsuits arising from negligence or ignorance.

Laws and ethics codes, by their very nature, tend to be reactive, emerging from what has occurred rather than anticipating what may occur. It is not wise to limit your behavior to merely obeying statutes and following ethical standards. Some professionals think mainly about practicing in ways that will protect them from a malpractice suit by their clients. If this legal perspective assumes primacy, helpers may limit their work with clients out of fear of a possible lawsuit and fail to provide effective services. Although it is essential to do what you can to avoid a malpractice action, do not let this overshadow your work as an ethical practitioner. We hope you will do what is best for your clients by working toward the best ethical standards of practice. It is important that you acquire this ethical sense at the beginning of your professional program. Remember that the basic purpose of practicing ethically is to advance the welfare of your clients.

Professional Codes and Ethical Decision Making

Various professional organizations have established codes of ethics that provide broad guidelines for professional helpers. These codes are not static; they are revised as new concerns arise. Some of the professional mental health organizations that have formulated codes of ethics are the National Association of Social Workers (2008), the American Psychological Association (2002), the American Counseling Association (2005), the American School Counselor Association (2004), the American Association for Marriage and Family Therapy (2001a), and the National Organization for Human Services (2000). Herlihy and Corey (2006a) identify several purposes that codes of ethics serve:

- Codes of ethics educate helpers about sound ethical practice. The application of these codes to particular situations demands a keen ethical sensitivity.
- Codes of ethics provide a mechanism for professional accountability. The ultimate end of a code of ethics is to protect the public.
- Codes of ethics serve as catalysts for improving practice. Codes can get us to critically examine both the letter and the spirit of ethical principles.

Ethics codes are necessary, but not sufficient, for the exercise of ethical responsibility. Although you have or will become familiar with the ethics codes of your specialization, you must still develop a personal ethical stance that will govern your practice. You have the ongoing task of examining your clinical practices to determine whether you are acting as ethically as you might. Ethics codes do not convey ultimate truth, nor do they make decisions for you. You may not find answers for the complex ethical dilemmas you will face in any single ethical decision-making model. In the process of weighing multiple and often competing demands and goals, you must use your professional judgment (Barnett, Behnke, Rosenthal, & Koocher, 2007).

In making ethical decisions, it will be necessary for you to grapple with the gray areas, raise questions, discuss your ethical concerns with colleagues, and monitor your own behavior. Reflection, collaboration, and consultation will set you on the path to a decision, but ultimately you must have the courage to make a decision without being certain of the outcome (Corey, Herlihy, & Henderson, 2008). When dealing with the uniqueness of each client, it is up to you to apply ethics codes to specific situations and to engage in a process of ethical decision making in determining the best course of action.

If you conscientiously practice in accordance with accepted ethics codes, you have some measure of protection in case of litigation. Compliance with or violation of ethics codes of conduct may be admissible as evidence in some legal proceedings. In a lawsuit, your conduct would probably be judged in comparison with that of other professionals with similar qualifications and duties.

The NASW *Code of Ethics* (2008) states that an ethics code cannot guarantee ethical behavior, nor can it resolve all ethical issues or disputes, nor can it capture the complexity involved in making responsible choices within a moral community. Instead, the code identifies ethical principles and standards to which professionals should aspire and by which their actions can be judged. The code reinforces the idea that ethical decision making is a process.

Practical application of ethics codes is often difficult. The issues you will encounter as a helper will require not only an understanding of the codes for your profession but also an educated interpretation of these codes to the real-life situations you face.

Codes of Ethics of the Various Professional Organizations

We suggest that you devote some time to reviewing the codes of ethics of one or more of the professional organizations. Examine the assets and limitations of these codes. As you think about these codes of ethics, look for the standards that you find most helpful. Also, identify any areas of possible disagreement that you might have with a particular standard. If your practice goes against a specific ethics code, be aware that you must have a rationale for your course of action. Realize also that there are consequences for violating the ethics code of your profession.

You can secure a copy of the codes of ethics of the different professional organizations by going to their websites:

American Counseling Association (ACA)
Code of Ethics (ACA, 2005)
Website: www.counseling.org

American Psychological Association (APA)
"Ethical Principles of Psychologists and Code of Conduct" (APA, 2002)
Website: www.apa.org

National Association of Social Workers (NASW)
Code of Ethics (NASW, 2008)
Website: www.socialworkers.org

American Association for Marriage and Family Therapy (AAMFT)
AAMFT Code of Ethics (AAMFT, 2001a)
Website: www.aamft.org

National Organization for Human Services (NOHS)
"Ethical Standards of Human Service Professionals" (NOHS, 2000)
Website: www/nationalhumanservices.org

Commission on Rehabilitation Counselor Certification (CRCC)
"Code of Professional Ethics for Rehabilitation Counselors" (CRCC, 2010)
Website: www.crccertification.com

National Association of Alcohol and Drug Abuse Counselors (NAADAC)
"NAADAC Code of Ethics"(NAADAC, 2004)
Website: http://naadac.org

Recognizing Unethical Behavior in Yourself

It is easier to see the shortcomings of others and to judge their behavior than to develop an attitude of honest self-examination. You can control your own professional behavior far more easily than you can that of your colleagues, so the proper focus is to look honestly at what you are doing. There is a tendency to think in terms of gross ethical violations while overlooking more subtle ways of being unethical. Consider for a moment these two scenarios, and ask yourself the degree to which you could picture yourself in each situation:

• You tell your clients that they can call you if they have a concern, and you give them your home phone number. One of your clients calls you frequently, often late at night. He tells you how appreciative he is of your offer that he can call you. Might you be flattered by being needed? Could you see yourself as fostering client dependency out of your need to be needed?

• A client who is in private therapy with you is ambivalent about continuing counseling sessions. She wonders whether it is time to terminate. Things are rather tight financially for you right now, and several other clients have recently terminated. Would you be inclined to support her decision? Might you be inclined to encourage her to continue, partly for financial reasons?

Unethical Behavior by Colleagues

You may occasionally encounter colleagues who appear to be behaving in unethical and unprofessional ways. Professional codes of conduct generally state that in such cases the most prudent action is to approach the colleague and share your concerns directly in an attempt to rectify the situation. If this step fails, you are then expected to make use of procedures established by your professional organization, such as reporting the colleague.

Koocher and Keith-Spiegel (2008) discuss the role of informal peer monitoring as a way to assume responsibility for watching out for each other. When ethically questionable acts are identifying, informal peer monitoring provides an opportunity for corrective interventions. Actions can be taken directly by confronting a colleague or indirectly by advising clients on how to proceed when they have concerns about another professional's actions.

Reflect for a few minutes on being in each of the following situations. What would you do in each case?

• A colleague frequently talks about his clients in inappropriate ways in places where others are able to hear him. The colleague says that joking about his clients is his way of "letting off steam" and preventing himself from taking life too seriously.

• A couple of female clients have told you that they had been sexually involved with another counselor at the agency where you work. In their counseling sessions with you, they are dealing with their anger over having been taken advantage of by this counselor. What are the legal and ethical ramifications of this situation for you?

• A colleague has several times initiated social contacts with her clients. She believes this practice is acceptable because she sees her clients as consenting adults. Furthermore, she contends that time spent socializing with these clients gives her insights into issues with which she can productively work in the therapy sessions.

• You see that one of your colleagues is practicing beyond what appears to be the scope of his competence and training. This person is unwilling to seek additional training and is not receiving adequate supervision. He maintains that the best way to learn to work with unfamiliar problems that clients present is simply to learn by doing.

The ethics codes generally address the matter of how to respond to unethical behavior of colleagues. For example, NOHS (2000) provides this standard:

> Human service professionals respond appropriately to unethical behavior of colleagues. Usually this means initially talking directly with the colleague and, if no resolution is forthcoming, reporting the colleague's behavior to supervisory or administrative staff and/or to the professional organization(s) to which the colleague belongs. (Statement 24)

Certainly, dealing with the unethical behavior of colleagues demands a measure of courage. If these people are in a position of power, you are obviously vulnerable. Even in the case of peers, such confrontations usually are difficult and require honesty and a willingness to deliver a difficult message.

An Ethical Decision-Making Model

The American Counseling Association's (2005) *Code of Ethics* states that when counselors encounter an ethical dilemma they are expected to carefully consider an ethical decision-making process. Various ethical decision-making models can guide you in working through ethical dilemmas, and it is a good idea to understand at least one model that you can apply in thinking about ethical practice. Having a systematic way of examining difficult ethical dilemmas increases your chances of making sound ethical decisions. We cannot overemphasize the importance of seeking consultation when deciding on the best course of action. It is good to consult with more than one colleague or supervisor; doing so can help you see various dimensions of a problem. Responsible and ethical practice requires you to do the following things:

• Base your actions on informed, sound, and responsible judgment.
• Consult with colleagues or seek supervision.
• Keep your knowledge and skills current.

- Engage in a continual process of self-examination.
- Remain open.

As much as possible, and when appropriate, include your client in the ethical decision-making process. Make ethical decisions *with* clients, not simply *for* them. Respecting the autonomy of your clients implies that you do not decide for them, nor do you foster dependent attitudes and behaviors. Cottone (2001) describes a **social constructivism model** of ethical decision making that is collaborative in nature. This model redefines the ethical decision-making process as an interactive rather than an individual or intrapsychic process and places the decision in the social context itself. This approach involves negotiating, consensualizing, and when necessary, arbitrating.

Garcia, Cartwright, Winston, and Borzuchowska (2003) describe a **transcultural integrative model** of ethical decision making that addresses the need for including cultural factors in the process of resolving ethical dilemmas. They present their model in a step-by-step format that counselors can use in dealing with ethical dilemmas in a variety of settings and with different client populations. Frame and Williams (2005) have developed a model of ethical decision making from a multicultural perspective, based on universalist philosophy. Their model recognizes cultural differences yet emphasizes common principles such as altruism, responsibility, justice, and caring that link cultures.

The ethical decision-making model we present here includes clients as collaborators whenever possible. The procedural steps we describe should not be thought of as a simplified and linear way to reach a resolution on ethical matters. It has been our experience that the application of these steps generally stimulates self-reflection and encourages discussion. Following these systematic steps will help you think through ethical problems.

1. *Identify the problem or dilemma.* Gather as much information as you can to clarify the situation you are facing. You might ask yourself these questions: "Is this an ethical, legal, professional, or clinical problem? Is it a combination of more than one of these?" If there are legal dimensions to the problem, seek legal consultation. Remember that many ethical dilemmas are complex, which means that it is best to examine the problem from various perspectives and to avoid looking for a one-dimensional solution. Ethical dilemmas often do not have "right" or "wrong" answers, so you will be challenged to deal with ambiguity. It may be helpful to seek consultation to determine whether there actually is an ethical concern—or to identify the exact nature of the problem. Including your client begins at this initial step and continues throughout the process of working through an ethical problem, as does the process of documenting your decisions and actions.

2. *Identify the potential issues involved.* After the information is collected, list and describe the critical issues and discard the irrelevant ones. Evaluate the rights, responsibilities, and welfare of all those who are affected by the situation. Good reasons can be presented that support various sides of a given issue, and different ethical principles may indicate different courses of action. Consider the cultural context of the situation, including any relevant cultural dimensions of the

client's situation. Ask yourself these questions: How can I best promote client independence and self-determination? What actions have the least chance of bringing harm to a client? What decision will best safeguard the welfare of the client? How can I create a trusting and therapeutic climate where clients can find their own solutions?

3. *Apply the relevant ethics code.* Once you have a clearer picture of the nature of the problem, review the code of ethics to see if the issue is addressed. If there are specific and clear guidelines, following them may resolve the problem. However, if the problem is more complex and a resolution is not apparent, you may need to employ additional steps to resolve the problem. Ask yourself whether the standards of your professional organization offer a possible solution to the problem. Consider whether your own values and ethics are consistent with or in conflict with the relevant codes. If you are in disagreement with a particular standard, do you have a rationale to support your position? Your state or national professional association may be able to provide you with guidance in resolving a dilemma. Such associations often make legal counsel available to their members.

4. *Know the applicable laws and regulations.* It is essential for you to keep up to date on relevant state and federal laws. This is especially critical in matters of keeping or divulging confidentiality, reporting child or elder abuse, dealing with issues pertaining to danger to self or others, parental rights, record keeping, assessment, and diagnosis. In addition, be sure you understand the current rules and regulations of the agency or organization where you work.

5. *Obtain consultation.* At this point, it is generally helpful to consult with a colleague or colleagues to obtain a different perspective on the problem. Poor ethical decisions often result from an inability to view a situation objectively. Prejudices, biases, personal needs, or emotional investment can distort the perception of the dilemma (Koocher & Keith-Spiegel, 2008). To increase your ability to be objective, consider consulting with more than one professional, and do not limit the individuals with whom you will consult to those who share your orientation. If there is a legal question, seek legal counsel. After you present your assessment of the situation and your ideas of how you might proceed, ask the person for feedback on your analysis. Reflect on questions such as these:

- What kinds of questions do you want to ask of those with whom you consult?
- How can you use the consultation process as an opportunity to test the justification of a course of action you are inclined to take?
- Are you considering all of the ethical, clinical, and legal issues involved in the case?
- Are there any questions you are afraid to ask?

Consultation can help you think about information or circumstances that you may have overlooked. It is imperative to document the nature of your consultation, including the suggestions provided by those with whom you consulted.

6. *Consider possible and probable courses of action.* Brainstorm as many possible courses of action as you can. In doing so, ask colleagues to help you generate potential courses of action. By listing a wide variety of courses of action, you may identify a possibility that looks most useful to you. Evaluate each option with reference to the potential consequences for all parties involved. Eliminate those options that do not promise to give the desired results or that may have problematic consequences. As you think about the many possibilities for action, discuss these options with your client, if or when appropriate, as well as with other professionals. Care needs to be taken to ensure that the client does not become the "helper" in cases where the client is included in these discussions. Determine which of the remaining options or combination of options is best suited to the situation. A good guideline in choosing your course of action would be the degree to which you would feel comfortable knowing your actions would be published in the newspaper or as a part of the news on radio or television. If your answer is "no," you have reason to reconsider your selected course of action.

7. *Explore the consequences of various decisions.* Ponder the implications of each course of action for the client, for others who are related to the client, and for you as the counselor. Again, a discussion with your client about consequences for him or her can be most important, when appropriate. Review the consequences of key decisions to determine if any new ethical problems might arise. If so, go back to the beginning and reevaluate each step of the process.

8. *Decide on the best course of action.* In making the best decision, carefully consider the information you have received from various sources. The more obvious the dilemma, the clearer is the course of action; the more subtle the dilemma, the more difficult the decision will be. In carrying out your plan, realize that other professionals might choose different courses of action in the same situation. However, you can only act in accordance with the best information you have. After you carry out your course of action, it is wise to follow up on the situation to evaluate whether your actions had the anticipated effect and consequences. Determine the outcomes and see if any further action is needed. Reflecting on your assessment of the situation and the actions you took is essential if you are to learn from your experience. This is where reviewing your notes can be particularly helpful in assessing the process. To obtain the most accurate picture, involve your client in this process, when appropriate.

Even if you follow a systematic model such as the one we have described, you may still experience some anxiety about whether you made the best possible decision in a given case. Many ethical issues are controversial, and some involve blending ethics and the law. An important sign of your good faith is your willingness to share concerns or struggles with colleagues, supervisors, and fellow students. It is essential that you keep abreast of the laws that affect your practice, maintain awareness of new developments in your field, and reflect on ways that your values will influence your practice. Developing a sense of professional and ethical responsibility is a task never completely finished.

Informed Consent

For most clients, asking for formal or professional help is a new experience. They are often unclear about what is expected of them and what they should expect from the helper. The ethics codes of most professional organizations require that clients be given adequate information to make informed choices about entering and continuing in the therapeutic relationship. The American Counseling Association (2005) standard regarding informed consent is one such example:

> Counselors explicitly explain to clients the nature of all services provided. They inform clients about issues such as, but not limited to, the following: the purposes, goals, techniques, procedures, limitations, potential risks, and benefits of services; the counselor's qualifications, credentials, and relevant experience; continuation of services upon the incapacitation or death of a counselor; and other pertinent information. Counselors take steps to ensure that clients understand the implications of diagnosis, the intended use of tests and reports, fees, and billing arrangements. Clients have the right to confidentiality and to be provided with an explanation of its limitations (including how supervisors and/or treatment team professionals are involved); to obtain clear information about their records; to participate in the ongoing counseling plans; and to refuse any services or modality change and to be advised of the consequences of such refusal. (A.2.b.)

Perhaps the best way to safeguard the rights of clients is to develop procedures to help them make informed choices. **Informed consent** involves the right of clients to be informed about what their relationship with you will entail and to make autonomous decisions pertaining to it. Informed consent is a shared decision-making process that will enable your clients to decide whether to participate in the helping relationship with you (Barnett, Wise, Johnson-Greene, & Bucky (2007). It is essential to give your clients an opportunity to raise questions and to explore the expectations they have in working with you.

How can you teach your clients about their rights and responsibilities from the outset of the helping relationship? Asking clients to sign a form at the initial session does not discharge your duty toward informed consent. It is best to conceptualize informed consent as an ongoing process rather than a single event. Although it is imperative that you secure informed consent at the outset of a helping relationship, realize that clients may not remember all that you tell them. Active informed consent is an ongoing process in the counseling relationship (Wheeler & Bertram, 2008).

Some mental health workers use written informed consent procedures. You will need to decide which approach works best for you and your clients. We suggest that you develop a comprehensive written statement to give to clients at the first session so that they can take the materials home and read them before the next session. In this way clients have a basis for asking questions and valuable time is saved. It is important to have clients sign the document indicating an understanding of these policies and procedures.

Getting informed consent involves a delicate balance between telling clients too little and overwhelming them with too much information at once. Do not assume that clients clearly understand what they are told initially about the helping process. Informed consent for treatment is a powerful clinical, legal, and ethical tool (Wheeler & Bertram, 2008). The more clients know about how the helping process works, including the roles of both client and practitioner, the more clients will benefit from this professional relationship. It is essential that you use clear and understandable language when you are discussing informed consent matters with clients. Furthermore, you need to take into account cultural implications of informed consent procedures and communicate in ways that are culturally sensitive (Corey & Herlihy, 2006a). Educating clients about the therapeutic process is an ongoing endeavor.

Although most professionals agree on the ethical duty to provide clients with relevant information about the helping process, there is not much consensus about what should be revealed and in what manner. Studies of therapists' informed consent practices have found considerable variability in the breadth and depth of the informed consent given to clients (Barnett, Wise, et al., 2007). In deciding what you would most want to tell a client, consider these questions:

- What are the goals of the helping relationship?
- What services are you able and willing to provide?
- What do you expect of your client? What can your client expect of you?
- What are the risks and benefits of helping strategies that are likely to be employed?
- What do you want to tell your client about yourself?
- What are the qualifications of the provider of the services?
- What are the financial considerations?
- What is the estimated duration of the professional relationship? How will termination be handled?
- What are the limitations of confidentiality? When does the law require mandatory reporting?
- Under what circumstances are you likely to consult with a supervisor or other colleagues about the case?
- Are there any alternatives to the approaches you might suggest?

If you are part of a managed behavioral health care program, you will also need to explain to your clients the number of sessions allowed, the limitations of confidentiality, and the narrower scope of short-term interventions.

Case example: Providing just enough information. During the initial interview, Simone asks the counselor, Allen, how long she might need to be in therapy. Allen tells Simone that the process will take a minimum of 2 years of weekly sessions. She expresses dismay at such a lengthy process. Allen says that this is the way he works and explains that in his experience significant change is a slow process that demands a great deal of work. He tells Simone that if she cannot commit to this time period he would be willing to give her a referral.

Your stance. Consider what you would do if Simone came to you for counseling. Did Allen take care of the need for informed consent? Explore the following questions:

- Did Allen have an ethical and a professional obligation to explain his rationale for the 2 years of therapy?

- Should Allen have been willing to explore alternatives to his approach to therapy, such as the possible values of short-term counseling?
- Given Allen's statement of the minimum length of therapy, would it have been ethical for him to offer short-term counseling to Simone?
- Would it be ethical for this practitioner to accept clients under a managed care system or with an insurance provider that paid for only a very limited number of sessions?

Discussion. When clients finally make an appointment, they are often anxious to get help on some pressing problem. Talking about the process in great detail could dampen the client's inclination to return for further sessions. Yet it is a mistake to withhold important information that clients need if they are to make wise choices. *What* and *how much* to tell a client is determined in part by the client. It is a good practice for helpers to employ an educational approach, encouraging clients' questions about evaluation or treatment and offering useful feedback as the helping process progresses. By providing your clients with adequate information, you are increasing the chances that they will become active participants and carry their share of the responsibilities in the relationship.

Confidentiality and Privacy

The helping relationship is built on a foundation of trust. If clients do not trust their counselor, they are unlikely to engage in significant self-disclosure and self-exploration. Trust is largely measured by the degree to which clients feel assured that what they say will be listened to and kept confidential. Mental health professionals have a dual ethical and legal responsibility to safeguard clients from unauthorized disclosures of information given in the context of the helping relationship. Helpers must not disclose this information except when required by law or authorized by the client to do so.

To explore all aspects of their lives without fear that these disclosures will be released outside the therapy room, clients need reasonable assurance that their confidentiality will be maintained. No effective therapy can occur unless clients trust that what they say is confidential. Counselors are ethically obligated to clearly assist clients in appreciating the meaning of confidentiality in language they can understand and in using an approach that respects the cultural experiences of the client (Barnett & Johnson, 2010).

Confidentiality is one of the most basic ethical obligations, yet it is also one of the most problematic issues for many practitioners. Helpers increasingly confront confidentiality issues that are created by complex legal requirements, new technologies, health care service delivery systems, and a culture that places increasing emphasis on consumer rights (Herlihy & Corey, 2006c).

Although your clients have every right to expect that their relationship with you will remain confidential, your obligation to safeguard client disclosures is not absolute. You need to develop the legal knowledge and an ethical sense for when you *must* break confidentiality. A major concern of counselors is confidentiality and its limits. This matter should be spelled out for clients in their informed consent. According to Herlihy and Corey (2006c), it is a good idea to discuss the following points with your clients:

- Do not reveal confidential information without client consent, or without sound legal or ethical justification.
- Some clients may want confidential information shared with members of their family or community.
- At times it is permissible to share information with others in the interest of providing the best possible services to the client.
- Confidential information may also be discussed with other helping professionals when the client requests it or gives permission.
- Confidentiality is not an absolute, and other obligations may override the helper's pledge. For example, it is required that confidentiality be breached to protect someone who is in danger.
- Confidentiality cannot be guaranteed when the client is a minor or when counseling couples, families, or groups.
- Confidentiality can be compromised if a client's records are subpoenaed.
- At the outset of a professional relationship, practitioners should clarify what, when, how, and with whom information can be discussed.

State law specifies the circumstances under which confidentiality must be compromised. You may have to reveal information when there is clear and imminent danger that clients will bring harm to others or to themselves. Know the laws in your state as there may be options other than breaking confidentiality available to you. Not all states have the same laws, but all states have mandatory reporting laws for incest and child abuse, and most states have mandatory reporting laws for elder abuse and dependent adult abuse. It is essential that you know how to assess signs of abuse and neglect. All states require reporting child abuse or neglect if it results in physical injury. In addition, you are expected to take action when clients are likely to harm themselves or others. If a client is suicidal, you have a responsibility to do what you can to protect this person.

Human services professionals are vulnerable to lawsuits if they improperly handle confidentiality issues, so it behooves you to know the laws of your state or jurisdiction, to follow them, and to be aware of the ethical standards of your profession. Seek help from your professional organization when dealing with complex ethical dilemmas.

To sharpen your thinking about issues surrounding confidentiality, think about what you would do in these cases:

- *Child abuse.* Two young girls are brought to a community agency by their aunt, who has gained custody of them in the last few months. One girl, age 11, is quite verbal, but the other, 13, is not. As they begin to talk and you ask about their history, they tell you of aunts and uncles who attempted to touch one of them and of an aunt who severely beat them. The 11-year-old tells of a suicide attempt by her sister after one such beating. If you were working with these girls, what action would you take and why? Do you have available the telephone number of Child Protective Services for the area in which you are working?

- *Runaway plan.* A student intern works with pupils in an elementary school. She says to the children in a group, "Everything you say here will stay here." Then a boy reveals a detailed plan to run away from home. The counselor, who has not talked about the exceptions to confidentiality with the children, does not know what to do. If she reports the boy, he may feel betrayed. If she does not report him, she may face a malpractice action for having failed to notify the parents. What might you suggest to her if she came to consult with you about this case?

- *Students' violation of confidentiality.* You are a counselor intern in a local agency. You are part of a training group of students that meets weekly to discuss cases. One day, while you are having lunch in a restaurant with some of the students, they begin to discuss their cases in detail, mentioning names and details of the clients loudly enough for others in the restaurant to overhear. What would you do in this situation?

It is tempting to talk about your clients and their stories, especially as others are usually curious about what you do. It may give you a sense of importance to be able to tell interesting anecdotes. You may talk more than you should when you feel overwhelmed by your clients and need to unburden yourself. As a professional helper, you must learn how to talk about clients and how to report without breaking confidentiality. Clients should know that confidentiality cannot be guaranteed absolutely, but they should have your assurance that you will avoid talking about them except when the law requires you to disclose information or it is professionally necessary to do so.

Confidentiality in Couples and Family Therapy

Generally speaking, from a *legal* perspective, confidentiality as applied to couples counseling, family therapy, group counseling, and counseling minors has limitations. However, from an *ethical* perspective, confidentiality is of the utmost importance and must be discussed so all parties are aware of what confidentiality involves in these forms of counseling. Kleist and Bitter (2009) maintain that when practitioners work with couples and families, confidentiality issues can become extremely complex and may involve determining who is the client, providing informed consent, and handling relational matters in an individual context. Some helpers contend that whatever information they get from one family member should never be divulged to the other members. By contrast, other helpers have a policy of refusing to keep any information private within the family. Their assumption is that secrets are counterproductive to helping family members be open with one another. These helpers encourage bringing all secrets out into the open. It is essential that you be clear in your own mind about how you will deal with disclosures obtained from family members and that you let your clients know your policy before they enter into a professional relationship with you.

Case example: Concealing information in couples counseling. Owen is involved in individual therapy, and later his wife, Flora, attends some of the sessions for marriage counseling. Owen discloses to the therapist that he became involved in a gay relationship a few months previously. He doesn't want his wife to know for fear that she will divorce him. In a later session in which the therapist is seeing the couple, Flora complains that she feels neglected and wonders if her husband is really committed to working on their marriage. She says that she is willing to continue marital counseling as long as she is sure that he wants to stay in the marriage and devote his efforts to working through their difficulties. The therapist knows about this gay relationship but decides to say nothing about it in the joint session and maintains that it is the husband's decision whether to mention it.

Your stance. What do you think of the therapist's ethical decision in this situation? If you were involved in a somewhat similar situation, what might you do differently? Suppose Owen confided that he was concerned that he had contracted AIDS and was very worried. What action might you take? Are you concerned about his withholding this information from Flora? Can a case be made for the duty to warn and protect an innocent party? (This is a topic we take up later in this chapter.)

Confidentiality in Group Counseling

When you lead a group, you will have to consider some special ethical, legal, and professional aspects of confidentiality. In a group setting, as is true for individual counseling, you must disclose the limitations of confidentiality. Because so many more people are privy to information shared in the group, you must also make it clear that you cannot guarantee confidentiality. Even if you continually emphasize to the members how essential it is to maintain confidentiality, there is still the possibility that some of them will talk inappropriately to others about what has been shared in the group. Leaders need to encourage members to bring up any fears about possible breaches of confidentiality. When members see it as their responsibility to talk about these concerns, this topic can be openly explored in the group.

Assume that members of a group you were co-leading brought up their reluctance to participate because they were concerned about the need for a firm commitment to keep in the group whatever was discussed. How would you deal with their concerns?

Confidentiality in School Counseling

In the context of school counseling, protection of confidentiality and privacy is a major concern. Children and adolescent clients have a right to know what information will and will not be kept confidential from their first contact with a school counselor. In cases involving minors who are unable to give informed consent, the parents or guardians will need to provide this informed consent and may need to be included in the counseling process. Parents and guardians have some legal right to request information about counseling sessions, as do school personnel, but this should be done in a manner that will minimize intrusion of the child or adolescent's privacy and in a way that demonstrates respect for the student. It is essential that school counselors clearly inform the students they see of the limitations of confidentiality and how and when confidential information may be shared.

When minor clients pose a danger to themselves or to others, school counselors must breach confidentiality. From both an ethical and legal perspective, any threat of suicide or of violence to others must be taken very seriously. Even if the risk of suicide is remote, the possibility may be enough to establish a duty to contact the parents and inform them of the potential for suicidal behavior. Courts have found that the burden involved in making a telephone call is minor considering the risk of harm to a student who is suicidal. In short, school personnel are advised to take every precaution to protect the student. The same is true in all cases where there is a potential for violent acts.

Continuing education is of the utmost importance, as is your willingness to seek appropriate consultation when you become aware of students who are at risk. You can be held legally accountable only for a judgment that is clearly negligent in light of the standard of care of other professionals with similar education and experience. As long as you act in an ethical and reasonable manner, you should not be overly concerned about legal sanctions related to student suicide or harm to others (Remley & Sparkman, 1993).

Case example: Informing parents and respecting confidentiality. Conrad, a 15-year-old high school senior, was referred to a psychologist, Andy, by his high school counselor for an evaluation for depression. Conrad currently lives at home with his parents and two younger siblings. He stated during the intake that for the past 2 years he has struggled academically and socially and has felt depressed for most of this time. His grades have suffered, and he has become more socially withdrawn. As a coping mechanism, he writes and plays music in his room, and he sometimes smokes marijuana with friends on weekends. He plans to remain home following graduation and will attend community college. Andy has met with Conrad for a total of four sessions, and he has been very responsive to talk therapy. Following the last session, Andy received a telephone message from Conrad's mother wanting an update on his progress and to share some information that she thinks is pertinent to his case.

Andy tells Conrad that his mother left a telephone message and that she seems to be interested in his progress. Conrad is not sure if he wants Andy to speak with his mother, because he doesn't trust what his mother might share with Andy. Andy and Conrad discuss the possibility of inviting both of his parents to a session. This approach would empower Conrad to remain active and in charge of his treatment decisions, and it would prevent trust issues from occurring between Conrad and Andy.

Your stance. What are the legal and ethical issues to examine? How do you navigate the needs of the client and the needs of his parents to be informed? Can you think of interventions that could be helpful to Conrad and his parents?

Confidentiality and Privacy in a Technological World

There are a host of ways to violate a client's privacy through the inappropriate use of various forms of technology. The use of the telephone, answering machines, voice mail, pagers, faxes, cellular phones, and e-mail can pose a number of potential ethical problems regarding the protection of privacy of clients. Mental health practitioners need to exercise caution in discussing confidential information with anyone over the telephone.

Using fax machines to send confidential material is another source of potential invasion of a client's privacy. It is the helper's responsibility to make sure fax transmissions arrive in a secured environment in such a way as to protect confidential information. Before sending a confidential fax, it is a good idea to make a telephone call to ensure that the appropriate person will be able to receive this information in a safe and sensitive manner (Cottone & Tarvydas, 2007).

Communication by way of electronic mail is fraught with potential privacy problems. Because e-mail messages can be accessed easily by people other than their intended recipients, you cannot count on privacy. Since there is no reasonable expectation of confidentiality for e-mail, clients need to have input regarding how they want communication to be handled so that their privacy is protected.

Although privacy and confidentiality of clients has long been a central issue, with electronic transactions things have become more complex. The **Health Insurance Portability and Accountability Act (HIPAA)** of 1996 was passed by Congress to promote standardization and efficiency in the health care industry. The **HIPAA privacy rule** was designed to give patients more rights and more control over their health information. Patients must be informed of their rights and are required to sign the appropriate forms authorizing a health care provider to obtain and provide information to other health care providers (Robles, 2009). The HIPAA privacy rule, which applies to both paper and electronic transmissions of protected health information by covered entities, developed out of the concern that transmission of health care information through electronic means could lead to widespread gaps in the protection of client confidentiality (Wheeler & Bertram, 2008). The new privacy regulations protect patients by limiting the ways that practitioners can use patients' medical information and other individually identifiable health information. The privacy rule requires health plans to establish policies and procedures to protect the confidentiality of protected health information about their patients.

This discussion of privacy may appear to be mere common sense. However, we have become so accustomed to relying on technology that careful thought is not always given to subtle ways that privacy can be violated. We emphasize the importance of using caution and paying attention to ways that you could unintentionally breach the privacy of your clients. As a part of the informed consent process, it is wise to discuss with your clients the potential problems of privacy regarding a wide range of technology and to take preventive measures so that both you and your clients have an understanding and agreement about these important concerns. Consider the following case pertaining to privacy issues in an agency setting.

Case example: Privacy issues and telecommunications. The agency you work for establishes a call center to take calls from clients and to schedule appointments for them. One of their new policies is to call clients to remind them of their upcoming appointment. A particular client has stated clearly that she does not want her husband to know that she is coming for counseling. However, a call center phone representative calls her residence to remind her of her next appointment, and in the process her husband gets the message about her upcoming appointment for counseling.

Your stance. Do you see an ethical issue pertaining to privacy or confidentiality in this case? How would you reconcile agency policy and client privacy in a situation such as this? How would you handle the client's phone call to you complaining about what has happened?

Privacy in a Small Community

I (Marianne) practiced for many years as a marriage and family therapist in a small community. This situation presented a set of ethical considerations involving safeguarding the privacy of clients. First, it was important that I choose an office that afforded privacy to clients as they entered and left. I considered leasing space in a small professional building in the center of town, but I quickly discovered that people would be uncomfortable making themselves that visible when seeking psychological help. A home office, which was remote from the center of the village, worked out well. However, I had to carefully schedule clients, allowing ample time between sessions so clients who might know each other would not meet in the office. When an office is located within a home, it is essential that a professional atmosphere be provided. Clients have a right to expect privacy and should not have to deal with intrusions by the therapist's family members.

I discussed with my clients the unique variables pertaining to confidentiality in a small community. I informed them that I would not discuss professional concerns with them should we meet at the grocery store or the post office, and I respected their preferences regarding interactions away from the office. Knowing that they were aware that I saw many people from the town, I reassured them that I would not talk with anyone about who my clients were. Another example of protecting my clients' privacy pertained to the manner of depositing checks at the local bank. Because the bank employees knew my profession, it would have been easy for them to identify my clients. Again, I talked with my clients about their preferences. If they had any discomfort about my depositing their checks in the local bank, I arranged to have them deposited elsewhere.

Your Obligation to Protect

Courts have created an exception to confidentiality when the mental health professional has a reasonable basis for believing that clients pose a danger either to themselves or to others. Counselors have a legal responsibility to protect their clients and others from harm, and they must breach confidentiality when necessary to provide this protection (Wheeler & Bertram, 2008).

Put yourself in this situation: A new client visits you at a college counseling center. He says he was severely abused by his father as a child and is now extremely angry. He is making threats to kill his father and tells you he is armed. How do you proceed?

How do you decide whether a particular client is dangerous? Although practitioners are generally not held legally liable for their failure to predict violent behavior of a client, an inadequate assessment of client dangerousness can result in liability for the therapist, harm to third parties, and inappropriate breaches of client confidentiality. Helping professionals faced with potentially dangerous clients should take specific steps designed to protect the public and to minimize their own liability. They should take careful histories, advise clients of the limits of confidentiality, keep accurate notes of threats and other client statements, seek consultation, and document steps they have taken to protect others.

It is extremely difficult to decide when breaching confidentiality to protect potential victims is justified. Mental health professionals are obligated to disclose when legal requirements demand it, thus, they must be familiar with the laws of their state regarding a duty to protect (Herlihy & Corey, 2006c). Practitioners are advised to consult with a supervisor, a colleague, or an attorney because they may be subject to liability for either failing to warn and protect those entitled to warnings or warning those who are not entitled. Most states either permit or require therapists to breach confidentiality to protect victims. In light of a number of court cases, mental health professionals have become increasingly conscious of a double duty—to protect other people from potentially dangerous clients and to protect clients from themselves. The responsibility to protect the public from potentially violent clients entails liability for civil damages when professionals neglect this duty by failing to diagnose or predict dangerousness, failing to protect potential victims of violent behavior, failing to commit dangerous individuals, and prematurely discharging dangerous clients from a hospital.

HIV issues. One of the more controversial ethical dilemmas pertaining to a helper's duty to warn and protect others involves working with people who have AIDS, or are HIV-positive, and who may be putting others at risk. As a helper, you may need to balance your client's right to confidentiality against warning a third party who may be at risk of being infected by your client's HIV status.

The ACA's *Code of Ethics* (2005) has the following standard pertaining to the helper's role in dealing with contagious, life-threatening diseases:

> When clients disclose that they have a disease commonly known to be both communicable and life-threatening, counselors may be justified in disclosing information to identifiable third parties, if they are known to be at demonstrable and high risk of contracting the disease. Prior to making a disclosure, counselors confirm that there is such a diagnosis and assess the intent of clients to inform the third parties about their disease or to engage in any behaviors that may be harmful to an identifiable third party. (B.2.b.)

At this time, there is no *legal* duty to warn, and it will take a court decision to resolve the legal questions. In the meantime, practitioners who work with HIV-positive clients will continue to wrestle with the *ethical* issues in deciding on a course of action with their clients. It is difficult to identify who in particular is at risk and to assess the degree to which individuals who have intimate relation-ships with persons with HIV are in serious and foreseeable harm. Disclosure requires a careful decision, and helpers should not take action until they have confirmed the diagnosis and have ascertained that the client has not informed the third party and has no intentions of doing so in the immediate future. Although the ACA's standard pertaining to communicable and life-threatening diseases gives practitioners *permission* to breach confidentiality, it does not state that they have a *duty* to warn, for such a provision could make them vulnerable to a malpractice suit. This example illustrates a situation that could represent a conflict for the helper regarding following a legal versus an ethical course of action. We know several colleagues who have specialized in seeing persons with HIV for many years, and they state that they have never broken confidentiality in this kind of case. They claim that there are many alternatives to breaking con-fidentiality and warning a third party.

Case example: Duty to inform and protect others. One of your male clients discloses to you that he is HIV-positive, but he says nothing about his sexual practices with a partner or partners. At a later session he discloses that he is not monogamous and that one of his partners is unaware of his condition. Since he has been engaging in unprotected sex with this person for some time, he sees no point in either disclosing his condition or changing his sexual practices.

Your stance. What might you do in this case? How useful is the ACA guide-line in determining your course of action? Would you initially address possible disclosure of information with others as part of the informed consent process? Why or why not? What do you see as your ethical and legal duty? How might you resolve potential conflicts between ethical and legal actions? How would you go about making your decision?

Harm-to-self. In addition to the duty to warn and to protect others from harm, helpers have a duty to protect clients who are likely to harm themselves. Many therapists inform their clients that they have an ethical and legal respon-sibility to break confidentiality when they have good reason to suspect suicidal behavior. Even if clients take the position that they are free to do with their lives what they want, therapists have a legal duty to protect them. The difficulty lies in determining when a client is serious about ending his or her life by suicide.

Cases have been made both for and against suicide prevention. Some mental health workers believe that many suicides can be prevented if those who work with suicidal clients learn to recognize, evaluate, and intervene effectively in crisis situations. Many clients who are in crisis may feel temporary hopeless-ness, yet if they are given help in learning to cope with the immediate problem, their potential for suicide can be greatly reduced. It is generally held that once mental health professionals determine that a significant risk does exist, appro-priate action is necessary. Practitioners who fail to act to prevent suicide can be held liable.

Szasz (1986) argues the case against suicide prevention. He presents the thesis that suicide is an act of a moral agent who is ultimately responsible. Therefore, he opposes coercive methods of preventing suicide such as forced hospitalization. He further contends that by attempting to prevent suicide, practitioners basically ally themselves with the police power of the state and resort to coercion. Clients are thus deprived of assuming responsibility for their own actions. Szasz agrees that helpers have an ethical and legal obligation to provide help to those clients who seek professional assistance for their suicidal tendencies. But for clients who do not ask for this help or who actively reject it, professionals have a duty either to persuade them to accept help or to leave them alone.

Although some have argued in favor of the right of clients to decide when and in what manner to end their lives, the codes of ethics of professional associations are in agreement that helpers must actively attempt to prevent suicide. In his article on working with suicidal clients, Wubbolding (2006) contends that counselors need to know how to handle suicide threats. They need practical skills that represent the highest level of ethical practice. The following questions can be useful in assessing the lethality of a threat and in determining whether further intervention is necessary:

- Is there a plan?
- Has the person attempted suicide in the past?
- Is the person seriously considered taking his or her life?
- Does the person have the means available?
- Who could stop the person?
- What kind of emotional support is available in the family, at home, or elsewhere?
- Have other family members committed suicide in the past?

If it is determined that a client is at risk of suicide, then it is the helper's ethical responsibility to take action outside the session. Possible interventions might include informing the parents, spouse, physician, or another significant person in the client's life.

Case example: Protecting a depressed client. A client is depressed and talks about putting an end to his life. He tells you that he is bringing this topic up only because he trusts you, and he insists that you not mention the conversation to anyone. He wants to talk about how desperate he feels, and he wants you to understand him and ultimately to accept whatever decision he makes.

Your stance. Consider your ethical and legal obligations in this case. What would you say to him? How would you proceed?

Case example: Acting on an informant's knowledge. A college counselor receives an e-mail message from a friend of a current client, Sadie. The friend wants to remain anonymous. The message reveals that Sadie is suicidal and already has a detailed plan to carry out suicide. The counselor telephones Sadie and asks her to come over to the counseling center as soon as possible.

Your stance. Do you believe counselors have an ethical obligation to respond to e-mail messages? Was the college counselor inappropriate in calling Sadie for an emergency session in response to an e-mail from her friend? Does the counselor have a duty to warn Sadie's family members? Do you think it was sufficient for the counselor to call the emergency session with Sadie?

Documentation and Keeping Records

From an ethical and legal perspective you are responsible to keep adequate records on your clients. It is considered below the standard of care to fail to keep current records for all your professional contacts. Record keeping serves multiple purposes. From a clinical perspective, record keeping provides a history that you can use in reviewing the course of treatment. Maintaining client records has a dual purpose: (a) to provide the best service possible for clients, and (b) to provide evidence of a level of care commensurate with the standards of the profession. From a legal perspective, state or federal law may require keeping a record, and maintaining adequate clinical records can provide an excellent defense against malpractice claims. Rivas-Vazquez and colleagues (2001) contend that the documentation of clinical services has taken on unprecedented importance for mental health professionals. From their perspective, the main objectives of documentation practices are (a) to structure quality care, (b) to decrease liability exposure, and (c) to fulfill requirements for reimbursement. According to Griffin (2007), writing client notes can be done in a simple, straightforward, and brief way. The complexity, length, and content will vary according to what happens in a particular session.

Practitioners keep two kinds of client records. **Progress notes**, or the client's clinical records, are required by law. These notes are *behavioral* in nature and address what people say and do. Progress notes contain client identifying information, the client's history, reason for seeking treatment, and documentation pertaining to the informed consent process; objective findings from the most recent physical examination; intake sheet; documentation of referrals to other providers, when appropriate; client's diagnosis, functional status, prognosis, symptoms, treatment goals, treatment plan, consequences, progress toward meeting goals, and alternative treatments; types of services provided; precise times and dates of appointments made and kept; and termination summary. Your client's clinical record should *never* be altered after you have documented information into the record. It is a good idea to enter notes into a client's record as soon as possible after a session and sign and date the entry.

Process notes, or psychotherapy notes, are different from progress notes. Process notes deal with client reactions such as transference and the therapist's subjective impressions of a client. These notes are not meant to be readily disclosed to others. They are intended for the use of the practitioners who created them. Information that is essential for treatment should not be included in the process notes. For example, excluded from process notes the diagnosis, treatment plan, symptoms, prognosis, and progress. It is important to note that the law requires clinicians to keep a separate clinical record (progress notes) on all clients, but the law *does not* require keeping psychotherapy (process) notes.

From both an ethical and legal perspective, it is of the utmost importance that you store client records in a secure place and take steps to maintain the privacy of your clients' records. Extra care should be taken if information is stored on computer disks. The length of time you are required to keep a client's records is determined by state law and the policies of your agency. Even when the record is discarded in a safe manner, a summary of a client's treatment should be retained.

Realize that clients have a legal right to view their clinical record, or a summary of their record. A client's record is not the place for your personal opinions or personal reactions to the client, and record keeping should reflect professionalism. If a client misses a session, it is a good practice to document the reasons. In writing client notes, it is important to use clear behavioral language. Focus on describing specific and concrete behavior and avoid jargon. When you write notes on your client, always assume that these records may be read by others. Although professional documentation is expected to be thorough, it is best to keep notes as concise as possible.

Be mindful of the dictum, "If you did not document it, then it did not happen." Record client and helper behavior that is clinically relevant. Include in clinical records interventions used, client responses to treatment strategies, the evolving treatment plan, and any follow-up measures taken. It is a wise policy for you to document your actions in crisis situations such as cases involving potential danger of harm to oneself, others, or physical property. However, it is not in the best interests of clients for you to be more concerned about record keeping as a self-protective strategy than you are to providing quality services to your clients.

Competent record keeping practices serve both the client and the counselor. Wheeler and Bertram (2008) suggest that practitioners who fail to maintain adequate clinical records put themselves at risk for malpractice suits because such failure breaches the standard of care expected of mental health practitioners. They add: "Well-organized and well-documented client counseling records are the most effective tool counselors have for establishing client treatment plans, ensuring continuity of care in the event of absence, and proving that quality care was provided" (p. 115).

Ethical Issues in a Managed Care Environment

A transformation has occurred in the delivery of helping services. As Cummings (1995) points out, there is a shift in values and a fundamental redefinition of the role of mental health practitioners in the transition from the traditional fee-for-service model to the **managed care model,** which is characterized by time-limited interventions, cost-effective methods, careful monitoring of services, and preventive more than curative strategies. This shift has implications for how you might view your role as a helper and how you may be expected to develop skills in brief interventions.

Key Ethical Issues

Helpers in a managed care system clearly have divided loyalties between doing what is best for the client and keeping their commitment to a system that demands cost containment through a reliance on short-term interventions. Many times clients need more than the very brief interventions that are available. MacCluskie and Ingersoll (2001) point out that there are new challenges for delivering services in a sensitive and ethical manner. They state that in the context of managed care the motives for decision making are primarily economic. This factor itself does not necessarily constitute unethical behavior, unless it sacrifices the quality of care of clients in the process. It is important that the welfare of the client does not get put on the back burner in the interests of preserving the financial integrity of the system.

Managed care demands that practitioners adopt a set of values congruent with limited interventions that mainly treat symptoms. This could raise ethical issues for practitioners who value growth and actualization more than remedial, short-term, solution-focused strategies. Those who work in a managed care context face a number of ethical issues that revolve around these concerns: informed consent, confidentiality, abandonment, utilization review, and competence.

Informed consent. Informed consent is an ongoing process that assumes particular importance under a managed care system. Prior to entering into a professional relationship with you, your clients have a right to know that a managed care company may request a diagnosis, results on any tests given, a wide range of clinical information, treatment plans, and perhaps even the entire clinical record.

From an ethical perspective, clients have a right to know that the focus on cost containment may have an adverse impact on the quality of care available to them. Clients have a right to know that other forms of treatment, possibly ones that may be more helpful, are being denied to them solely for cost-containment reasons. They have a right to know if you are versed in brief therapy, that an outside person is likely to judge what kind of treatment will be given and how many sessions will be allowed, the specific limitations of the plan they are participating in, and who decides the time of termination of therapy.

Confidentiality. Although confidentiality has traditionally been considered to be an ethical and legal duty imposed on helping professionals to protect client disclosures, managed care has redefined the scope of confidentiality. Confidentiality concerns are more complex because of demands for detailed case information by reviewers of managed care programs (Koocher & Keith-Spiegel, 2008). Because managed care providers take an active role in treatment planning, client confidentiality is compromised. Treatment is monitored by the third-party payer, who may influence decisions pertaining to interventions used, access to assessments, and access to outcomes of treatment (Cooper & Gottlieb, 2000).

Although there have always been exceptions to confidentiality, the demand for client information inherent in a managed care framework far exceeds previous limitations to confidentiality to the extent that the confidential nature of the therapist–client relationship is threatened. Clients should be aware that the managed care plan may require practitioners to reveal sensitive client information to a third party who is in a position to authorize initial or additional treatment. Practitioners can no longer assure their clients of confidential treatment at any level because they have no control over confidential information once it leaves their offices. Because of these restrictions on confidentiality, helpers have an obligation to inform clients from the outset of the therapeutic process about the relevant limits of confidentiality under their managed care policy (Acuff et al., 1999; Cooper & Gottlieb, 2000). If clients want to protect their confidentiality, they may decide to seek treatment that does not involve third-party reimbursement.

Abandonment. The codes of ethics of the various professional organizations state that mental health practitioners do not abandon clients. Traditionally, the matter of termination of therapy is a collaborative effort involving both the client and the helper. Under managed care programs, termination generally does not come out of a collaborative process but from company policy. Clients may have a sense of abandonment if their treatment ends abruptly. It is a helper's responsibility to inform clients that the request for additional sessions may or may not be granted by the managed care company. Managed care guidelines often limit treatment to a specific number of sessions annually with lifetime cost caps. Clients may be denied the care they need if it extends beyond their benefits and they are unable to pay for additional care. Although time limitations may make financial sense, this situation can become ethically problematic, forcing the practitioner to refer a client if continued therapy is needed.

It is clear that managed care presents both ethical and legal issues for professional practice. Ethically, professional helpers must not abandon their clients, and they have a responsibility to render competent services. But under managed care, many critical decisions are made for the client and the practitioner by the program.

Utilization review. Under managed care programs, all treatment is monitored by someone other than the practitioner. **Utilization review** refers to the use of predefined criteria to evaluate treatment necessity, appropriateness of therapeutic intervention, and therapy effectiveness. This process can take place before, during, and after treatment (Cooper & Gottlieb, 2000). Utilization review of clients is generally done by way of a written document that is periodically sent to the company.

Competence. Those who work in a managed care system need to have special knowledge and skills competencies to deliver a variety of brief services in a flexible and holistic manner with a diverse range of client populations and client problems. This requires helpers to acquire an eclectic or integrative theoretical orientation. Mental health practitioners are forced to become more proficient in time-limited and effective treatment approaches. Treatment plans need to be formulated rapidly, goals must be limited in scope, and the emphasis must be on attaining results. If helpers are not trained in brief treatment methods, and if clients will not be well served by a limited number of sessions, then helpers need to have skills in making appropriate referrals.

Legal Aspects of Managed Care

Practitioners are ultimately responsible to their clients, even if the decisions are made by the managed care system. Legally, practitioners employed by managed care units are not exempt from malpractice suits if clients claim that they did not receive the standard of care they required. Professionals cannot use the limitations of the managed care plan as a shield for failing to render crisis intervention services, make appropriate referrals, or request additional services from the plan. Practitioners are sometimes caught in conflicting roles when they attempt to offer what the client needs versus what is covered by the managed care plan. Increasingly, mental health providers may feel pressure by third-party payers to limit the amount of care provided to the degree that the needs of clients may be compromised (Koocher & Keith-Spiegel, 2008). Regardless of the structure underlying the delivery of services, ethical practice requires that practitioners put the best interests of their client first.

The Future of Managed Care

The debate on how to best deliver human services will continue, and the reality of managed care may have a profound influence on how you work with your clients. Overall, experts agree that managed care is here to stay (Cooper & Gottlieb, 2000). Many of you will be faced with finding a way to maintain your integrity while working within the constraints imposed by managed care programs. Accountability is being given increased emphasis in many work settings. Managed care requires that agencies and practitioners be accountable by demonstrating the efficacy of the services they provide. Increasingly, you will be expected to quickly assess the salient problems of your clients, formulate a short-term treatment approach, and demonstrate the degree to which your interventions were effective.

Malpractice and Risk Management

Malpractice is generally defined as the failure to render proper service, through ignorance or negligence, resulting in injury or loss to the client. Malpractice is a legal concept involving negligence that results in injury or loss to the client. **Professional negligence** consists of departing from the usual standard of practice or not exercising due care in fulfilling one's responsibilities. The primary problem in a negligence suit is determining which **standards of care** apply to determine whether a clinician has breached a duty to a client. Practitioners are judged according to the standards that are commonly accepted by the profession; that is, whether a reasonably prudent counselor in a similar circumstance would have acted in the same manner (Wheeler & Bertram, 2008). As a helper, you will be judged according to the standards that are commonly accepted by your profession. You are expected to abide by legal standards and adhere to the ethics codes of your profession in providing care to your clients. Unless you take due care and act in good faith, you are liable to a civil lawsuit for failing to do your duty as provided by law. Although you need not be perfect, you are expected to possess and exercise the knowledge, skill, and judgment common to other members of your profession.

For a malpractice suit to be filed against you, these four conditions must be present: (1) you must have a duty to the client (there must be a professional relationship between you and another person); (2) you must have acted in a negligent or improper manner or have deviated from the "standard of care" by not providing the expected level of services; (3) your client must have suffered harm or injury, which must be demonstrated; and (4) there must be a causal relationship between that negligence and the damage claimed by the client.

Grounds for Malpractice Actions

In their study of the reasons for disciplinary actions against counselors, Kirkland, Kirkland, and Reaves (2004) found that the major offenses were related to sexual misconduct and unprofessional conduct/negligent practice. Other specific areas that constituted grounds for disciplinary actions included conviction of crimes, fraudulent acts, inadequate record keeping, breach of confidentiality, improper or inadequate supervision, impairment, failure to comply with continuing-education requirements, and fraud in applying for a license. In their review of the literature on grounds for disciplinary actions against psychologists, Knapp and VandeCreek (2003) identify the following issues: violations of sexual boundaries, nonsexual multiple relationships, incompetence, breaches of confidentiality, abandonment, inadequate supervision, inadequate record keeping, and child custody disputes.

As a student, you may think that you have no worries about being sued for malpractice. Unfortunately, student practitioners are vulnerable to such action. At this time in your professional development, you might well give serious consideration to ways in which you can lessen your chances of being sued for failing to practice in a professional manner. The reality of today is that even if you abide by the ethics codes of your profession and practice within the boundaries of the law, you can still be sued. No matter how careful you are, you can still be accused of wrongdoing. Even if the suit does not succeed, it is likely to be highly stressful, and it can take a toll on you in terms of time, energy, and money. You will have to spend many hours preparing and supplying documents and responding to requests for information. The best defense against becoming embroiled in a malpractice action is to practice quality client care and to know and follow the ethical standards of your profession.

Case example: Who is to blame? A teenage client takes the step of suicide despite the therapist's best efforts to be of help. The child's parents fault the therapist for not having known more and done more to prevent this final action.

Your stance. Consider your own stance on the duty to protect. Do you have to be able to predict a possible suicide? Assuming that you are able to identify a suicidal client, will you always know the best course of action to take?

Discussion. Although you do not have to prove that you are a perfect being, you do have to demonstrate that you possess and exercised the knowledge and skill required for the services you provided. You must be able to demonstrate that you acted in good faith, that you have been willing to seek supervision and consultation when needed, and that you have practiced within your competence. It is also essential that you can produce documentation to support your claims.

Ways to Prevent Malpractice Suits

It should be clear that you would be wise to know your limitations in working with clients, to accept them, and to act only within the scope of your competence. Never hesitate to seek consultation, regardless of your professional experience. Consultation with colleagues often sheds light on a subject by providing a new and different perspective. Even if you are able to make wise decisions, it is validating to get support for your position from other professionals. If you are involved in litigation, it will be helpful to be able to demonstrate that your interventions were in accord with the standard of care exercised by other practitioners. It cannot be emphasized enough that adequate documentation is essential in defending yourself in any malpractice action. If you employ unusual therapeutic techniques with little rationale behind them, you are likely to find yourself the loser in a civil action. Contending that you were following your instincts and doing what "felt right" is not likely to get you very far if you are asked to defend your therapeutic practices.

Risk Management

Risk management is the practice of focusing on the identification, evaluation, and treatment of problems that may injure clients, lead to filing of an ethics complaint, or lead to a malpractice action. Bennett and colleagues (2006) contend that good risk management should involve more than simply following the minimal legal requirements; good risk management practices require that clinicians work to fulfill their highest ethical ideals. One of the best precautions against malpractice is personal and professional honesty and openness with clients. Providing quality professional services to clients is the best preventive step one can take. You need to know your limitations and remain open to seeking consultation in difficult cases, and of course, it is essential that you document the nature of any consultations.

If you want a guarantee that you will not be sued for professional negligence, you probably should think about another career. There are no absolute protections in the mental health professions, but some risk management practices can significantly lessen your chances of becoming involved in a legal action. The following are some additional guidelines:

- Make use of informed consent procedures. Do not attempt to mystify the helping process; professional honesty and openness with clients will go a long way in establishing genuine trust.
- Consider ways to define contracts with your clients that clearly structure the helping relationship. Clarify your role with your clients. What are your clients coming to you for? How can you best help them obtain their goals?

- Because you can be sued for abandonment, take steps to provide coverage for emergencies when you are going away.
- Restrict your practice to client populations for which you are prepared by virtue of your education, training, and experience. Refer clients who are clearly not within the scope of your competence and take steps to maintain your competence.
- Keep up-to-date and accurate records of clients and carefully document a client's treatment plan. Develop a diagnostic profile, and keep relevant notes on each client.
- Become aware of local and state laws that limit your practice, as well as the policies of the agency you work for. Keep abreast of legal and ethical developments by becoming involved in professional organizations.
- Be aware of the limits of confidentiality, and clearly communicate these to your clients. Attempt to obtain written consent whenever disclosure becomes necessary.
- Report any case of suspected child, elder, or dependent adult abuse as required by law.
- If you make a professional determination that a client is a danger to self or others, take the necessary steps to protect the client or others from harm.
- Treat your clients with respect by attending carefully to your language and your behavior. This practice generally leads to good relationships.
- Present information to your clients in clear language and check to make sure they understand this information.
- Obtain written parental consent when working with minors. This is generally a good practice, even if not required by state law.
- Make it a practice to consult with colleagues or clinical supervisors whenever there is a potential ethical or legal concern. Find sources of ongoing supervision.
- Establish and maintain appropriate professional boundaries. Learn to anticipate problems and set ground rules.
- Pay attention to how you react to your clients and monitor your countertransference.
- Avoid imposing your values on your clients and avoid making decisions for them.
- Before engaging in any multiple relationships, seek consultation and talk with your client about the potential advantages and disadvantages of such a relationship.
- Have a clear rationale for the techniques you use. Be able to intelligently and concisely discuss the theoretical underpinnings of your procedures.
- Have a clear standard of care that can be applied to your services, and communicate this standard to your clients.
- Do not promise clients anything that you cannot deliver. Help them realize that their effort and commitment will be key factors in determining the outcomes of the helping process.
- If you work for an agency or institution, have a contract that specifies the employer's legal liability for your professional functioning.

- Abide by the policies of the institution that employs you. If you disagree with certain policies, first attempt to find out the reasons for them. Then see if it is possible to work within the framework of institutional policies.
- At the outset of therapy, clearly define issues pertaining to fees. Adhere to billing regulations and paperwork requirements as prescribed.
- Make it a practice to assess the progress your clients are making, and teach them how to evaluate their progress toward their goals.
- Let your clients know that they have the right to terminate professional services at any time they choose.
- Carry malpractice insurance. Students are not protected against malpractice suits.

These guidelines will lessen the chances of a malpractice suit, but we encourage you to continually assess your practices and keep up to date on legal, ethical, and community standards affecting your work setting and client populations.

A Word of Caution

Students sometimes burden themselves with the unrealistic expectation that they should have clear answers for the ethical issues we raise in this chapter. Quite the contrary is true. Indeed, seasoned professionals are aware that the complex nature of their work with people defies neat and absolute answers. They have an appreciation of the necessity for continuing learning, for ongoing consultation and supervision, and for remaining humble.

Our intention has not been to overwhelm you but to stimulate you to develop habits of thinking and acting that will enhance your ability to base your practice on ethical and professional principles. Working in the helping professions is sometimes a risky as well as a rewarding venture. You probably will make mistakes from time to time. Be willing to acknowledge those mistakes and learn from them. Make full use of supervision; you will not only learn from what may seem like mistakes but you will also minimize the chances of harming clients.

Don't be frozen with anxiety over needing to know everything at all times—or be afraid to intervene for fear of becoming embroiled in a lawsuit. Perhaps the best way to prevent a malpractice action is by having a sincere interest in doing what is going to benefit your client. Ask yourself these questions throughout your professional career: "*What* am I doing, and *why* am I doing it? Would I be doing the same thing if my colleagues were observing me?"

By Way of Review

- One of the trends in the helping professions is an increased interest in ethical and professional practice. This trend stems, at least in part, from a rise in malpractice actions against mental health practitioners.

• Ethical decision making is a continuing process. Issues that you look at as a student can be examined from another perspective as you gain experience in your professional specialty.

• It is essential that you be familiar with the professional codes of ethics. However, knowledge of ethical standards is not sufficient in solving ethical problems.

• Ethical issues rarely have clear-cut answers. Ethical dilemmas, by their very nature, involve the application of professional judgment on your part.

• Ultimately, you will have to make many difficult decisions as a practitioner. Responsible practice entails basing your actions on informed, sound, and responsible judgment. Be open to consulting with colleagues and supervisors throughout your professional career.

• Many clients have not even thought about their rights or responsibilities. As a helper, you can do much to safeguard your clients by developing informed consent procedures to help them make wise choices.

• Confidentiality is the cornerstone of the helping relationship. Although clients have a right to expect that what they talk about with you in the professional relationship will remain private, there are times when you will have to breach confidentiality. Clients have a right to know from the outset of the relationship the specific grounds for divulging confidences. It is essential that you know and follow the laws pertaining to confidentiality.

• Confidentiality takes on special meaning if you work with couples, families, groups, and minors.

• At times you will have a professional and legal obligation to warn or to protect clients. It is essential that you know your duties in this area.

• Your job is to teach clients how to help themselves and thus decrease their need to continue seeing you. Encouraging dependency in your clients is unethical, and it does not lead to client empowerment.

• It is essential to keep adequate clinical records for all clients. Documentation is critical, both for the client's benefit and for the protection of the professional rendering the services.

• Managed behavioral health care programs have had a major impact on the kinds of psychological and social services that can be delivered and the quality of those services. Ethically, it is important that helpers do what they can to inform their clients about the services available and about potential limitations on the helping relationships due to the focus on cost-effective methods.

• Although it is important to know how to deal with unethical behavior on the part of your colleagues, it is even more important to recognize your own potential unethical behaviors. These unethical acts are often subtle. Maintain a stance of honest self-exploration to ensure ethical behavior.

• Understand what can lead to becoming involved in a malpractice suit, and learn practical ways to lessen the chances of this happening.

What Will You Do Now?

1. Find at least one person in the helping professions to interview about ethical issues in practice. Focus on the major ethical problem that this person has faced. How did this helper deal with this ethical concern? What are their concerns, if any, about malpractice suits?

2. Visit a community agency (such as a Child Protective Services agency) and ask about ethical and legal situations that are being reported. What are some key ethical concerns with which this agency has to cope? Are the staff members concerned about malpractice issues? How does the current malpractice crisis influence what they do in their agency?

3. Think about a particular ethical dilemma that you have experienced in one of your field placements. How did you deal with the situation? If you could replay the situation, would you do anything differently?

4. Identify what you consider to be the most pressing ethical issue you expect to face, and write about your concerns and ideas in your journal. If you are involved in fieldwork, keep journal entries about any potential ethical dilemmas and bring your concerns to your supervision sessions or class meetings. You might write down specific ways for you to increase your likelihood of becoming an ethical practitioner. What can you do now to move in this direction?

5. Structure a class debate around the arguments for and against suicide prevention. Failure to prevent suicide can be one of the grounds for successful malpractice suits against mental health professionals. Consider debating a specific case of a client who is terminally ill with AIDS and decides that he wants to end his life because of his suffering and because there is no hope of getting better. Divide the class into teams for an exchange on the therapist's responsibility to prevent this suicide.

6. In small groups discuss specific circumstances in which you would break confidentiality, and see whether you can agree on some general guidelines. In your groups, explore ways you might teach clients about the purposes of confidentiality and the legal restrictions on it. Discuss how you would do this in various situations, such as school counseling, group work, couples and family counseling, and counseling with minors.

7. For the full bibliographic entry for each of the sources listed here, consult the References at the back of the book. A useful guide to legal and ethical practice is Wheeler and Bertram (2008). For a casebook geared to the ACA's code of ethics, see Herlihy and Corey (2006a). For practical desk references for interpreting and applying ethics codes, see Barnett and Johnson (2008) for APA codes and Barnett and Johnson (2010) for ACA codes. For a comprehensive handbook that deals with a wide range of topics in ethics, see Bersoff (2003). For a concise guide for helpers in managed care, see Davis and Meier (2001). For a useful discussion of duty to protect issues pertaining to harm to others, harm to self, and end-of-life decisions, see Werth, Welfel, and Benjamin (2009). For a book on ethics and the law in counseling practice, see Remley and Herlihy (2010). Consult Corey, Corey, and Callanan (2011) and Welfel (2010) for textbooks dealing with ethical issues in the helping professions.

8. We recommend that you familiarize yourself with the basic standards for ethical practice of the various mental health professions. Refer to the list of websites provided in this chapter or see Chapter 1, which has contact information for various professional organizations. You can contact these organizations directly to obtain specific ethics codes. Alternatively, 17 ethics code documents have been compiled in a supplement to this textbook titled *Codes of Ethics for the Helping Professions* (2011), which is available at a nominal price when ordered as a bundle option with this textbook.

Ethics in Action *CD-ROM Exercises*

9. In role-play segment 1, Teen Pregnancy, in Part One (Ethical Decision Making), the client is a 13-year-old who just found out she is pregnant. She begs the counselor not to tell her parents. In this situation, what are the rights of the minor client? What rights do the parents have for access to certain information? What ethical and legal issues are involved in this case? What kind of informed consent process would you implement if you were counseling minors?

10. In role-play segment 4, The Divorce, the client says that she has decided to leave her husband and get a divorce, and the counselor's line of inquiry is about who will look after the welfare of her children. This case raises some interesting points about the rights of clients to know about your values as a counselor if these values influence your approach to counseling them. If you were counseling couples or families, what would you want to tell clients about your values pertaining to matters such as faithfulness in relationships and divorce? In class, role-play a situation in which you are meeting a client (or a couple) for the first session. What would you want to tell them about your role as a counselor? Would you discuss core values you hold that could either enhance or interfere with therapeutic progress?

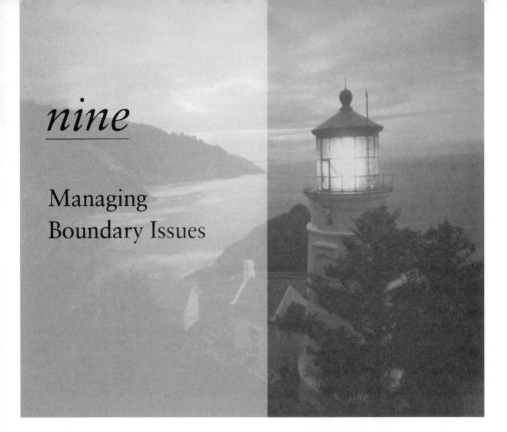

nine

Managing
Boundary Issues

Focus Questions

1. What problems might you expect to encounter in establishing boundaries with your clients?

2. If a client lost her job and could no longer afford to pay you for counseling services, would you be willing to enter into a bartering arrangement if she suggested bartering as an alternative to terminating her sessions? What other alternatives can you think of?

3. If a client offered you a gift at the termination session and explained how important it was to him that you accept this gift as a token of his appreciation for your help, what would you be inclined to do?

4. Multiple relationships exist when professionals assume two or more roles simultaneously or sequentially with a person seeking help. Do you believe multiple relationships are fundamentally unethical, or are such relationships inevitable and not always problematic?

5. What kinds of multiple relationships do you believe are problematic, and why? Can you think of any multiple relationships that you might be willing to engage in with a counseling client?

6. How might you deal with an unavoidable multiple relationship with your clients?

7. If a client were interested in forming a social relationship with you, what would you say? If this person were a former client, would that make a difference?

8. If a client expressed sexual attraction to you, what would you be likely to do or say? What would you do if *you* experienced sexual attraction to a client?

9. What ethical, legal, and clinical issues would you consider before entering a multiple relationship (social, sexual, business, professional) with a *former* client?

10. How effective are you at establishing and maintaining boundaries in your personal life? How do you think this affects your ability to create effective boundaries in your professional relationships?

Aim of the Chapter

Regardless of which helping profession you enter, you will be faced with learning to define and maintain appropriate boundaries with your clients. As will become clear in this chapter, part of becoming a helper involves being able to establish both personal and professional boundaries in a variety of situations. If you are not able to establish and maintain good boundaries in your personal life, you may have trouble with boundaries in your professional life. In this chapter we introduce you to an array of ethical concerns that helpers encounter in keeping relationships professional with their clients. In many ways, the topics covered in this chapter are a continuation of the discussion of ethical decision making in Chapter 8. Learning to deal with a range of boundary concerns are key ethical and clinical issues that practitioners in all settings have to address.

It is sometimes difficult to understand the rationale behind prohibitions and boundary limitations that may seem arbitrary. Codes alone will not keep helpers from behaving in unethical ways. Good judgment, the willingness to reflect on your practices, and being aware of your motivations are critical dimensions of being an ethical practitioner. Mental health professionals oftentimes get into trouble by not heeding warning signs in their relationships with clients. They may not have paid sufficient attention to potential problems involved in boundary crossings. Practitioners may innocently cross boundaries that lead to problems for both the client and themselves.

The underlying theme of this chapter is the need for helpers to be honest and self-searching in determining the impact of their behavior on clients. Some of the issues and cases we present may seem clear-cut, but others are not. Resolving the ethical dilemmas we pose requires personal and professional maturity and a willingness to continue questioning your motivations.

Self-Inventory on Managing Boundaries

What are some of your major concerns about establishing appropriate boundaries with clients? Perhaps at this point you have not raised or reflected on this question. We hope you will broaden your awareness of the importance of creating and maintaining appropriate boundaries in the helping relationship. For each of the following statements, indicate the response that most closely identifies your beliefs and attitudes. Use this code:

5 = I *strongly agree* with this statement.
4 = I *agree* with this statement.
3 = I am *undecided* about this statement.
2 = I *disagree* with this statement.
1 = I *strongly disagree* with this statement.

____ 1. It will be relatively easy for me to establish clear and firm boundaries with my clients.
____ 2. At times I am concerned about my ability to keep relationships with my clients professional.

____ 3. I am not sure how I would respond to a *current* client who asked me for a date or wanted some other social involvement with me.

____ 4. I might be willing to consider a social relationship with a *former* client if both of us were interested in meeting on a social basis.

____ 5. I don't think my training has prepared me to deal with sexual attractions in the helping relationship.

____ 6. Because multiple relationships are so widespread, they should not be considered as either inappropriate or unethical in all circumstances but should be decided on a case-by-case basis.

____ 7. Multiple relationships are almost always problematic and therefore should be considered unethical.

____ 8. If I were a truly ethical professional, I would never be sexually attracted to a client.

____ 9. If I were counseling a client who was sexually attracted to me, I might refer this client to another counselor.

____ 10. I might be inclined to barter my therapeutic services for goods if a client could not afford my fees.

____ 11. If a client initiated the possibility of exchanging services in lieu of payment, I would consider bartering as an option.

____ 12. Sexual involvement with a client is never ethical, even after therapy has ended.

____ 13. I would never accept a gift from a client because doing so constitutes crossing appropriate boundaries.

____ 14. It is essential to consider the cultural context in deciding on the appropriateness of bartering, accepting gifts, and the helper assuming multiple roles with a client.

____ 15. I would have no trouble accepting a close friend as a client if we had a clear understanding of how our personal relationship could be separated from our professional one.

Once you have finished this inventory, spend a few minutes reflecting on any ethical concerns you have at this time. This reflection can help you read the chapter more actively and raise ethical questions. Identify a few of the areas where you are uncertain about your position, and bring this ambiguity up in class discussions.

Multiple Relationships and the Codes of Ethics

Ethical problems are often raised when helpers blend their professional relationship and another kind of relationship with a client. **Multiple relationships** occur when professionals assume two or more roles simultaneously or sequentially with a person seeking their help. Helpers establish a multiple relationship in cases where they have another, significantly different relationship from the professional one they have with one of their clients, students, or supervisees. In these situations, the potential for a conflict of interest and for exploiting those seeking help cannot be ignored.

The terms *dual relationships* and *multiple relationships* (APA, 2002) have been used interchangeably, and some codes of ethics continue to use both terms The ACA (2005) ethics code refers to these as *nonprofessional relationships.* In this chapter we use the term *multiple relationships,* which encompasses both dual and nonprofessional relationships. The scope of multiple relationships may involve assuming more than one professional role (such as instructor or super-visor and therapist) or blending a professional and a nonprofessional relation-ship (such as counselor and business partner). Other multiple relationships result from providing therapy to a relative or a friend's relative, socializing with clients, becoming emotionally or sexually involved with a client or former client, borrowing money from a client, or loaning money to a client. Mental health pro-fessionals must learn how to effectively and ethically manage multiple relation-ships, including dealing with the power differential that is a basic part of most professional relationships, managing boundary issues, and striving to avoid the misuse of power (Herlihy & Corey, 2006b).

Codes of ethics deal specifically and extensively with setting appropriate boundaries, recognizing potential conflicts of interest, and taking steps to manage multiple relationships. Examples of codes of ethics that address these issues include those of the American Counseling Association (2005), the American Psy-chological Association (2002), the National Association of Social Workers (2008), and the National Organization for Human Services (2000). Although codes may function as guidelines, multiple relationships are frequently not a clear-cut matter. Ethical reasoning and judgment come into play when ethics codes are applied to specific situations. Consider the following examples of ethics codes addressing multiple relationships.

NASW's *Code of Ethics* (2008) focuses on the risk of exploitation or potential harm to clients:

> Social workers should not engage in dual or multiple relationships with clients or former clients in which there is a risk of exploitation or potential harm to the client. In instances when dual or multiple relationships are unavoidable, social workers should take steps to protect clients and are responsible for setting clear, appropriate, and culturally sensitive boundaries. (1.06.c.)

NOHS's (2000) ethical standards highlight the power and status differential between helper and client:

> Human service professionals are aware that in their relationships with clients power and status are unequal. Therefore they recognize that dual or multiple relationships may increase the risk of harm to, or exploitation of, clients, and may impair their professional judgment. However, in some communities and situa-tions it may not be feasible to avoid social or other nonprofessional contact with clients. Human service professionals support the trust implicit in the helping relationship by avoiding dual relationships that may impair professional judg-ment, increase the risk of harm to clients or lead to exploitation. (Statement 6)

The APA (2002) code states that multiple relationships that are unlikely to cause impairment or risk exploitation or harm are not unethical:

> A psychologist refrains from entering into a multiple relationship if the multiple relationship could reasonably be expected to impair the psychologist's objectivity,

competence, or effectiveness in performing his or her functions as a psychologist, or otherwise risks exploitation or harm to the person with whom the professional relationship exists.

Multiple relationships that would not reasonably be expected to cause impairment or risk exploitation or harm are not unethical. (3.05.a.)

The ACA (2005) code cautions counselors about nonprofessional relationships:

Counselor–client nonprofessional relationships with clients, former clients, their romantic partners, or their family members should be avoided, except when the interaction is potentially beneficial to the client. (A.5.c.)

The ACA's (2005) code places the responsibility on the counselor for exercising good judgment, even in the case of potentially beneficial nonprofessional interactions:

When a counselor–client nonprofessional interaction with a client or former client may be potentially beneficial to the client or former client, the counselor must document in case records, prior to the interaction (when feasible), the rationale for such an interaction, the potential benefit, and anticipated consequences for the client or former client and other individuals significantly involved with the client or former client. Such interactions should be initiated with appropriate client consent. . . . Examples of potentially beneficial interactions include, but are not limited to, attending a formal ceremony (e.g., a wedding/commitment ceremony or graduation); purchasing a service or product provided by a client or former client (excepting unrestricted bartering); hospital visits to an ill family member; mutual membership in a professional association, organization, or community. (A.5.d.)

Zur (2007) observes that none of the codes of ethics of any of the professional organizations refer to boundary considerations such as home visits, meeting outside the office, self-disclosure, home office, and nonsexual touch. None of the codes state that nonsexual dual relationships are unethical, and most of them acknowledge that some are unavoidable (Lazarus & Zur, 2002). Zur (2007) writes that the APA's (2002) code of ethics now provides more flexible guidelines regarding multiple relationships and places emphasis on the importance of context in making ethical decisions.

Multiple relationships are prohibited by most ethics codes, and professionals are mandated to avoid relationships that are harmful, exploitive, or are likely to negatively affect the professional relationship (Herlihy & Corey, 2008). When multiple relationships harm or have the significant potential to harm clients, they are unethical. Helpers should be very cautious about entering into more than one role with a client and avoid this unless there is a sound clinical justification for doing so.

The Multiple Relationship Controversy

The helping professions have become increasingly concerned about the ethics of multiple relationships. During the 1980s, the issue of sexual dual relationships was given considerable attention in the professional literature. There is no doubt that sexual dual relationships are unethical, and all of the ethics codes of the professional organizations prohibit sexual relationships between client and therapist. This prohibition extends at least 2 to 5 years after termination of a professional relationship. Furthermore, most codes of ethics warn against any activities on the helper's part that could lead to the risk of exploitation.

Nonsexual multiple relationships, sometimes referred to as **nonprofessional relationships,** came under increased scrutiny in the 1990s. Examples of nonsexual multiple relationships include accepting clients who are family members or friends, combining the roles of supervisor and therapist, forming business arrangements with therapy clients, or combining personal counseling with consultation or supervision. Nonsexual multiple relationships are generally discouraged, however, and helpers are cautioned about the dangers of exploitation of and harm to clients.

Nonprofessional relationships tend to be complex, and few of the questions surrounding them have simple and absolute answers. Helpers cannot always perform a single role when working with clients or in the community, nor is it always desirable that they limit themselves to one role. Many times, helpers will be challenged to balance multiple roles in their professional relationships. Helpers are advised to reflect carefully on problems that could arise from engaging in multiple relationships before becoming involved in them. Counselors need to take steps to safeguard clients and themselves through informed consent, consultation, supervision, and documentation (Glosoff, Corey, & Herlihy, 2006).

Moleski and Kiselica (2005) view multiple relationships on a continuum that ranges from therapeutic to destructive. Although some multiple relationships are harmful, other secondary relationships complement, enable, and enhance the counseling relationship. Moleski and Kiselica encourage counselors to examine the potential consequences that a secondary relationship might have on the primary counseling relationship. They suggest that counselors should consider forming multiple relationships only when it is clear that such relationships are in the best interests of the client.

Some behaviors that helpers engage in have a potential for creating a multiple relationship, but they are not, by themselves, multiple relationships. For example, neither bartering for services nor accepting small gifts from clients necessarily involve multiple relationships, but both can be potentially problematic. Other examples include accepting a client's invitation to a graduation ceremony or engaging in nonerotic touching when this is appropriate. Some writers (Gabbard, 1995; Gutheil & Gabbard, 1993; Smith & Fitzpatrick, 1995) suggest that these incidents might be considered boundary *crossings* rather than boundary *violations.* A **boundary crossing** is a departure from standard practice that could potentially benefit clients, whereas a **boundary violation** is a serious breach that causes harm to the client. Interpersonal boundaries are fluid; they may change over time and may be redefined as counselors and clients continue to work together. Even though boundary crossings may not be harmful to clients, these crossings can lead to blurring of professional roles and can result in multiple relationships that do have a potential to be harmful. It is critical to take steps to prevent boundary crossings from becoming boundary violations.

Barnett (Barnett, Lazarus, Vasquez, Moorehead-Slaughter, & Johnson, 2007) states that even well-intentioned clinicians must thoughtfully reflect on their actions to determine when crossing a boundary may result in a boundary violation. If a therapist's actions result in harm to a client, this would be viewed as a boundary violation. Failing to practice in accordance with prevailing community standards, as well as other variables such as the role of the client's diagnosis, history, values, and culture, can result in a well-intentioned action being perceived as a boundary violation.

There is considerable disagreement about the appropriateness of multiple relationships. Some in the helping professions want to see stricter laws and ethics codes prohibiting multiple relationships. Others argue that certain forms of multiple relationships are clearly beneficial (Lazaruz & Zur, 2002; Zur, 2007). Not all multiple relationships can be avoided, and some believe these relationships are not necessarily harmful, unethical, or unprofessional (Herlihy & Corey, 2006b; Herlihy & Corey, 2008). This is particularly true in small, isolated communities. In many rural communities there is a high likelihood that helpers will be involved in multiple relationships.

Schank and Skovholt (1997) conducted interviews with psychologists who lived and practiced in rural areas and small communities. They found that all of the psychologists in their study acknowledged concerns involving professional boundaries. Some of the major themes were the reality of overlapping social or business relationships, the effects of overlapping social relationships on members of the psychologist's own family, and the dilemma of working with more than one family member as clients or with clients who have friendships with other clients. Although the psychologists knew the content of the ethics codes, they admitted that they often struggled in choosing how to apply those codes to the ethical dilemmas they faced in rural practices.

Sleek (1994) describes some ethical dilemmas that plague rural practice. The local pharmacist, physician, mechanic, banker, carpenter, or beautician might be a client of a particular helper. Furthermore, rural professionals see clients in the local store and ponder whether to acknowledge the person in the presence of others. If they are in local organizations such as the Chamber of Commerce or if they attend the same church, they may worry about conflicts with some fellow members who are also clients. They may be concerned if clients have children in the same school who are friends with their children or are on the same sports team. There is also the problem of mixing business with the therapeutic endeavor in rural communities. For example, if a therapist shops for a new tractor, he or she risks violating the letter of the ethics code if the only person in town who sells tractors happens to be a client. However, if the therapist were to buy a tractor elsewhere, this could strain relationships with the client because of the value rural communities place on loyalty to local merchants. Or consider clients who wish to barter goods or services for counseling services. Some communities operate substantially on swaps rather than on a cash economy. This does not necessarily have to become problematic, yet the potential for conflict exists in the therapeutic relationship if the bartering agreements do not work well. In rural settings, helpers typically play multiple roles and are likely to experience more difficulties maintaining clear boundaries than do their colleagues who practice in urban areas.

Campbell and Gordon (2003) address some of the unique aspects of rural practice and offer strategies for evaluating, preventing, and managing multiple relationships in rural practice. They point out that the APA (2002) ethics code offers three helpful criteria in making decisions about multiple relationships: (1) risk of exploitation, (2) loss of therapist objectivity, and (3) harm to the professional relationship. Campbell and Gordon (2003) also mention that in the everyday professional practice in rural areas, prospective multiple relationships do not often fit precisely into a single ethical category and that they are inevitable.

Smith, Thorngren, and Christopher (2009) contend that even though there are inherent challenges in working in a rural setting, the work can be rewarding and exciting. They encourage helpers to "tap into the strengths of their rural clients and allow themselves to be taught about the culture in which these people survive and thrive"(p. 270). Due to the demands rural practitioners face, consultation with peers and colleagues, even via distance communication, is recommended to help prevent burnout.

Establishing Personal and Professional Boundaries

We find it useful to frame the discussion of multiple relationships within the context of boundaries. If you have developed clear boundaries in your personal life, you are less likely to have trouble with multiple relationships professionally. If your boundaries are poorly defined or if you attempt to blend roles that do not mix well, such as therapy and friendship or therapy and business, you are likely to stumble into an ethical dilemma.

We do not think that prohibiting all forms of multiple relating is a realistic answer to the problem of exploitation of clients; rather, helpers need to learn how to establish and maintain appropriate and useful boundaries. We appreciate Lazarus's (2001, 2006) reasonable perspective on therapeutic boundaries. Lazarus contends that a general prohibition against multiple relationships has led to unfair and inconsistent decisions by state licensing boards, brought sanctions against practitioners who have done no harm, and often impeded a practitioner's ability to perform optimum work with a client. Lazarus contends that some well-intentioned ethical standards can be transformed into artificial boundaries that result in destructive prohibitions and undermine clinical effectiveness. Moreover, he believes some multiple relationships can enhance treatment outcomes. Lazarus argues for a case-by-case, nondogmatic evaluation of boundary questions that involves a selective process of deciding when it may be appropriate to enter into a secondary relationship. He contends that it is essential to consider individual client differences rather than to be subjugated to rigid standards. From his perspective, great benefits can accrue when therapists are willing to think and venture outside the proverbial box.

Lazarus (2001) admits that some well-intentioned guidelines can backfire. He has socialized with some clients, played tennis with others, taken walks with some, respectfully accepted small gifts, and given gifts (usually books) to some of his clients. Lazarus makes it clear that he is opposed to any form of disparagement, exploitation, abuse, harassment, or sexual contact with clients. He is not advocating elimination of all boundaries, for he sees certain boundaries as being essential. Rather than being driven by rules, however, Lazarus calls for a process of negotiation in many areas of nonsexual multiple relationships that some would contend are in the forbidden zone. Lazarus (2006) emphasizes that transcending boundaries should not be undertaken without serious consideration. He believes that a clear rationale for crossing a boundary is necessary, roles and expectations should be quite clear, and possible power differentials must be kept in mind.

Guidelines for Setting Boundaries

Although there are divergent viewpoints on multiple relationships, most professionals will agree that blending the roles of counselor and employee or counselor and lover is not appropriate. Whenever helpers play multiple roles, there is a potential for a conflict of interests, loss of objectivity, and exploitation of persons who have sought help. Ethical practitioners must take appropriate precautions to ensure that the best interests of their clients are maintained. Herlihy and Corey (2006b) provide these guidelines in cases where professionals are operating in more than one role:

• Set healthy boundaries from the outset. In your informed consent document, it is wise to state your policy pertaining to professional versus social or business relationships.

• Involve the client in setting the boundaries of the professional relationship. Discuss with clients what you expect of them and what they can expect of you.

• Informed consent is essential when you are playing more than one role with a client. Clients have a right to know about any potential risks associated with multiple relationships. Informed consent and discussion of unforeseen problems and conflicts is an ongoing process.

• Consultation with colleagues is most useful in obtaining an objective perspective and identifying unanticipated difficulties. If you are functioning in more than one role or engaging in multiple relationships, it is a good policy to consult on a regular basis.

• When multiple relationships are particularly problematic, or when there is a high degree of risk for harm, it is wise to work under supervision.

• It is essential that counselor educators and supervisors discuss with students and supervisees topics dealing with balance of power issues, boundary concerns, appropriate limits, purposes of the relationship, potential for abusing power, and subtle ways in which harm can result from engaging in multiple and sometimes conflicting roles.

- From a legal perspective, it is good practice to document any discussions about multiple relationships with your clients. Include in your notes any actions you have taken to minimize the risk of harm.

- If necessary, refer the client to another professional.

The controversy surrounding nonsexual multiple relationships is likely to continue. As with any complex ethical issue, complete agreement may not be reached. Prohibiting all forms of multiple relationships does not seem to be the best answer to the problem of exploitation of clients. Barnett (2007) claims that avoiding certain multiple relationships could be potentially harmful to some clients and that therapists should use their professional judgment to determine which multiple relationships should be avoided, which are acceptable, and which are necessary. Zur (2007) contends that rigid avoidance of all boundary crossings could result in a weakening of the therapeutic alliance. He adds that therapists should avoid crossing boundaries if doing so would likely harm the client or would be expected to impair the therapist's objectivity, judgment, competence, or interfere with his or her therapeutic effectiveness. Helping professionals need to clarify their stance to a host of boundary issues they will face in their practice and develop a systematic way of making ethical decisions.

Lamb, Catanzaro, and Moorman (2003) suggest that nonsexual overlapping relationships be evaluated by considering factors such as context, history, current status of the professional relationship, the reaction of the client to the multiple relationships, and how the therapist explains the purpose of the boundary crossing within the context of the goals of the professional relationship. Lamb and colleagues raise a significant question: How do therapists determine whether a particular action is likely to cause impairment, exploitation, or harm?

Herlihy and Corey (2006b) present a decision-making model that can be applied when helpers are confronted with multiple relationship issues. If the potential multiple relationship is *unavoidable,* helpers would do well to (1) secure informed consent of clients, (2) seek consultation, (3) document and monitor their practices, and (4) obtain supervision. If the potential multiple relationship is *avoidable,* helpers should first assess the potential benefits and risks in the case. If the benefits outweigh the risks, the multiple relationship may be justified. However, if the risks outweigh the benefits, helpers might decline to enter the relationship, explain the rationale to the client, and, if necessary, offer a referral to another professional.

In your struggle to determine what constitutes appropriate boundaries, you are likely to find that some blending of roles is inevitable in certain situations. Therefore, it is crucial to learn how to manage boundaries, how to keep boundary crossings from turning into boundary violations, and how to develop safeguards that will prevent exploitation of clients. Even seasoned professionals are often challenged to follow the most ethical course when it comes to crossing boundaries and establishing appropriate roles. Managing multiple relationships can be even more challenging to students, trainees, and inexperienced helpers. For those with relatively little clinical experience, the wisest course might well be to avoid engaging in multiple relationships whenever possible. Think about these general themes and the guidelines we have discussed, and apply them to each situation presented in this chapter. Ask yourself how you would proceed in resolving any ethical dilemmas over conflicting roles with your clients.

Combining Professional and Personal Relationships

You may be tempted to form social relationships with clients who admire you excessively and who invite you to develop a friendship. This lure can be especially strong if you like your client and if you have a limited circle of friends. You may also be afraid to deal with your clients' potential feelings of rejection if you tell them that a personal or social relationship is not possible.

Balancing a professional and a personal relationship with a client is complex. As a helper you may not be inclined to challenge such clients lest you endanger your personal relationship with them. Or you may experience difficulty in separating yourself from your clients. Even if you are able to maintain your objectivity, provide an optimal balance between confrontation and support, and still be a therapeutic agent, your clients may have difficulty keeping the two relationships separate. One factor to consider is that no matter how you look at this issue, the relationship is bound to be unequal. The client/friend pays you for your time and attention. Even if you don't charge a fee, the relationship is still unequal because you are likely to be doing more of the listening and giving. In an equal friendship, both partners are typically giving and receiving.

At times, social relationships between helpers and their clients may occur. When you find yourself in this position, here are some questions to ponder: "Does the social relationship get in the way of working effectively with my client?" "Does the friendship get in the client's way of working with me?" "Am I retaining enough objectivity to determine any possible negative effects?" We do have concerns about helpers who rely on their clients to make social and personal contacts. If most of your social acquaintances are people whom you serve professionally, we question whether you are using your role as a helper to meet your personal needs.

Case example: Going to lunch with a client. A therapist, Roberta, has been seeing a client for some time. The male client, Joel, asks Roberta if she would be willing to meet for lunch. When asked about the reason for the out-of-office meeting, Joel says that he would like to talk in an informal setting and would like to take Roberta to lunch as an expression of appreciation for the help she has provided. The situation is complicated by the fact that one of Joel's personal issues is the fear of being rejected. Joel tells Roberta that he is taking a risk with this invitation.

Your stance. How would you handle this situation? Would it make a difference whether the client was of the same or the opposite sex? Would your own feelings toward the client influence your decision?

Case example: Attending group functions outside of therapy. Bill has been facilitating a men's group in an agency setting. The members discuss how men in our culture are isolated, and to deal with this isolation they decide to establish a once a month potluck meeting outside of the regular weekly group meeting time at the agency. They invite the group leader, Bill, to join them in this out-of-group meeting.

Your stance. Do you think it is appropriate for Bill to attend these potlucks? What are your ethical concerns about this situation? What are the pros and cons of socializing with group members? How would you respond to them, and why? Would your gender make a difference in your decision?

The cultural context. The cultural context can play a role in evaluating the appropriateness of blending friendships with a helping relationship. In writing about multiple relationships from an African perspective, Parham and Caldwell (2006) question the Eurocentric ethical standards that discourage multiple relationships and claim that such standards can prove to be an obstacle or hindrance in counseling African American clients. From an African perspective, the helping relationship is not limited to the office. Instead, counseling involves multiple activities that might include conversation, playful activities, laughter, shared meals and cooking experiences, travel, rituals and ceremony, singing or drumming, storytelling, writing, and touching. Parham and Caldwell view each of these activities as having the potential to bring a "healing focus" to helping experiences.

In a similar spirit, Sue (2006) makes it clear that some cultural groups may value multiple relationships with helping professionals. In some Asian cultures it is believed that personal matters are best discussed with a relative or a friend. Self-disclosing to a stranger (a professional helper) is considered taboo and a violation of familial and cultural values. According to Sue, some Asian clients may prefer to have the traditional helping role evolve into a more personal one.

Socializing With Former Clients

Although combining personal and professional relationships with current clients is problematic at best, at least one study suggests that friendships between counselors and clients may be acceptable after termination of counseling (Salisbury & Kinnier, 1996). Seventy percent of counselors in this study believed friendships with former clients were acceptable 2 years after termination, and 33% reported that they had engaged in such friendships. The most important concern expressed by counselors in determining the circumstances under which posttermination friendships would be appropriate related to avoiding potential harm to the client.

In their study of nonromantic, nonsexual, posttherapy relationships between psychologists and former clients, Anderson and Kitchener (1996) found little consensus regarding how ethical these contacts are. Some therapists believe the client–therapist relationship continues in perpetuity. However, many of the participants in Anderson and Kitchener's study did not hold to the concept of "once a client, always a client" when it comes to nonsexual posttherapy relationships. The majority of therapists in this study described nonsexual relationships with former clients as being ethical, especially if some time had elapsed after termination. Others proposed that such relationships were ethical if the former client decided not to return to therapy with the former therapist and the posttherapy relationship did not seem to hinder later therapy with another therapist.

Although making friends with former clients may not be unethical, the practice may be unwise. The safest policy would be to avoid developing social relationships with former clients. In the long run, former clients may need you more as a therapist at some future time than as a friend. If you develop a friendship with a former client, he or she is no longer eligible to use your professional services.

Additionally, it is possible that in many situations the imbalance of power never changes. Even in the social relationship, you may be seen as the provider of help, or you may behave as the person in the helping role. You need to be aware of your own motivations, as well as the motivations of your clients, before allowing a professional relationship to evolve into a personal one. If you are in the habit of developing relationships with former clients, you may find yourself overextended and come to resent the relationships you sought out or consented to. What is central in this situation is your ability to establish clear boundaries regarding what you are willing to do and not do.

What are your thoughts about developing friendships with present or former clients? Would you be willing to form such personal or social relationships with clients? Why or why not? What issues would you want to discuss with a former client before entering a personal relationship?

Bartering in Counseling

The practice of bartering psychotherapy for goods or other services has the potential for conflicts. Glosoff, Corey, and Herlihy (2006) maintain that counselors who engage in bartering or exchanging goods or services for counseling services are often motivated by benevolent reasons, typically to help clients who are unable to afford professional counseling. When clients are unable to afford the professional services of a counselor, they may suggest a barter arrangement—for example, cleaning house for the helper, performing secretarial services, or doing other personal work. Clients can easily be put in a bind when they are in a position to learn personal information about their counselor. This can interfere with the counselor–client relationship.

Bartering is an accepted practice in many cultures, but bartering for counseling services can be especially problematic. Clients may believe their counseling is not progressing well and resent the helper for not following through on his or her agreement. Likewise, helpers may be dissatisfied with the lack of timeliness or the quality of goods and services delivered by clients, which can lead to resentment and ultimately interfere with the therapeutic relationship.

Ethical dimensions of bartering. At the present time, most professional ethics codes have a specific standard pertaining to bartering. Although bartering is not prohibited outright, there are stipulations to the practice. The *ACA Code of Ethics* (ACA, 2005) provides this guideline on bartering:

> Counselors may barter only if the relationship is not exploitive or harmful and does not place the counselor in an unfair advantage, if the client requests it, and if such arrangements are an accepted practice among professionals in the community. Counselors consider the cultural implications of bartering and discuss relevant concerns with clients and document such agreements in a clear written contract. (A.10.d.)

In some cultures and in certain communities, bartering is an accepted practice. Bartering is an example of a multiple relationship that we think allows some room for helpers to use their professional judgment and to consider the cultural context in which they practice.

If you are considering some form of bartering in lieu of payment for your professional services, consult with experienced colleagues or a supervisor. This type of consultation is likely to reveal alternatives that you and your client have not considered. After reflecting on the relevant issues involved in a situation and consulting others, we highly recommend a straightforward discussion with your client about the pros and cons of bartering in your particular situation. This collaborative discussion with your client, as well as the opinions of others, might assist you in identifying potential problems associated with certain kinds of proposed bartering arrangements. Ongoing consultation and discussion of cases, especially in matters pertaining to boundaries and multiple roles, provide a context for understanding the implications of certain practices. Of course, all of the discussions with those whom you consult and with your clients should be documented.

Before bartering is entered into, both parties should talk about the arrangement, gain a clear understanding of the exchange, and come to an agreement. It is also important that potential problems that might develop be discussed and that alternatives be examined. Using a sliding scale to determine fees or making a referral are two possible alternatives to bartering that might have merit. Perhaps the safest course to follow as a general rule is to refrain from accepting goods or services in exchange for professional services because of the potential for conflicts, exploitation, and strain on the helping relationship. However, you will have to assess the real-life situations that confront you in your professional practice.

Legal aspects of bartering. Bartering is not prohibited by ethics or law. As a helper, you may face situations where you will need to decide whether you will use bartering as an alternative, especially when clients can no longer afford to pay for services. If you were to consult with Robert Woody, who is a counselor educator and an attorney, he would likely advise you to stay clear of any bartering arrangements. Woody (1998) argues against the use of bartering for psychological services, saying that a case could be made that bartering is below the minimum standard of practice. If you enter into a bartering agreement with your client, you will have the burden of proof to demonstrate (a) that the bartering arrangement is in the best interests of your client; (b) that it is reasonable, equitable, and undertaken without undue influence; and (c) that it does not get in the way of providing quality psychological services to your client. Because bartering is so fraught with risks for both client and therapist, Woody believes prudence dictates that it should be an option of last resort. He concludes that bartering is a bad idea and should be avoided.

Other perspectives on bartering. Koocher and Keith-Spiegel (2008) contend that bartering can be a reasonable and humanitarian practice when people require psychological services but do not have insurance coverage and are experiencing financial difficulty. They suggest that bartering arrangements may prove satisfactory to both parties. Thomas (2002) views bartering as a legitimate means of helping a person with financial difficulties. He maintains that bartering should not be ruled out simply because of the slight chance that a client might initiate a lawsuit against the therapist. However, Thomas believes that venturing into any multiple relationship requires careful thought and judgment. He contends that the vast majority of professional work should be paid by the usual monetary means, yet he adds that when this is not possible due to a client's economic situation, allowances should be made so that psychological services might be available. Bartering can be one way of providing help to those in financial straights who do not qualify for insurance reimbursement. Thomas recommends a written contract that spells out the nature of the agreement between therapist and client, which should be reviewed regularly.

Case example: Bartering for therapy services. For several months Carol has been counseling Wayne, who has consistently paid for her services and who is currently making excellent progress in counseling. Wayne comes to a session very depressed because he lost his job as an auto mechanic at a large dealership. He can see no way of continuing to see Carol because of his other pressing financial commitments. He proposes that he do a complete engine overhaul on Carol's vintage car as a way of paying for some counseling sessions. He asks if Carol would be willing to go along with this arrangement because he really does not want to interrupt counseling at this point. On top of his other problems, he is now unemployed.

Your stance. Would you be inclined to enter into some form of bartering arrangement with Wayne? Why or why not? Besides bartering, what other options might you present to Wayne? Would you consider seeing him without payment due to his circumstances? Consider what you would do as you address the following issues:

- Would your decision be dependent on whether you were practicing in a large urban area or a rural area?
- How might you take the cultural context into consideration when making your decision?
- If you engaged in this exchange of services and Wayne did not do a good job on the engine, how might this affect your work with Wayne?
- If you told Wayne that you did not feel comfortable bartering and he responded that he felt you were abandoning him in a time of need, how might you respond?

Giving and Accepting Gifts in the Therapeutic Relationship

Few professional codes of ethics specifically address the topic of giving or receiving gifts in the therapeutic relationship. However, the AAMFT (2001a) ethics code does address this issue: "Marriage and family therapists do not give or receive from clients (a) gifts of substantial value or (b) gifts that impair the integrity or efficacy of the therapeutic relationship" (3.10.). The latest version of the *ACA Code of Ethics* (ACA, 2005) also added a standard on receiving gifts:

> Counselors understand the challenges of accepting gifts from clients and recognize that in some cultures, small gifts are a token of respect and showing gratitude. When determining whether or not to accept a gift from clients, counselors take into account: the therapeutic relationship, the monetary value of the gift, a client's motivation for giving the gift, and the counselor's motivation for wanting or declining the gift. (A.10.e.)

Lavish gifts certainly present an ethical problem, but you might have mixed feelings about accepting a small gift from a client or giving a client such a gift. Some practitioners include a policy statement that they do not accept gifts from clients in their informed consent document. Our preference is to evaluate the circumstances of each case because a number of factors need to be considered. Koocher and Keith-Spiegel (2008) believe that accepting a small gift typically does not raise ethical problems although practitioners may want to inquire what meaning even a small gift has for the client. Accepting certain kinds of gifts (highly personal items) would be inappropriate and requires an exploration of the client's motivation. Zur (2007) suggests that a number of factors need to be considered in making a decision of whether to accept gifts from clients, some of which are monetary value, timing, frequency, motivation of the giver, content, the effect on the giver or receiver, the cultural dimensions, and clinical implications. He emphasizes the importance of understanding and evaluating the meaning of a gift within the context that it is given. Here are some questions you might explore in deciding whether to accept a gift from a client:

• *What is the monetary value of the gift?* Most helping professionals would probably agree that accepting a very expensive gift would be inappropriate and unethical. It could also be problematic if a client offered tickets to the theater and wanted you to accompany him or her to this event.

• *What are the clinical implications of accepting or rejecting the gift?* It is important to know when accepting a gift from a client is clinically contraindicated and be willing to explore this with your client. You would also want to explore with the client his or her motivation for presenting you with a gift. A client might be seeking your approval, in which case the main motivation for giving you a gift is to please you. Accepting the gift without adequate discussion would not be helping your client in the long run.

• *At what phase in the helping process is the offering of a gift occurring?* It makes a difference if a client wants to give you a gift during the early stage of the relationship or whether this occurs at the termination of the professional relationship. Small gifts given by either the client or therapist as part of a termination process may be appropriate and valuable from a clinical perspective. It is more problematic to accept a gift at the early stage of a counseling relationship because doing so may be a forerunner to relaxing needed boundaries.

• *What are your own motivations for accepting or rejecting a client's gift?* Would you be inclined to accept a gift simply because you do not want to hurt a client's feelings, even though you are not personally comfortable doing so? It could be that you would accept a gift because you are unable to establish firm and clear boundaries. You might also accept a gift because you actually want what a client is offering. Zur (2007) recommends that therapists carefully consider the risk/benefit ratio as it applies to accepting or not accepting a gift, or as it applies to giving or not giving clients gifts. He also suggests that gifts given by clients or therapists should be documented in a client's record.

• *What are the cultural implications of offering a gift?* In working with culturally diverse client populations, clinicians often discover that they need to engage in boundary crossing to enhance the counseling relationship (Moleski & Kiselica, 2005). The cultural context does play a role in evaluating the appropriateness of accepting a gift from a client. Giving gifts has different meanings in various cultures. In some cultures, if you were not to accept a gift, it is likely that your client would feel insulted. For example, an Asian client may offer a gift to show gratitude and respect and to seal a relationship. Although such actions are culturally appropriate, some helpers believe accepting the gift would distort boundaries, change the relationship, and create a conflict of interest.

Brown and Trangsrud (2008) conducted a survey to assess the ethical decision making of 40 licensed psychologists regarding accepting or declining gifts from clients. This survey indicated that psychologists were more likely to accept gifts from clients in cases where the gift was inexpensive, was culturally appropriate, and was given as a sign of appreciation at the end of treatment. They were more likely to decline gifts that were expensive, that were offered during treatment rather than at the end of treatment, and that had sentimental or coercive value. This survey revealed that cultural considerations are important in weighing the benefits of accepting the gift against the risk of jeopardizing the therapeutic relationship by refusing the gift.

If you find a pattern of clients wanting to give you gifts, reflect on the possibility that you might be, in some way, promoting a sense of indebtedness on your clients' part. If, however, it is rare that clients offer you a gift, you still need to determine a therapeutic way to address the situation. Consider what you feel comfortable doing and what is in the best interests of your client. If you decide not to accept the gift, we recommend that you discuss your reasons with your client. An open discussion is more fruitful and sensitive than simply giving your client a rule or a policy. As is the case with discussions about bartering, it is wise to document your reasons either for accepting or not accepting a gift from a client.

Case example: Giving and receiving gifts. A Chinese client, Lin, presents her therapist with a piece of jewelry after five therapy sessions, and it is likely that they will continue for another five sessions. Lin says she is grateful for all that the therapist is doing for her and that it would mean a lot to her for the therapist to accept this jewelry, which has been in her family for many years. This is her way of expressing her appreciation.

Your stance. Consider your stance on giving or receiving gifts in the client–therapist relationship. Do you see a difference between accepting a gift during the therapy or at the end of therapy? What aspects would you want to explore with Lin before accepting or refusing her gift? To what extent would you consider Lin's cultural background and the meaning giving a gift holds for her in making your decision? What might you say to Lin if she told you that in her culture it is expected that you will reciprocate in some way if you accept her gift?

Dealing With Sexual Attractions

Some helpers feel guilty over an attraction toward a client, and they feel uncomfortable if they sense that a client is attracted to them. There is a tendency to treat sexual feelings as if they shouldn't exist, which makes it difficult for helpers to recognize and accept them. Pope, Sonne, and Holroyd (1993) maintain that the lack of research, theory, training, and opportunity to discuss sexual attractions has created a context that does not encourage helpers to explore such feelings when they occur. They add that the topic of sexual feelings in psychotherapy is surrounded by a taboo, which has created a sinister context for the helper's experience of sexual attraction. Typical reactions to sexual feelings in the helping relationship include surprise, startle, and shock; guilt; anxiety about unresolved personal issues; fear of losing control; fear of being criticized; frustration at not being able to speak openly; frustration at not being able to make sexual contact; confusion about tasks; confusion about boundaries and roles; confusion about actions; and fear over frustrating the client's demands.

In *Sexual Feelings in Psychotherapy*, Pope, Sonne, and Holroyd (1993) break the silence surrounding the taboo of acknowledging and dealing with sexual feelings in therapy and offer these guidelines:

- Exploring helpers' sexual feelings and reactions should be a key aspect of training programs and continuing professional development.
- Sexual feelings must be clearly distinguished from sexual intimacies with clients.

- It is never permissible for helpers to exploit clients.
- Most helpers have experienced sexual attraction to a client, which can result in their feeling anxious, guilty, or confused.
- It is essential that helpers do not avoid recognizing and dealing with sexual attraction in the helping relationship.
- Helpers are best able to explore their feelings in a context with others that is safe, nonjudgmental, and supportive.
- Understanding sexual feelings is not a simple matter, which means that helpers need to be willing to engage in a personal, complex, and often unpredictable process of exploration.

Being emotionally or sexually attracted does not mean that you are guilty of therapeutic errors or that you are perverse. It is important, however, that you acknowledge your feelings and avoid developing inappropriate sexual intimacies with a client. Although transient sexual feelings are normal, intense preoccupation with clients is problematic. Gill-Wigal and Heaton (1996) identify some warning signs that may indicate you are exceeding appropriate boundaries and should take preventive actions:

- Wanting increased time with a particular client
- Feeling powerful when this particular client is present
- Experiencing increased pleasure with the client
- Enjoying discussion of sexual content
- Persistently engaging in sexual fantasies about the client
- Feeling sexually aroused when the client is present
- Wanting the client's approval
- Desiring physical contact with the client
- Feeling that you are the only one who can help this client
- Experiencing anxiety and guilt when thinking about the client
- Denying harm from turning a professional relationship into a sexual one

Part of learning how to deal effectively with emotional reactions or attractions to clients involves recognizing your own feelings and taking steps to minimize the chances of an attraction interfering with the client's welfare. Gill-Wigal and Heaton (1996) suggest that responsible management of attractions requires acknowledging that attractions must never be acted out, encouraged, or nurtured, and they recommend these strategies for managing an attraction to a client:

- Do not deny feelings of attraction, for responsible management is not possible if these feelings are disowned.
- Seek out a supervisor, a trusted colleague, or a therapist to discuss and come to a clearer understanding of your sexual attractions.
- Accept the responsibility of attending to your own therapeutic needs before your sexual feelings interfere with the progress of a client.
- Recognize that you have the responsibility for maintaining appropriate boundaries by setting clear limits.

Koocher and Keith-Spiegel (2008) advise therapists to discuss feelings of sexual attraction toward a client with another therapist, an experienced and trusted colleague, or an approachable supervisor. Getting a fresh perspective on the situation can help therapists clarify the risk, become aware of their vulnerabilities, and explore some options on how to proceed. Seeking professional consultation is always a good idea, but we caution against sharing your feelings of attraction with your client directly. Such disclosures often detract from the work of therapy and may be a confusing burden for the client. Koocher and Keith-Spiegel emphasize that therapists are always responsible for managing their feelings toward clients and that shifting blame or responsibility to clients is never an excuse for unprofessional or unethical conduct.

As you read the case examples that follow, consider what you would do in each situation.

Case example: A therapist's attraction to a client. A single female colleague of yours tells you that she is having a problem with one of her female clients, whom she is very much attracted to. She finds herself willing to run overtime in the sessions. If she were not a client, your colleague confides to you that she would most likely ask this person out for a date. Your colleague is wondering if she should terminate the professional relationship and begin a personal one. She has shared with her client that she is sexually attracted to her, and the client admits finding her attractive too.

Your stance. Your colleague comes to you for your suggestions on how she should proceed. What would you say to her? What do you think you would do if you found yourself in a similar situation?

Case example: A client's attraction to a therapist. In a counseling session, one of your clients discloses "finding you sexually attractive." The client is uncomfortable making this admission and now wonders what you are thinking and feeling.

Your stance. If you heard this, how do you imagine it would affect you? What might you say in response to your client's concern?

Case example: Discussing sexual feelings. One of your clients describes in detail sexual feelings and fantasies. As you listen, you begin to feel uncomfortable. The client notices this and asks, "Did I say something that I shouldn't have?"

Your stance. How would you respond to this client's question? Would you pursue this issue in your own therapy or talk with colleagues to gain some perspective on your own feelings? How much of this would you share with your client?

Case example: A personal request by a client. A client whom you find attractive tells you how accepting, kind, gentle, and understanding you are. This client expresses a desire to hear more about your life.

Your stance. Do you think your self-disclosure could help this client? Might you take the focus off the client and engage in self-disclosure for your own needs? Could you see yourself engaging in personal conversations that are really not relevant to the therapeutic purpose of your relationship? If this happened, what actions might you take?

Training in Managing Attractions

Seeking help from a colleague, supervision, or personal therapy can give students and trainees access to guidance, education, and support in managing their feelings of attraction toward clients. Pope, Sonne, and Holroyd (1993) maintain that practice, internships, and peer supervision groups are ideal places to discuss sexual feelings about clients. Deliberate attention to sexuality issues during training is essential for the development of competent mental health professionals. This training should involve accurate information and opportunities for experiential practice, such as role-playing difficult situations (Wiederman & Sansone, 1999). Hamilton and Spruill (1999) believe it is crucial to increase student awareness of sexual attraction issues before students begin seeing clients. They recommend the inclusion of how to deal with sexual attractions as a basic component of a preparatory clinical skills course.

In light of the challenges of dealing with sexual attractions in the helping process, Herlihy and Corey (2006b) recommend that training programs in the helping professions place increased emphasis on the issue of sexual attraction. Helpers need to be assured that their feelings are natural and that with awareness they can learn to provide professional assistance to clients, even if they might experience sexual attraction at times. Herlihy and Corey stress the value of learning to monitor your own countertransference, consulting with colleagues, and being alert to the subtle ways that sexual attractions can cross the boundary into inappropriate multiple relationships. We recommend Irvin Yalom's (1997) book, *Lying on the Couch: A Novel,* for an interesting case and discourse on the slippery slope of sexual attraction between therapist and client.

Sexual Relationships With Current Clients

Sexual misconduct is one of the major causes for malpractice actions against mental health providers. Those who have studied the sexual relationships between helpers and clients generally report that such misconduct is more widespread than is commonly believed. Studies demonstrate that sexual contact in the helping relationship can potentially cause severe harm to clients (Knapp & VandeCreek, 2003). Sonne and Pope (1991) report that clients who had been sexually involved with their therapists tended to exhibit reactions similar to those of survivors of incest and rape, including intense feelings of betrayal, confusion, and guilt.

Sexual misconduct is one of the more serious allegations in malpractice suits. Most mental health professionals take the position that erotic contact with clients is totally inappropriate and is an exploitation of the relationship by the therapist. They view sexual contact with clients as unprofessional, unethical, and clinically harmful.

Therapist–client sexual contact is highly disruptive and is the most potentially damaging boundary violation (Smith & Fitzpatrick, 1995). The literature shows that sexual relationships with clients carry serious consequences in both ethical and legal terms. These consequences include being the target of a lawsuit, being convicted of a felony, having a license revoked, being expelled from a professional organization, losing insurance coverage, and losing a job. Therapists may also be placed on probation, be required to undergo their own psychotherapy, be closely monitored if they are allowed to resume their practice, and be required to obtain supervised practice.

As you read this, you may think that you would never become involved in sexual misconduct with any of your clients. The chances are that those practitioners who have engaged in sexual intimacies with clients made the same assumption. Realize that you are not immune to the possibility of becoming sexually involved with those you help. Remain alert to your own needs and motivations and how they could get in the way of your work when you find yourself attracted to a client.

Clients are usually with you for a short time, and they are probably seeing the best side of you. You are likely to receive respect and adulation and to be perceived as someone who has no faults. This unconditional admiration can be very seductive, especially for beginning helpers, and you may come to depend on this feedback too much. If clients tell you how understanding and how different you are from anyone else they have met, it may be difficult to resist believing what they say. You are heading for trouble as a helper if you cannot keep the feelings that your clients express to you in proper perspective. Without self-awareness and honesty, you may direct the sessions toward meeting your needs and may eventually become sexually involved.

The reason erotic contact is unethical centers on the power that helpers have by virtue of their professional role. Because clients are talking about very personal aspects of their lives and making themselves highly vulnerable, it is easy to betray this trust by exploiting clients for helpers' own personal motives. Sexual contact is also unethical because it fosters dependency and makes objectivity on the part of the helper impossible. But perhaps the most important argument against sexual involvement with clients is that most clients report harm as a result. Clients typically become resentful and angry at having been sexually exploited and abandoned and generally feel stuck with both unresolved problems and unresolved feelings relating to the traumatic experience.

Sexual Relationships With Former Clients

Most of the codes of ethics of the various professions do not currently have an absolute ban on sexual relationships after the end of a professional relationship, but helpers are cautioned against forming romantic relationships with former clients for a specified time period, usually 2 to 5 years after termination. However, this does not imply that such relationships with clients are ethical or professional after the specified number of years has elapsed. The ethics codes of the ACA (2005), NASW (2008), CRCC (2010), AAMFT (2001), and APA (2002) are quite specific about conditions pertaining to relationships with former clients. For example, it is not considered ethical to terminate with a client because of an attraction, wait the time period, and then begin a romantic relationship. Even after 2 to 5 years, it is incumbent on helpers to examine their motivations, to continually consider what is best for the former client, and to be extremely careful to avoid any form of exploitation.

In the exceptional circumstance of a sexual relationship with a former client, the burden of demonstrating that there has been no exploitation clearly rests with the practitioner. The factors that must be considered include the amount of time that has passed since termination of therapy; the nature and duration of therapy; the circumstances surrounding termination of the helper–client relationship; the client's personal history; the client's competence and mental status; the foreseeable likelihood of harm to the client or others; and any statements or actions of the helper suggesting a romantic relationship after terminating the professional relationship.

The *ACA Code of Ethics* (ACA, 2005) standard pertaining to sexual contact with former clients is explicit:

> Sexual or romantic counselor–client interactions or relationships with former clients, their romantic partners, or their family members are prohibited for a period of 5 years following the last professional contact. Counselors, before engaging in sexual or romantic interactions or relationships with clients, their romantic partners, or client family members after 5 years following the last professional contact, demonstrate forethought and document (in written form) whether the interactions or relationship can be viewed as exploitive in some way and/or whether there is still potential to harm the former client; in cases of potential exploitation and/or harm, the counselor avoids entering such an interaction or relationship. (A.5.b.)

Most in the helping professions agree that termination of a helping relationship, in and of itself, does not justify changing the professional relationship to a sexual one. If a helper were to consider getting romantically involved with a former client after 5 years had passed, it would be wise to consult with a colleague or seek a therapy session conjointly with the former client to explore mutual transferences and expectations. It is essential to remain aware of the potential harm that can result from sexual intimacies that occur after termination, of the aspects of the therapy relationships that can influence the new relationship, and of the continuing power differential (Herlihy & Corey, 2006b).

By Way of Review

- A multiple relationship may occur whenever you interact with a client in more than one capacity. Be aware of your position of power and avoid even the appearance of conflict of interest.

• It helps to keep your relationships with your clients on a professional, rather than a personal, basis. Mixing social relationships with professional relationships often works against the best interests of both the client and the helper.

• It is probably a good idea to avoid bartering, except when this is the best available option and when it is the cultural norm. Exchanging services can lead to resentment on both your part and your client's.

• In deciding whether to accept a gift from a client, consider the cultural context, the client's motivations for offering a gift, and the stage of the helping process.

• Sexual attractions are a normal part of helping relationships. It is important to learn how to recognize these attractions and to develop strategies to deal with them appropriately and effectively.

• Sexual misconduct is the leading cause of malpractice actions against mental health providers. Sexual intimacies between helpers and clients are unethical for a number of reasons. One of the main reasons is that they entail an abuse of power and trust.

What Will You Do Now?

1. Some say that multiple relationships are inevitable, pervasive, and unavoidable and have the potential to be either beneficial or harmful. In small groups explore both the potential benefits and the risks of multiple relationships. Come up with guidelines as a group for how you might assess the balance between the benefits and risks of multiple relationships.

2. Review the discussion on sexual relationships with former clients. Form two teams and debate the issue of whether sexual and romantic relationships with former clients should be allowed a specific length of time after termination of the counseling relationship.

3. Assume that you are a member of a committee with the task of revising an ethics code. What input would you have regarding the appropriateness of social, sexual, business, and professional relationships with former clients? Should these relationships be considered unethical under some or most circumstances? Can you think of exceptions? Can you think of situations where you might accept a social invitation from a former client? Would you see it as appropriate to engage in a business relationship with a former client? Can you think of any times when you might form professional relationships with former clients?

4. In small groups spend some time discussing what you learned about the importance of creating personal and professional boundaries. What difficulties

might you expect to encounter in establishing and maintaining certain boundaries with some clients?

5. For the full bibliographic entry for each of the sources listed here, consult the References at the back of the book. For a treatment of many facets of the multiple relationship controversy, see Herlihy and Corey (2006b), Lazarus and Zur (2002), and Zur (2007).

Ethics in Action *CD-ROM Exercises*

6. Complete the self-inventory on Boundary Issues and Multiple Relationships before viewing role-play segments 8 through 12. Bring your completed responses to class for discussion.

7. In video role-play segment 8, The Picnic, the client (Lucia) would like to meet with the counselor (John) at the park down the street for their counseling sessions so she can get to know him better and feel closer to him. She suggests that she could bring a lunch for a picnic. John is concerned about creating an environment that would help Lucia the most, and she says "that [meeting in the park] would really help me." Through role playing, demonstrate how you would establish and maintain boundaries with this client.

8. In role-play segment 9, The Friendship, at their last therapy session the client (Charlae) says she would like to continue their relationship because they have so much in common and she has shared things with the counselor (Natalie) that she has not discussed with anyone else. Natalie informs Charlae that this puts her in a difficult situation and she feels awkward. Charlae says, "What if we just go jogging together a couple of mornings a week?" Via role playing, demonstrate how you would handle such a request from a former client who is interested in developing a social relationship with you.

9. In role-play segment 10, The Disclosure, the counselor (Conrad) shares with the client (Suzanne) that he has been thinking about her a lot and that he is attracted to her. Suzanne responds with, "You're kidding, right?" She says she came to him because of having problems with men taking advantage of her and not respecting her. She has bared her soul to him and now she feels devalued. Suzanne suggests possibly seeing another counselor, but Conrad thinks they can work it out. Role-play the way you would deal with a client who disclosed to you that he or she found you "quite attractive." Assume that you also found this client "quite attractive."

10. In role-play segment 11, The Architect, the client (Janice) lost her job and can no longer pay for counseling sessions. She suggests providing architectural services for the counselor (Jerry). Jerry suggests they discuss the pros and cons and that he wants to be sure that this is in her best interests. He mentions the code of ethics that discourages bartering. Jerry talks about issues of value

and timeliness of services. In a role play, demonstrate how you would deal with this client. What issues would you want to explore?

11. In role-play segment 12, Tickets for Therapy, the client (John) shows his appreciation for his counselor (Marianne) by getting tickets to the theater for her. John says, "I got tickets for you so you can go and enjoy it and have a good time." Marianne talks about why she cannot accept the tickets, in spite of the fact that she is very appreciative of his gesture. What issues would you explore with John? Might you accept the tickets under any circumstances? Why or why not? Demonstrate, through role playing, what you would say to the client.

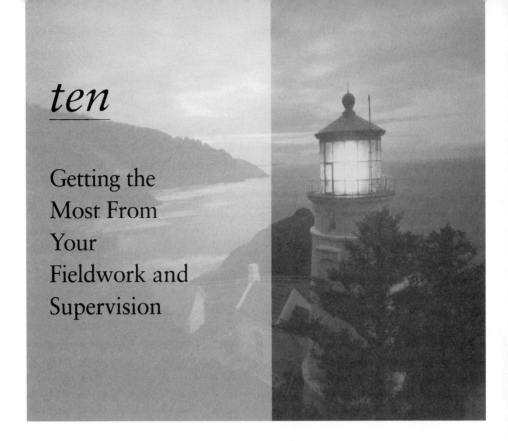

ten

Getting the Most From Your Fieldwork and Supervision

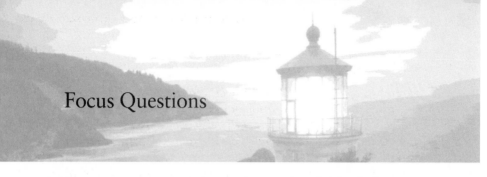

Focus Questions

1. What can you do to maximize your learning from fieldwork placements?

2. How can you better profit from your supervision? If you are not getting the quality of supervision you need, what steps can you take?

3. What are some ways to challenge your self-doubts in your fieldwork placement? How can you change your fears into assets and opportunities for learning?

4. What specific steps can you take to confront any difficulties you are experiencing in your field placement? What are some possible benefits of staying with a field placement that is not to your liking?

5. In meetings with your supervisor, what attitudes and behaviors of yours are most likely to lead to maximizing your learning?

6. What are your thoughts about receiving personal counseling as part of your program? Why do you think ethical practice dictates that the supervisory relationship should not be turned into personal therapy sessions with your supervisor?

7. What would you look for in a field placement? What kinds of questions would you ask before accepting a field placement assignment?

8. What personal characteristics do you think are associated with an effective supervisor?

9. What are your thoughts about informed consent in supervision? What would you want to know about what supervision entails from the beginning of the relationship?

10. What are some possible advantages of group supervision?

Aim of the Chapter

You will get far more from your program of studies and your fieldwork activities by assuming an *active stance*. At times students are disillusioned with their department, their professors, and their supervision. There are negative aspects to any educational system, yet it is more useful and productive to focus on how you can get the most from both your course work and your fieldwork experiences. Rather than concentrating on what you cannot do, think of what you can do and the advantages of taking a more active role in all aspects of your educational program. In this chapter we encourage you to take steps to ensure that you will be involved in meaningful fieldwork placements and that you will take an active role in getting adequate supervision.

Making the Most of Your Fieldwork

In the helping professions of counseling, social work, psychology, and couples and family therapy, most graduate programs have fieldwork and internship placements at their core. Most undergraduate programs in human services have a comprehensive fieldwork component, which is often the heart of the program. These activities provide a bridge between theory and practice. Actual experience in a field placement gives students opportunities to learn firsthand about paperwork, agency policies and procedures, and the challenge of working with a wide range of client populations and problems. These are some of the goals of a fieldwork instruction program:

- Provide students with knowledge of the varied approaches and methods used in human services programs
- Help students extend self-awareness and achieve a sense of professional identity
- Broaden students' sociocultural understanding of the individual, the family, the community, and relevant social systems
- Assist students in recognizing and respecting cultural diversity and offer ways to use this understanding in practice
- Help students expand their awareness of professional role relationships within their organization as well as the agency's role in the community

Before you can meaningfully participate in fieldwork and internship placements, you need theory courses, specific knowledge, and a range of helping skills. You can enhance your academic learning by volunteering to work in a community agency. It is the combination of academic course work, fieldwork placement, skills training, and personal development that makes for a sound program.

Take an Active Role in Getting a Meaningful Placement

If you have some choice in selecting the place where you will be gaining supervised practical experience, take an active role in securing the best placement possible. One way of actively participating in securing a quality fieldwork placement is by asking questions of potential agency settings when you are going through the interviewing process for a field placement. Here are some questions you might ask:

- What are the goals and purposes of your agency or organization? What services are provided?
- Have you worked with student interns before? If so, what have been some of their activities?
- How does the agency and professional staff view the role of interns? Are they viewed as members of the team or more as peripheral observers?
- What internship opportunities are now available at this agency?
- Are interns ever employed at this agency once they complete their internship?
- What would be my specific responsibilities?
- Are there any special skills or requirements for the placement?
- To whom would I report? Who would supervise me? How many hours per week would I meet for supervision?
- Are there training or staff development opportunities at the agency? What kinds of training might I receive prior to and during my placement?
- Is there any videotaping equipment available?
- Would I be covered by the agency for malpractice liability?

We hope you will assume an active role in selecting a meaningful placement that will enhance your learning. This can take considerable thought, time, and preparation on your part. Strive for a placement where you will receive adequate supervision and where you will be able to profit from learning how to cope with a variety of problems that clients bring to the agency.

If you are employed at a community agency and want to use this agency for your fieldwork placement, we suggest that you branch out to get as much variety as possible in your placements. If you already have volunteer or paid work experience in a particular setting, try doing something different for your internship: do different tasks, occupy a different role, or work with another client population. Your fieldwork experience should provide you with a variety of settings in which to work and also with various supervising environments. A wide range of opportunities exists within most agencies. Secure training in areas new to you as a way to acquire new knowledge and skills. Internships and supervised fieldwork placements provide practical experiences that can help you learn how to work meaningfully within a system. The more practical and supervised experience you can get the better. Commit yourself to becoming the most competent practitioner you can be.

When we talk with graduates of human services programs, they typically mention that they found their current job as a result of contacts they established at their fieldwork placement. In fact, most graduates report wishing they had been able to participate in even more fieldwork activities. Some regret not having had a broader range of experience in their internships. We recommend that you visit as many sites as possible before making your selection, if that is allowed in your program. Review job descriptions and arrange interviews with selected agencies.

Knowledge and Skills Required for Successful Job Performance

When we asked practitioners about the skills they most need in their present jobs, they listed counseling skills, supervisory skills, consulting skills, communication skills, the ability to interact with different levels of management, the ability to write a proposal, organizational skills, the ability to deal with crisis intervention, and networking skills. A number of professionals pointed out the value of self-exploratory experiences, especially groups aimed at personal and interpersonal growth. These therapeutic experiences gave them opportunities to look at themselves and to deal with their own feelings and problems, activities that were seen as especially helpful in preparing them to relate to clients. Even those professionals who were primarily engaged in the administration of human services programs commented on the value of self-awareness and the understanding of interpersonal dynamics as tools they used in their managerial functions. Those in management pointed out that they would not be able to develop and coordinate their programs if they did not know how to work effectively with people.

A view from community agencies. As part of the self-study program conducted by our department at the university, community agencies that offer fieldwork placements to our students were contacted and asked a number of questions regarding what they were looking for in hiring employees as well as their views on other relevant issues. Here are some of the questions we posed to agency personnel along with a representative sample of their responses to these questions.

1. What special knowledge and skills do our students need in order to work effectively at your agency?

   - Ability to work with diverse cultures
   - Understand ethics and confidentiality issues
   - Ability to connect with others
   - Resourcefulness and ability to direct and give referrals
   - Listening skills, case management skills, and counseling skills
   - Ability to be proactive rather than reactive

2. What knowledge, skills, and competencies do you consider most important for employees in your agency?

   - A good deal of independence combined with responsible reporting of treatment plans, incidents, and therapeutic progress
   - Ability to identify and maintain clear personal and professional boundaries
   - An outreach person who can organize a program from start to finish
   - Must be creative, adaptable, and open-minded with an eagerness to serve the community in a nonjudgmental way
   - Awareness and acceptance of cultural diversity, including the immigrant experience
   - Self-motivated and hard-working

- Good organizational skills
- Ability to work with a disabled population in an educational environment
- Flexibility and ability to work as a team
- Good problem-solving skills and a good innovator
- Crisis intervention skills

3. What trends do you foresee in the future for the field of human services?

- Family preservation and preventive programs
- Expansion in services for the upcoming senior population explosion
- Short-term interventions aimed at psychoeducational goals
- More community outreach to assist multiethnic communities with access to health care services
- Managed care models

How to Profit From Your Fieldwork Experiences

For a variety of reasons, students often do not derive the maximum benefit from fieldwork and supervision. Here are some practical strategies for getting the most value out of your fieldwork placements:

- Instead of limiting yourself to one kind of population, seek a variety of placements. Stretch your boundaries to help you to discover where your talents lie and the kind of population you would eventually like to work with. Through your internships you may learn what you do not want to do as well as what you would like to do. Some students who initially want to practice counseling exclusively later find themselves in the role of administrator or supervisor.

- Take courses and workshops that will prepare you for the type of work expected of you in your placement. These workshops can be a useful resource for staying on the cutting edge of new developments with specialized populations.

- Let yourself fit into the agency, instead of trying to make it fit you. Be open to learning from the staff and the clients who come to the agency. Attempt to suspend your preconceived judgments about what you should be learning and focus instead on the lessons that are available to you. Learn as much as you can about the politics of the agency by talking with people who work there, by attending staff meetings, and by asking questions.

- Be aware of the toll that your work can have on you both emotionally and physically. Certain aspects of your life may surface as you get involved with clients, which can lead to more anxiety in your life. Consider the value of personal therapy as a part of self-care.

- Practice within the boundaries of your training and put yourself in situations where you will be able to obtain supervised experience. It is essential to learn the delicate balance between being overly confident and constantly doubting yourself.

• Strive to be flexible in applying techniques to the different client populations, but do so under supervision. Be open to fitting your theory to your clients rather than your clients to your theory. Realize that diverse client backgrounds necessitate diverse communication approaches. Although it is essential to learn therapeutic skills and techniques, they should be applied in appropriate ways.

• Do not write off as a waste of time a placement that you do not particularly like. At least you are learning that working in a particular agency or with a specific clientele may not be what you want for a career. Identify what you don't find productive about the placement and ask yourself why you feel that way.

• Make connections in the community. Learn how to use community resources and how to draw on support systems beyond your placement. Talk to other professionals in the field, ask fellow students about their connections in the community, and develop a network of contacts. This kind of networking may well lead to a range of job opportunities.

• Keep a journal; record your observations, experiences, concerns, and personal reactions to your work. Your journal is an excellent way to stay focused on yourself as well as to keep track of what you are doing with clients.

• Be open to trying new things. If you have not worked with a family, for example, observe a family session or, if possible, work with a supervisor who is counseling a family. Avoid setting yourself up by thinking that if you do not succeed perfectly in a new endeavor you are a dismal failure. Give yourself room to learn by doing, at the same time gaining supervised experience.

• Look for ways to apply what you are learning in your academic courses to your experiences in the field. For example, one professional recalls having taken abnormal psychology as part of her graduate program and also having served as an intern in a state mental institution. Through this internship she was able to see some of the concepts she was studying come to life.

• Be prepared to adjust your expectations. It is unlikely that you will be asked to provide direct services to clients before the agency staff get to know you. You will probably start your fieldwork in an observing role. However, be aware that some agencies may give interns jobs without adequate preparation.

• Treat your field placement like a job. Approach fieldwork in much the same way as you would if you were employed by the agency. Demonstrate responsibility, be on time for your appointments and meetings, follow through with your commitments, and strive to do your best.

• Learn as much as you can about the structure of the agency where you are placed. Ask about agency policies, about the way the programs are administered, and about management of the staff. At some point, you may be involved in the administrative aspects of a social program.

• Try to gain a global perspective of the agency as well as seeing it as clients might view it. Learn how agency systems work, and assess how you can work successfully within the system. Identify others in the agency who are successfully working within the system: talk to them, learn from them, and use them as a support system. Find out what keeps them motivated to do a good job.

• Think and act in a self-directed way by involving yourself in a variety of activities. Take the initiative to get involved in meaningful assignments.

The Challenge of Working With Differences

As we have suggested, it is a good idea to seek a placement where you will be expected to work with a variety of clients and tasks. By working with diverse populations, you can explore your interests and develop new ones. If you focus narrowly on the population or problem area you have chosen as a specialization, you are likely to close off many avenues of learning and limit yourself professionally.

As a part of your fieldwork for internship placement, you usually receive on-the-job training and supervision. Therefore, you might not need expertise in counseling rape victims before being accepted for such a placement. Your coworkers and supervisors will teach you some interventions in working with such clients. Thus, more important than knowing how to work with a specific population or a specific problem is having a general background of knowledge and skills and being open to acquiring more specific abilities.

Helping someone different from you. One of our colleagues told us that her client who was paralyzed became upset and angry when she said to him, "I understand how you feel." His reply was: "How would you know? You can walk out of here, and I can't." On reflection, our colleague thought that a better response might have been the following: "You're right, I don't fully understand your situation. I can imagine your frustration and pain over being paralyzed at such a young age. But I haven't been in your situation, so I don't know what you're thinking and feeling. I hope you will help me understand what this is like for you, and I hope I can help you work with your feelings about being paralyzed."

Some interns make the mistake of clinging to the conviction that to help a person they must have had the same life experience. Thus, a male clinician may doubt his capacity to effectively counsel an adolescent girl who is struggling with what she wants to do about a pregnancy. A helper may doubt that she can work with a client of a different race. Or a practitioner who has not experienced trauma may wonder about her ability to empathize with clients who have had pain and trauma in their lives. A helper who works with people with addictions may doubt his ability to effectively reach his clients if he has not had an addiction problem. When these helpers are confronted by a client, they often backtrack and become apologetic. We hope that you can see the value of drawing on your own life experience in working with clients who are different from you. You may not have had the same problem, but you have some experience with pain. It is more important to be able to understand the client's world than to have had an identical problem. It is crucial that you realize that some of your clients will view the world from a different perspective than you do (see Chapter 7 for a more detailed discussion on understanding diversity).

Profiting From Your Supervision

Most professionals question their competence at certain times and in certain situations. We hope you can be patient with your feelings of incompetence rather than denying them. The purpose of your supervised fieldwork is to provide you with a varied and meaningful learning opportunity. This is a place where you can acquire specific knowledge and where you can develop the skills to translate the theories you have learned into practice. Be clear in your own mind about what you expect from your supervisors, and discuss your desires with them from the outset. This section suggests how to approach your supervision and actively participate in this process.

Be Open to Multiple Sources of Supervision

Be open to input not only from supervisors but also from teachers, peers, colleagues, and clients. Take advantage of your role: as a student, you are not expected to know everything. If you understand that making mistakes provides you with an opportunity for self-reflection, critical thinking, and, ultimately, learning and change, you will be less likely to feel frozen in an attempt to avoid making mistakes. Talk openly with your supervisor about your presumed mistakes and discuss what to do in various situations when you feel uncertain of your abilities. Believing that you must already have the knowledge and skills you need to be successful puts undue pressure on you; this attitude can get in the way of your ability to learn from your supervisors, peers, and clients.

In our training of group facilitators we typically find that the students approach workshops with considerable anxiety over looking incompetent in the eyes of their peers and supervisors. Early in the workshop we tell them this: "Be as active as you can. Stretch yourself past the point at which you typically stop. No matter what happens, there is something to be learned. If a group session is unproductive, you can explore what specific factors contributed to that outcome."

When we give students these instructions, they usually react with relief and acknowledge feeling much less anxious. We let them know that we understand and empathize with their difficulty in being observed by their peers and by supervisors. It is not possible to escape from being watched by clients, supervisors, and coworkers. Talking about our experience of being observed allows us to be in control of this process rather than being controlled by what others might think of us. Students often find it helpful to openly share their fears. Paradoxically, their fears are diminished by this act of acknowledgment.

Dealing with challenge and self-doubts. Trainees may be unsure, apologetic, and unwilling to credit themselves with the ability to be helpful. Ask yourself how you typically deal with any self-doubts you may have about your ability as a helper.

Consider how you might deal with a client who challenged you. At the initial session your client is surprised at your age. "How can you help me?" he asks. "You look so young, and I wonder if you have the experience to help me." Assume that this challenge reflects your own fears and doubts. Can you imagine saying any of the following things silently to yourself?

- "He's right. There are many years separating us. I wonder if I can understand his situation?"
- "This man's attitude makes me angry. I feel judged before I've even had a chance to know him."
- "I don't feel comfortable with this confrontation, but I don't want to back down. I feel like letting him know that even though we differ in age we might have many similarities in our struggles. I'd like an opportunity to at least explore whether we can form a relationship."

Certainly as individuals we are all affected when someone challenges us, yet we need to learn how to deal with these situations. Helping is not about proving that we are "right." By staying focused on the best interests of our clients, we can address any challenges in a direct and honest manner. If you feel that you might have done something more effectively or sensitively, it helps to simply acknowledge this.

It's okay not to know. Be willing to admit a lack of knowledge or understanding about a situation with both your supervisor and your clients. Don't be afraid to say you don't know something and to ask for help. You are at your placement to learn, not because you already have all the knowledge and skills you need. If you feel intimidated because you do not have an answer to a client's problem, you can say something like this: "Carla, I am struck by how much you want me to have answers for you. Yet I think I need to take some time to think about your situation and to consult my colleagues and supervisor so that I can help you in the best possible way." In this way you acknowledge your limitations to Carla, but you keep the door open to providing her with information she can use in resolving her problem. Your role as helper is not to provide answers or to tell people what to do but to teach them how to examine options and apply problem-solving skills.

Think out loud. In working with both students and professionals, we often find that they have many powerful reactions that they keep to themselves. We typically encourage our trainees to talk out loud rather than engaging in an internal monologue. Telling us what they were thinking but not saying helps them to get unstuck. Most of the time we find that what they are not saying could be extremely helpful to themselves and their clients if they were to share it. In a recent workshop one trainee, Victoria, was quiet throughout the group session. The supervisor asked Victoria what was going on. She replied, "I feel inhibited in following my hunches, and I fear that you might be judging me and not liking what you see." Her supervisor encouraged her to more frequently say aloud these kinds of thoughts. Victoria reported that by simply making this statement she felt much less self-conscious and less frightened over her supervisor's reactions.

In another instance one trainee, Lee, continually suggested one exercise after another during a particular group-training session. Later, when Lee was asked why he had introduced so many different exercises in such a short session, he replied: "Well, the group seemed to be going nowhere. People seemed to lack energy, and I felt responsible for making something happen! I was hoping to bring the group alive by trying some interactive exercises." We told Lee that it would have been good to describe what he saw happening in the group, rather than trying techniques without explaining what was going on. We are not suggesting that you express every fleeting reaction you have to your clients, but in your supervision meetings it is appropriate to talk about your thoughts and feelings about some of your observations.

Finding your voice while listening to others. We have observed that some trainees limit their own development by trying too hard to copy the style of a supervisor or teacher. You are likely to observe supervisors whom you respect, and you may tend to adopt their style. It is important, however, to avoid becoming a copy of another person. To get the most from your supervision, try different styles, but continually evaluate what works for you and what does not.

You might ask yourself: "What fits my belief system, both personal and theoretical? Do I have any conflicts between the theory or application of my supervisor's way and my own?" If you pay too much attention to another person, you are likely to blur your own unique approach to helping people. The more experience you gain, the easier it will become to listen to your own intuitive voice and to respect your inner hunches. Eventually, you will have less need to look to outside experts.

Focus of supervision. Some approaches to supervision emphasize the client's dynamics and teach you strategies for intervening in specific problems. Others focus on your dynamics as a helper and as a person and on your behavior in relation to your client. In our opinion, comprehensive supervision takes both of these elements into consideration. You need to understand models of helping clients, and you need to understand yourself if you hope to form truly therapeutic alliances. If your supervision is focused solely on what your client is doing or on teaching you specific techniques for what to do next, we think your supervision will be lacking a significant dimension. A critical focus for discussion in supervision sessions is the degree to which you are as present as possible for your clients. If you are overly concerned about what to do about a client's problem, this concern is likely to distract you from making connections with the person. A useful focus of supervision is the quality of the relationship between you and your clients. In supervision, you can talk about what you are experiencing as you work with different clients. This focus will reveal a good deal about both you and your clients.

Our style of supervision. When we supervise, we pay attention to the relationship between our supervisees and ourselves, as well as the dynamics and relationships between supervisees and their clients. Here we see a parallel process operating between a practice model and a supervisory model. Supervisees can learn ways to conceptualize what they are doing with their clients by reflecting on what they are learning about interpersonal dynamics in the supervisory relationship.

Rather than placing emphasis exclusively on assessing and treating a client's problems, we are very concerned with the interpersonal aspects that are emerging between the supervisee and his or her clients. In our view, supervisors do well to look beyond the cases that trainees bring to the supervisory sessions and focus on the interpersonal dimensions.

In our role as supervisors we attempt to help our supervisees develop their own insights and refine their clinical hunches. Rather than placing the emphasis on direct teaching with supervisees by giving them information, we strive to help them learn how to conceptualize a case and think about how they are likely to proceed with a given client and why. Instead of using our words with supervisees' clients, we hope supervisees will discover their own words and find their own voice. Our style of supervision is reflected by the following questions we typically explore:

- What are you wanting to say to your clients?
- What direction do you think is most appropriate to take with your clients?
- How are you affected by your clients?
- How is your behavior affecting them?
- Which clients are difficult for you to work with, and what might this say about you?
- How are your values manifested by the way you interact with your clients?
- How might our relationship, in these supervisory sessions, mirror your relationships with your clients?
- Are you feeling free enough to bring into these supervisory sessions any difficulties you are having with your clients?

Many of the points we are making about supervision reflect our particular philosophy and style of supervision. Other styles of supervision may operate from a different set of assumptions. From what you have read in this section, consider these questions: What style of supervision do you think would be most useful for you at this stage of your development? What kind of supervisor do you think would be the most difficult for you to work with, and why? If it were impractical to change positions or change supervisors, what strategies could you use in constructively dealing with this supervisor?

Maximize your time in supervision. You will get the most from your supervision if you take an active stance as a supervisee. Here are a few suggestions for benefiting from your supervision:

- Know the general purpose of supervision.
- Recognize that different supervisors will attempt to achieve the purpose of supervision in a variety of ways.
- Accept that a certain level of anxiety is normal to the supervision process.
- Clarify any aspects of your contract with your supervisor regarding the content of the supervision sessions.

- Strive to be as honest and open as possible during your supervision sessions.
- If you are not able to select your supervisor, do your best to work within the framework of the supervisory style of the supervisor assigned to you.
- Clarify for yourself what you most want and need from supervision, and inform your supervisor of your needs.
- Take the time to prepare for your supervision session by identifying questions you want to explore and by bringing in examples you want to discuss with your supervisor.

Get the Supervision You Deserve

The assertion skills you practice in getting adequate supervision will be useful in your relationships with both clients and colleagues. Being assertive does not mean being aggressive. An aggressive approach will needlessly put others on the defensive. Being passive is not useful either because your supervisor will have no idea what you want or need. Being aggressive or passive will shut you off from many opportunities to learn.

Get a clear picture of how you want to spend your time in an agency. Identifying what you want may not be easy, especially if this is your first fieldwork placement. You can begin by thinking about what you would most like to learn and what skills you would like to acquire. A placement typically involves a written contract signed by the student and the supervisor of the agency. This contract usually spells out the number of hours to be worked per week, the activities that will be performed, the learning objectives, the opportunities for training, the expectations for the intern, and the expectations for the supervisor. A written supervisory contract also typically addresses the number and frequency of supervision sessions, when and how contact will be established, and guidelines for how both supervisor and supervisee should prepare for each session (Brislin & Herbert, 2009). Before signing your contract with your supervisor, discuss in some detail what you want and the kinds of opportunities available to you. In collaboration with your supervisor, spell out what you would like to experience and learn before you leave. Although you may not always get what you want, if you have a clear idea of what that is, you will have a better chance of obtaining it.

It helps to realize that supervisors are people too. They have demands placed on them. As their client load grows and pressures increase, they may not initiate the regular supervision sessions that you have been promised. Furthermore, some practitioners do not volunteer to become supervisors but are told that they should add interns to their already heavy workload. At times their training for being a supervisor is minimal, and they find they must take continuing education course work to learn how to effectively supervise. If you are able to understand the predicament of your supervisors, you are more likely to be able to establish a basis of communication with them. Within a climate of open communication, you can sensitively and assertively let your supervisor know that you need help. If you have a difficult case, you can say something like this: "I really think I am at an impasse with Kristen. For several weeks now, we have made little progress. Every suggestion I make seems to go nowhere. I suggested termination, and she got angry with me. Now I don't know what to do. Can I meet with you to talk about some alternatives?" By being clear, specific, and persistent, you are more likely to have your needs met.

If you approach your supervisors with a genuine attitude of informing them of what you need from them, supervisors are more likely to respond positively than if you keep your distance from them. If you learn to ask for what you want and need from your supervisors without being aggressive, you will be going a long way toward creating a positive fieldwork experience and using supervision to its fullest extent.

Unfortunately, some students have negative experiences with fieldwork and with supervisors. At a conference of human service educators, Tricia McClam of the University of Tennessee made a presentation on effective field supervision. The relationship between the field supervisor and the student seems to be a key variable in determining whether the student's reactions are positive or negative. Supervisors certainly play a key role in the student's learning, and it is part of the student's responsibility to communicate with the assigned supervisor, even if he or she is less than ideal.

Students with positive reactions to supervisors made comments such as these: "She was available." "She was involved in my cases." "My supervisor clearly stated what he expected of me and what I could expect of him." "My supervisor was both supportive and flexible." Students with negative reactions to supervisors observed the following: "He was too busy to properly supervise." "My supervisor did not meet with me regularly." "My supervisor was not organized." "My supervisor expected me to do things her way and gave me little encouragement to find my own style."

When students begin their fieldwork activity, McClam states that students do best with supervisors who are clear about their expectations and who provide support and guidance. Firmness coupled with flexibility is useful for beginning trainees. When students have gained some fieldwork experience, they still need support and guidance, along with feedback from their supervisors, but they can profit from experiences that will demand more intuition and skill. Most important is establishing regular communication between supervisors and supervisees. Take the initiative to communicate with your supervisor. This is particularly difficult in cases where you perceive your supervision to be inadequate, a topic we explore shortly. Your program is responsible for providing you with regular and competent supervision. As an intern, you deserve to have a meaningful supervision experience.

Case example: Duties outside an intern's area of competence.

A supervisor asks an intern to counsel a family, consisting of mother, father, and two young boys. The supervisor tells the intern that the parents are primarily interested in learning how to manage their problem children and want to learn disciplinary techniques. In the supervisor's view, a more important problem consists of the conflicts between the wife and husband. The intern has had very little course work or training in working with families and feels lacking in the competencies to do family counseling.

Your stance. If you were the trainee in this situation, what might you do? Might you give into pressure from the supervisor, especially with the offer of some supervision? How could you look for ways on the job to acquire the knowledge base that would enable you to work with a family? How would you like to be able to respond to this supervisor?

It is important to let your supervisor know of your concerns, so the two of you can talk about alternatives. Consider the following dialogue, and see how you might say some of the same or different things as the trainee.

SUPERVISOR: We are short on personnel in the agency, and we really need you to work with some families.

TRAINEE: I feel flattered that you think enough of me to ask for my help in seeing families. Yet at this stage of my professional development, I am going to have to decline.

SUPERVISOR: Look, it is you or no treatment at all. Most of us have hesitations when we begin working with new populations. Just jump in and get involved.

TRAINEE: In my case it is more than feeling anxious and having self-doubts. I have yet to take a single course in family therapy. It just does not seem ethical for me to undertake this task now.

SUPERVISOR: Well, I don't want you to do something that doesn't seem ethical to you. But I would be available for supervision, so you won't be without any guidance.

TRAINEE: I appreciate your offer for supervision. Perhaps I could observe your work with a family, with their permission of course, and then we could talk about your interventions after the session.

SUPERVISOR: If I had the time that would be great, but that would be adding one more thing to an already overbooked schedule.

TRAINEE: After I take the family therapy course next semester, perhaps I'll be in a better position to assist in this kind of work. For now, I need to work within my own limits.

Discussion. This case example is realistic in the sense that some organizations use interns as relatively "free" staff. The problem is not so much using interns to fill critical service needs but being unwilling to provide adequate supervision for trainees. Student interns do need some minimal theoretical foundation and knowledge competencies in working with families before they are able to effectively participate in actual clinical work with families. Certainly, when trainees are moving into a new area, they will need to acquire practical skills that will enable them to work effectively in this new setting. Good supervision enables trainees to apply their knowledge while acquiring these intervention strategies. If trainees take on work that is new for them, they can learn and gain competence through supervision.

The Effective Supervisor

Although there is no one right way of conducting clinical supervision, there are established standards for counseling supervisors. The "Ethical Guidelines for Counseling Supervisors" (Association for Counselor Education and Supervision [ACES], 1993, 1995) are designed to help supervisors (1) observe ethical and legal protection of clients' and supervisees' rights; (2) provide training for supervisees in ways that are consistent with clients' welfare and requirements of the program; and (3) establish policies, procedures, and standards for implementing programs. The supervisor's main functions are to teach trainees, to foster their personal and professional development, and to assist in the provision of the effective delivery of counseling (helping) services.

Based on input from practicing clinical supervisors, Corey, Haynes, Moulton, and Muratori (2010) compiled this list of personal characteristics of an effective supervisor:

- Is aware of clinical, legal, and ethical issues
- Possesses good clinical skills
- Behaviorally demonstrates empathy, respect, genuineness, and listening
- Establishes an accepting supervisory climate
- Creates a supervisory relationship characterized by trust and respect
- Is flexible in determining the developmental level of the supervisee and providing supervision methods that will best serve the training needs of the supervisee
- Has a sense of humor
- Develops clear boundaries
- Encourages appropriate risk-taking on the part of supervisees
- Supports a collaborative supervisory process
- Respects the knowledge that supervisees bring to the supervisory relationship
- Appreciates individual differences among supervisees and differing opinions about theoretical viewpoints
- Is open, approachable, and supportive
- Has a keen interest in training and supervision
- Shows sensitivity to the anxieties and vulnerabilities of supervisees
- Values supervision as a "protected" time
- Provides honest and constructive feedback

In a nutshell, good supervisors tend to be available, accessible, affable, and able.

The picture of the effective supervisor that emerges from the research is derived primarily from findings regarding supervisee satisfactions and preferences. The effective supervisor is one the supervisees respond to positively, find satisfactory, and are able to trust. The general picture of the effective supervisor is a technically competent professional with good human relations skills and effective organizational and managerial skills (Corey, Haynes, et al., 2010).

Barnett, Cornish, Goodyear, and Lichtenberg (2007) report that numerous studies have found that the quality of the supervisory relationship is a key component in determining outcomes, much as it is for the client–therapist relationship. Effective clinical supervisors provide constructive feedback to their supervisees in a supporting and nonjudgmental environment. They are well trained, knowledgeable, and skilled in the practice of clinical supervision. They limit their supervision to those areas in which they are competent, and they delegate portions of supervision when necessary to make sure that supervisees receive the best quality of supervision possible.

You may meet and work with supervisors who demonstrate effectiveness and others who seem ill equipped to do what is expected of them. Some may be as insecure in their supervisory role as you are in your new role as an intern. We hope that you will remember that getting the most from supervision is a shared responsibility between you and your supervisor.

Dealing With Supervision That Is Less Than Ideal

From time to time you may encounter supervision that is far from ideal. How can you recognize inadequate supervision? What can you do to ensure that you get the quality of supervision you need and have a right to expect?

Accepting different styles of supervision. You can benefit from learning how to function under a range of supervisory styles, both now as a student and later as a helping professional. One supervisor may believe confrontation is a way to cut through a client's defenses. Another may provide frequent advice for clients and promote a problem-solving orientation for client problems. Some supervisors foster a supportive and positive orientation with clients exclusively. Some supervisors may work very hard at establishing collegial relationships with their interns, whereas others may be more professionally distant. Be open to supervisors with various orientations and styles, and be open to incorporating some of their viewpoints in your practices. Do not be too quick to criticize a style different from yours, but consider it as an opportunity for learning. As a supervisee, recognize that at different stages in your professional development you may require different styles of supervision.

If you do have trouble with a supervisor, the answer is not always merely finding a new one. You can learn a great deal by working with supervisors who have perspectives different from yours and from supervisors who may initially appear to be difficult for you to make contact with. When you experience conflicts with a supervisor, it is a good idea to talk about these conflicts and do all that you can to work them out. Rather than telling yourself that your supervisor will not be cooperative, assume that he or she will be open to your suggestions. Later, when you accept a position in an agency, you typically will not have the option of changing supervisors. What is more, you often do not choose who your coworkers will be. Thus, it is important to learn the interpersonal skills necessary in working out differences.

Solving problems in your supervision. You may encounter a number of problems in working with a supervisor. Communication may not be open or encouraged. Some supervisors may poorly define what they expect of you. Some may fail to show up for appointments. Others may delegate their responsibilities to their secretary. There is also the supervisor who is insecure but disguises this insecurity by being overly controlling and autocratic. Some supervisors put too much responsibility on an intern too soon or delegate menial work. Supervisors may be guilty of unethical practices. One supervisor had her supervisee do her work and then wrote up the proceedings as though she had seen the client. Some supervisors misuse power through a need to be seen as always right. Others give little feedback, keeping the student intern in the dark and offering very little direction. Although most supervisors have good intentions and strive to provide quality supervision, many of them feel overwhelmed with the multitude of responsibilities expected of them. This can lead to supervisors not being attentive to those in their charge.

Supervisory roles and functions themselves can be detrimental to efforts to create an open relationship. Supervisors are responsible for your work with clients and will evaluate you. It is understandable that you might be anxious about being observed and evaluated. It may help to accept that performance anxiety goes with the territory of being a supervisee. However, you can face and deal with your fears rather than allowing yourself to be caught up in performance expectations.

If you are very dissatisfied with your supervisor and believe that you are not getting the quality of supervision you have a right to receive, consider discussing this with the supervisor in question as an initial step. If you decide this is not a good alternative, bring the matter to your university supervisor for help in exploring your options.

Informed consent in supervision. Informed consent is a basic part of the supervisory relationship (ACES, 1993, 1995). McCarthy and colleagues (1995) provide a practical guide to **informed consent** in clinical supervision. They conclude that informed consent is an essential ingredient of effective supervision that must be clearly articulated through written documents and a discussion between the supervisor and supervisee. Accountability is increased by developing a written contractual agreement for supervision. When expectations are discussed and clarified at the beginning of a supervisory relationship, the relationship will be enhanced, promoting quality client care. McCarthy and her colleagues identified seven topic areas that are significant to informed consent: purpose, professional disclosure, practical issues, supervision process, administrative issues, ethical and legal issues, and statement of agreement. When these issue areas are addressed in the informed consent process in supervision, both supervisors and supervisees have a clear idea of the nature of their respective roles, rights, and responsibilities. Written informed consent documents, along with a discussion of their contents, are excellent ways for supervisors to teach supervisees an approach they can use with their clients. Written contracts for supervision inform the supervisee of the expectations and responsibilities of both parties in the supervisory relationship and serve to benefit both the supervisor and the supervisee. **Supervisory contracts** can increase the quality of care for the clients of the supervisee as well (Sutter, McPherson, & Geeseman, 2002).

Thomas (2007) reports that it is only in recent years that supervisors have more formally incorporated the principles of informed consent into their work with supervisees. It is now considered the standard of practice to incorporate clear informed consent material for supervisees, both orally and in writing. The goal of informed consent is to enhance the quality of the supervision experience. It is beneficial to discuss the rights of supervisees from the beginning of the supervisory relationship, in much the same way as the rights of clients are addressed early in the therapy process. If this is done, the supervisee is empowered to express expectations, make decisions, and become an active participant in the supervisory process.

Participating in Group Supervision

The value of group supervision is sometimes overlooked. In groups, trainees benefit by listening to others and by discussing cases with their peers as well as with a supervisor. Our approach is to combine individual and group supervision when this is practical and possible. **Group supervision** is a time-efficient and unique format that assists trainees in developing skills in conceptualizing cases and in implementing a variety of treatment interventions. One study suggests that group supervision is not only complementary to individual supervision but may be interchangeable with individual supervision (Ray & Altekruse, 2000). Crespi, Fischetti, and Butler (2001) contend that group supervision, using a case model approach, is a viable way to conduct supervisory sessions with school counselors. Group supervision using audio recordings of a session may be more efficient than individual supervision in terms of rate of learning (Calhoun, Moras, Pilkonis, & Rehm, 1998). Although group supervision will cut into other service responsibilities of school counselors, Calhoun and colleagues (1998) believe group supervision can lead to greater accountability, improve outcomes and, in the long run, be more cost-effective than individual supervision. Like individual supervision, there are various theoretical orientations to group supervision. Melnick and Fall (2008) describe a Gestalt approach to group supervision: "The challenge of group supervision involves the ability to balance the individual and group needs, while at the same time holding the well-being of the client as central" (p. 59).

If you participate in group supervision, you learn not only from your supervisor but also from fellow trainees. You learn that you are not alone with your anxiety and concerns surrounding clinical work, and you are exposed to different perspectives of the helping relationship. You can benefit from learning about issues that other supervisees are facing. This social learning dimension of group supervision can assist you to expand in areas that could be potentially problematic in the future (Brislin & Herbert, 2009). In group supervision you will have many opportunities to role-play challenging clients and to try on a variety of helper roles in a given situation. Role playing offers many possibilities, not only for you to become aware of potential countertransference issues but as a way to acquire alternative perspectives in working with clients you sometimes perceive as being "difficult." You can assume the role of your client by "becoming" the client while the supervisor demonstrates other approaches for dealing with your client. Later, the supervisor can switch roles and become the client while you try another way of dealing with your client. Of course, in a group context your peers can assume various roles, which can enhance learning. Role-playing techniques tend to bring to life a situation that all can witness, as opposed to merely talking about problems with clients.

The group supervision model is enhanced when you make the process a personal one. You can do this by focusing on your own reactions and sharing them in your supervision group. What clients trigger you? What clients do you hope won't show up next week? What clients threaten you? What clients do you like more than others? By focusing on your relationships with your clients and your own dynamics, you can increase your self-awareness through the feedback you get from others in the group.

It is also helpful to explore your values and attitudes in conjunction with your supervision. If you become aware of a tendency to seek gratitude or approval from clients, for example, it could be useful to explore your own need for approval and your fear of rejection, either in your own personal therapy or in a group supervision session.

Multiple Roles and Relationships in Supervision

Those who teach or supervise students in the helping professions have an obligation to trainees to openly discuss appropriate boundaries and to work with trainees to solve problems involved in these multiple roles and relationships. The *Code of Ethics* of the ACA (2005) deals directly and clearly with boundary issues in teaching and supervisory relationships. It is the responsibility of clinical supervisors to create and maintain appropriate relationship boundaries with supervisees. One of these boundary areas pertains to blending supervision and personal therapy. A serious boundary violation occurs when the supervisory relationship becomes sexualized. We consider each of these topics in the sections that follow.

Supervision Versus Personal Therapy

Supervisors play multiple roles in the supervision process, functioning as teachers, consultants, mentors, and at times, counselors. This complexity of roles means that the boundaries are always changing. It may not be possible for supervisors to function in a singular role, so supervisors must demonstrate responsible behavior in managing multiple roles and relationships. The process of supervision has some similarities with instructor–student and therapist–client relationships, but there are also distinctions. The therapeutic role of the supervisor is certainly not the same as the role of the counselor, yet the distinction between these two roles is not always clear. Supervisors should not serve as counselors to supervisees over whom they have administrative, teaching, or evaluative roles *unless* this is a brief role associated with a training experience. The ACES (1993, 1995) ethical guidelines state that "supervisors should not establish a psychotherapeutic relationship as a substitute for supervision. Personal issues should be addressed in supervision only in terms of the impact of these issues on clients and on professional functioning" (2.11).

The primary role of clinical supervision is to maximize a supervisee's ability to become a skilled, competent, and ethical practitioner (Stebnicki, 2008). The central focus of supervision is to protect each client's welfare (Brislin & Herbert,

2009). Because clinical supervision often includes personal and professional concerns that have an impact on the helping relationship, discussion of the supervisee's thoughts and feelings often occurs during a supervision session. Supervisees need to understand that the supervision process can be emotionally charged and challenging (Brislin & Hebert, 2009). It is the supervisor's responsibility to help trainees identify how their personal dynamics are likely to influence their professional work, but it is not the supervisor's task to serve as a personal counselor to supervisees. In the supervisory relationship, it is appropriate to identify a supervisee's personal problems that are interfering with effectively working with clients. However, once a problem is identified and briefly discussed in supervision, it is the responsibility of the trainee to explore this problem area in his or her personal therapy.

One study suggests that exploring supervisees' personal issues in an appropriate manner does not necessarily affect the supervisory relationship negatively. Such supervisors confront their supervisees with personal issues that influence their work with clients, but in a warm and supportive instructional manner. As supervisees gain experience, they may be more able to benefit from identifying and exploring personal issues that affect their relationships with clients (Sumerel & Borders, 1996).

Supervisors are in a good position to recognize some of your blocks and countertransferences. They can help you identify attitudes, feelings, and behaviors that could interfere with your handling of certain clients. If further exploration is needed, and if your difficulties with certain clients are rooted in your own dynamics, a supervisor may encourage you to get involved in personal therapy. This does not mean that you are personally unfit for the profession. Getting involved in the lives of clients is likely to open up some of your own psychological wounds, and unresolved conflicts are likely to surface. We strongly encourage personal therapy along with your supervision as an ideal combination (provided your supervisor and your therapist are not the same person). This arrangement prevents blurring of boundaries and allows the proper focus to be either on working with clients (in supervision) or on dealing with your personal issues (in personal therapy). We address the importance of personal therapy for trainees in more detail in Chapter 3.

When Sex Enters the Supervisory Relationship

Those who are in charge of supervising student trainees must avoid engaging in sexual relationships with trainees and avoid subjecting trainees to any form of sexual harassment. You have a right to expect a learning environment free from sexual harassment, both in the classroom and at your field placement. Ideally, you should not be expected to deal with situations involving unwanted sexual advances from those who function in teaching or supervisory roles. Realistically, however, you need to know what to do in the event that you are faced with sexual harassment. Most agencies and institutions of higher education have specific policies regarding sexual harassment, as well as procedures to follow to report such abuse. Find out what the procedures are at your institution and be prepared to use them should the need arise.

By Way of Review

- Your fieldwork courses are likely to be among the most important experiences you will have in your program. Select these experiences wisely and arrange for diversity in your placements. Realize that these placements can help you decide on your professional specialization.

- Treat your field placement like a job, even if you don't get paid for your internship.

- Don't try to be a perfect intern. Fieldwork experiences are designed to teach you about the skills of helping, and you can learn much from your mistakes.

- Learn how to ask for what you need from your supervisor. It is important that you learn your limits and communicate them to your supervisor.

- Supervisors have different styles, and no one way is right. You can learn a great deal from various supervisors.

- The ideal supervisor may be hard to find. Supervisors are sometimes assigned to this role with little preparation or training. If your supervision is inadequate, be assertive in doing something about it by taking an active stance in asking for what you need from your supervisor.

- Even though supervision is similar to therapy in some ways, there are important differences. Supervision sessions should not evolve into personal therapy sessions. Personal therapy can be a useful adjunct to supervision, but the supervisor and the therapist should not be the same person.

- Sexual relationships between supervisors and supervisees (or professors and students) are unethical because of the harm that they typically do to supervisees (or students). Such relationships represent a clear misuse of power and also confound the supervisory or learning process.

What Will You Do Now?

1. If you have a supervisor (for your fieldwork or in your job), make up a short list of questions that you would like to discuss with him or her. What would you like to gain from supervision? Approach your supervisor before the end of the semester to discuss your goals.

2. Make it a point to visit several community agencies where you might work as an intern. Interview the director of the agency or the supervisors who make decisions about accepting fieldwork students. Learn to ask questions

that will help you select a placement that will teach you about various client populations and a range of problems. Each student in your class could visit just one agency and then present the findings to the rest of the class.

3. Reflect on some of the following issues and use this as a basis for your journal writing. Remember to write whatever comes to mind rather than censoring your thoughts and the flow of your writing.

- Write about the kind of learner you see yourself as being. What does the concept of active learning imply to you? How can you become a more active learner as you read this book and take this course?
- Write about the ideal kind of fieldwork experience you would like to obtain. What can you do to get that kind of field placement?
- If you are already in a field placement, write briefly about the work you are doing. What are your reactions to the staff at the agency? How are you being affected by your clients? Are any personal issues emerging as a result of your work with clients? What are you learning about yourself?
- If you are in supervision currently, what is most satisfying about it? What kind of relationship do you have with your supervisor? What ideas do you have for improving the quality of your supervision sessions?

4. The full bibliographic entry for each of these sources can be found in the References at the back of the book. For a comprehensive book on clinical supervision, see Bernard and Goodyear (2009); for a practical approach to doing and making use of supervision, see Corey, Haynes, Moulton, and Muratori (2010). Useful introductory texts in the human services field include Neukrug (2008) and Woodside and McClam (2009). For a practical and concise guide to the internship experience, see Faiver, Eisengart, and Colonna (2004). Refer to Kiser's (2008) human service internship handbook as a way to get the most from your internship experience, and see Russell-Chapin and Ivey (2004) for useful discussions on how to maximize your supervised practicum and internship experiences. For an excellent treatment of the successful internship, see Sweitzer and King (2009). Refer to Alle-Corliss and Alle-Corliss (2006) for a most useful book on orientation to fieldwork.

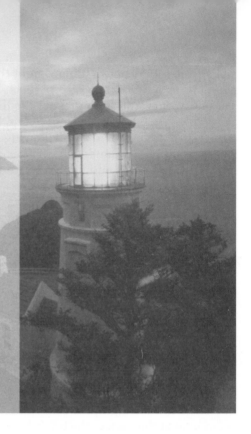

eleven

Stress, Burnout, and Self-Care

Focus Questions

1. To what degree are you willing to seek help from others when you experience difficulties?

2. What are your major stressors, both at home and at work?

3. What specific strategies do you use to cope with stress? Do you effectively manage stress in your personal life? in your professional life?

4. It has been said that either you control stress or stress controls you. How would you apply this maxim to yourself at this time in your life?

5. Are you aware of self-defeating attitudes and beliefs you may hold? To what extent do you engage in self-defeating internal dialogues?

6. If you have experienced burnout, what have you done about it?

7. What do you do to decrease the likelihood that you will experience burnout?

8. How do you retain your vitality, both in your personal and professional life?

9. How satisfied are you with your self-care practices?

10. If you can project yourself one year hence, what are some changes you would most like to make in the way you are taking care of yourself?

Aim of the Chapter

In your career as a professional helper, you may be looking forward to helping people resolve problems they face and to assisting them in dealing constructively with pain in their lives. You may be thinking about the satisfaction that comes with knowing that you can be an agent of change for your clients and that you are taking part in making the world a better place. We support you in your journey to become an effective helper. There are many rewards associated with being a helper, and we hope you bring your enthusiasm and idealism to your work. At the same time, it is important to be aware of the potential stress involved in your work and how these stressors may affect you. The aim of this chapter is to provide some ideas for managing stress more effectively so you can prevent burnout and can develop self-care practices that will keep you vital both personally and professionally.

A major part of this chapter addresses factors that contribute to stress. It is unrealistic to think that you can have a stress-free personal or professional life, but stress can be managed. You can recognize the signs of stress and make decisions about how to think, feel, and behave in stressful situations. You can become aware of ineffective reactions to stress and learn constructive ways of coping with it. In short, you can learn to manage and control stress rather than being controlled by it.

When you become a licensed professional and begin practicing full time, new stresses will emerge from the nature of your work and from professional role expectations. Too often, helpers in a training program are not given enough warning about the potential hazards of the profession. Becoming aware of sources of stress and learning strategies to cope with stress will enable you to maintain your optimism and belief in what you are doing in the service of others.

In this chapter the emphasis is on developing attitudes, thought patterns, and specific action plans to help you maintain your devotion and enthusiasm for your career choice. We also discuss the effects of stress and how prolonged stress can lead to burnout and professional impairment. Retaining vitality as a person and as a professional requires **self-care**, and we address this topic as a basis for utilizing your strengths to deal effectively with the stresses of your work and prevent some of the risk factors leading to burnout. If you read this chapter in a personal way, you can begin to reflect on how you plan to take care of yourself so you can make a significant difference in the lives of others throughout your career.

Individual Sources of Stress for Helpers

The sources of work-related stress for helping professionals fall into two categories: individual and environmental. To understand stress, you must understand both the external realities that tend to produce stress and the ways you contribute to your stress by your perceptions and interpretations of reality.

If you personalize and internalize these stressors, you will diminish your effectiveness as helper.

Individual stressors can be discovered by examining your attitudes and personal characteristics as a helper. Think about client behaviors (as well as behaviors of colleagues and supervisors) that would make the following situations stressful for you. Look over the checklist of behaviors and rate them according to this scale:

1 = This would be *highly stressful* to me.
2 = This would be *moderately stressful* to me.
3 = This would be *mildly stressful* to me.
4 = This would *not be a source of stress* to me.

_____ 1. I am seeing a client who seems unmotivated and is coming to the sessions only because he was ordered to attend.

_____ 2. One of my clients wants to terminate counseling, but I don't think she is ready for termination.

_____ 3. A client is very depressed, sees very little hope that life will get better, yet keeps asking me for help.

_____ 4. One of my clients makes suicidal threats, and I have every reason to take his threats seriously.

_____ 5. A colleague in my agency is upset with me for not adequately supporting her at meetings.

_____ 6. I feel a great sense of identification with a client, almost to the point of overidentifying with him.

_____ 7. A colleague at my agency is frequently critical of my work at case conference meetings.

_____ 8. A client tells me that she (he) is sexually attracted to me, and I am sexually attracted to her (him).

_____ 9. My client is very demanding and wants to call me at home for advice on how to deal with every new problem that arises.

_____ 10. My supervisor at my place of work does not give me the recognition and appreciation that I deserve.

Once you have made your ratings, assess the patterns that emerge. What specific behaviors seem to be the most stressful for you? How does this stress affect you, both on a personal and a professional level?

Cognitive Approaches to Stress Management

Our beliefs largely determine how we interpret events. Therefore, events themselves are not necessarily the cause of our stress; it is the meaning we give to these events that regulates our stress level. **Rational emotive behavior therapy (REBT)** is a theory of personality and psychotherapy that places emphasis on the role thinking plays in influencing feelings and behavior. Albert Ellis, the founder of REBT, cites the Stoic philosopher Epictetus: "Men are disturbed not by things, but by the views that they take of them." **Cognitive therapists** help people become aware of their cognitions—the dialogue that goes on within—and how their thinking affects how they feel and act. The cognitive approaches offer specific strategies to clients for challenging and changing self-defeating cognitions and for developing sound thinking that leads to less stressful living. In this section we draw heavily from the writings of Ellis and other cognitive therapists, especially Aaron Beck, in presenting the strategies cognitive therapists use that can help you manage stress.

We are all prone at some time to engage in self-defeating thinking and ineffective self-talk. If you can recognize the nature of your faulty beliefs and understand how they lead to problems, you can begin to defuse self-defeating cognitions. Because you have the capacity to escalate the stress you experience, you also have the means to lessen it. Cognitive strategies can be employed to retain vitality on both personal and professional levels. In discussing these strategies, our examples are geared primarily to situations that you are likely to encounter in your work as a helping professional.

The A-B-C Theory

Ellis has developed the **A-B-C theory of irrational thinking** (Ellis, 2001b, 2008). This theory explains the relationship among events, beliefs, and feelings. According to Ellis, your interpretations of events are frequently more important than what occurs in reality. He calls *A* an Activating event, *B* one's Belief system, and *C* the emotional Consequence. Consider the situation of going through an interview. Let's imagine the worst outcome: The director of the agency interviewed you and said that you lack the necessary experience for a placement in this agency. You do not get the job you badly wanted. The activating event (A) in this case is the situation of being rejected. The emotional consequences (C) you experience may include feeling depressed, hurt, and maybe even devastated. Chances are that you hold what Ellis would term "irrational beliefs" about not having been accepted. Ellis would say that your beliefs (B) about this rejection might be some combination of the following thoughts: "It is absolutely horrible that I didn't get this job, and it surely proves that I'm incompetent." "I should have gotten this job, and this rejection is unbearable." "I must succeed at every important endeavor, or I'm really worthless." "This rejection means I'm a failure."

REBT and other cognitive-behavioral therapies are grounded on the premise that emotional and behavioral disturbances are originally learned by the incorporation of irrational beliefs from significant others during our childhood, as well as by our own creative invention of inflexible thinking. We actively and continually reinforce these false beliefs by the processes of autosuggestion and self-repetition (Ellis, 1999, 2001b). It is largely our own repetition of these faulty thoughts, rather than a parent's repetition, that keeps dysfunctional attitudes alive within us.

To complete Ellis's (2001b, 2008) A-B-C model, we look briefly at the final element, *D* (Disputing), which is the process of actively and forcefully disputing irrational beliefs. If you are successful in this process of disputing and in substituting constructive thinking for destructive thinking, you have a basis for thinking, feeling, and acting differently. Thus, instead of feeling depressed about a loss, you can put it in a new perspective and feel appropriately disappointed. Instead of feeling devastated by the lack of approval, you can feel appropriately hurt if a significant person rejects you. By changing your beliefs, you also change your feelings, which is a useful way of reducing stress.

Ellis (2001b, 2004b, 2008) contends that we have the power to control our emotional destiny. He suggests that when we are upset it is well to look to our hidden dogmatic "musts" and absolutistic "shoulds." We have the ability to observe how our absolutistic demands and musts largely *create* our destructive feelings and behaviors. We have the power to change these demands into strong *preferences* instead of grandiose, unrealistic commands. Because we have the capacity for self-awareness, we can observe and evaluate our goals and purposes and change them (Ellis, 1999, 2001a, 2001b, 2008; Ellis & Dryden, 1997; Ellis & Harper, 1997; Ellis & MacLaren, 2005).

Identifying Self-Defeating Internal Dialogue

Those of us who are human services providers often incorporate a wide range of dysfunctional beliefs that impair our capacity to function effectively when people seek our assistance. At times we may distort the processing of information, which can easily lead to faulty assumptions and misconceptions. As a helper, you can complicate your life by telling yourself that you *must* be all-knowing and perfect. If you feel depressed or agitated about the job you are doing, it is essential that you examine your basic assumptions and beliefs to determine how they are influencing what you are doing and how you are feeling. As you become more aware of your faulty thinking, you are in a position to change these patterns (Beck, 1976, 1987; Corey, 2009c; Ellis & Dryden, 1997).

Our negative thoughts tend to produce stress. By becoming aware of the quality of our language, we can get some idea of how our self-talk influences us. Here are some examples of negative thinking:

- I *must* act competently in all situations, and I *must* win people's approval.
- If I make a mistake, it proves I am a *failure.*
- I *must* perform well at all times. If I'm ever less than perfect, I am *inadequate.*
- I *should* always put the interests of other people before my own. My job is to help others, and I *shouldn't* be selfish.
- I *ought* to be available when anybody needs me. If I'm not, this shows that I'm not a caring person and that I've probably chosen the wrong profession.
- If a client discontinues, it is *most likely* my fault.
- If clients are in pain, I *should always* be able to alleviate their pain.

Statements such as these can be repeated endlessly in our self-talk, and as you can see, most of these statements refer to feelings of inadequacy, a nagging belief that we should be more, and a chronic sense of self-doubt.

By assuming the major share of responsibility for your clients, you relieve them of the responsibility to direct their own lives, and in addition create stress for yourself. Reread these faulty belief statements, and underline the statements that you hear yourself making. Do you tend to make other related statements, especially with regard to your role in assuming responsibility for being the "perfect" helper? What are some examples of things you say to yourself that create stress for you?

Changing Distorted and Self-Defeating Thinking

Aaron Beck developed an approach known as cognitive therapy, which has a number of similarities to rational emotive behavior therapy. Beck (1976, 1987) contends that people with emotional difficulties tend to commit characteristic "logical errors" that tilt objective reality in the direction of self-deprecation. **Cognitive therapy** perceives psychological problems as stemming from commonplace processes such as faulty thinking, making incorrect inferences on the basis of inadequate or incorrect information, and failing to distinguish between fantasy and reality. A number of systematic errors in reasoning may lead to such faulty assumptions and misconceptions, which are termed **cognitive distortions** (Beck & Weishaar, 2008). Let's examine a few of these errors.

• **Arbitrary inferences** refer to making conclusions without supporting and relevant evidence. This includes "catastrophizing," or thinking of the absolute worst scenario and outcomes for most situations. You might begin your first job as a counselor with the conviction that you will not be liked or valued by either your colleagues or your clients. You may be convinced that you somehow just managed to get your degree, but now you are certain that you do not have the skills to be successful in your profession.

• **Selective abstraction** consists of forming conclusions based on an isolated detail of an event. In this process other information is ignored, and the significance of the total context is missed. The assumption is that the events that matter are those dealing with failure and deprivation. As a counselor, you might measure your worth by your errors and weaknesses, not by your successes.

• **Overgeneralization** is a process of holding extreme beliefs on the basis of a single incident and applying them inappropriately to dissimilar events or settings. If you have difficulty working with one adolescent, for example, you might conclude that you will not be effective in counseling any adolescents. You might also conclude that you will not be effective in working with *any* clients!

• **Magnification** and **minimization** consist of perceiving a case or situation in a greater or lesser light than it truly deserves. You might make this cognitive error by assuming that even minor mistakes you make in counseling a client could easily create a crisis for the individual and might result in psychological damage.

- **Personalization** is a tendency for individuals to relate external events to themselves, even when there is no basis for making this connection. If a client does not return for a second counseling session, you are absolutely convinced that this absence is due to your "inadequate performance" during the initial session. You might tell yourself, "I really let that client down, and now she may never seek help again!"

- **Dichotomous thinking** involves thinking and interpreting in all-or-nothing terms, or categorizing experiences in either/or extremes. You might give yourself no latitude for being an imperfect person and imperfect counselor. You might view yourself as either being the perfectly competent helper or as a total failure if you are not at all times fully competent.

The most direct way to change dysfunctional emotions and behaviors is to modify inaccurate and dysfunctional thinking (Beck, 1976). Cognitive therapy teaches people how to identify their dysfunctional cognitions through a process of evaluation. Through a collaborative effort, individuals learn to discriminate between their own thoughts and events that occur in reality. They learn the influence that cognition has on their feelings and behaviors and even on environmental events. People are taught to recognize, observe, and monitor their own thoughts and assumptions, especially their negative automatic thoughts.

Learning how to answer and to dispute your self-defeating thinking entails identifying your core negative thoughts. Review the common cognitive distortions we have discussed, and think about statements you might be inclined to make that contain these errors. How often do you create stress in yourself with such thoughts? After you have identified a few core self-defeating beliefs, begin to challenge them through vigorous disputation. One method for disputing unfounded beliefs is illustrated in these examples wherein we provide a dysfunctional belief, a disputation, and a constructive belief.

SELF-STATEMENT: I should always be available for anyone who needs me. If I'm not, this shows that I'm not a caring person.
DISPUTATION: Why must I always be available? I must stop telling myself that if I am not always there when a client wants me, I am not a caring person.
CONSTRUCTIVE BELIEF: Although I want to be responsible, I also want to set limits. Sometimes clients want and demand too much.

SELF-STATEMENT: I should be able to do everything well. Either I'm the perfect helper, or I am worthless.
DISPUTATION: Where did I pick up this belief? Does it make any sense that I should always do everything well? Can I do some things less than perfectly and still be outstanding in other areas?
CONSTRUCTIVE BELIEF: Although I like doing well, I can at times accept imperfection in myself. I can tolerate mistakes. I do not have to be perfect to be capable. Perfection is an unrealistic ideal.

SELF-STATEMENT: I should always put the interests of other people before my own.

DISPUTATION: Is it really wrong to be concerned about myself? Can't I have self-interests and still be interested in others?

CONSTRUCTIVE BELIEF: I can't show more interest in others than I have for myself. If I don't take care of myself, the chances are that I'll not be able to help others take care of themselves.

Awareness is the first step in self-change, followed by learning how to deal with self-defeating thinking. However, merely identifying faulty beliefs and learning to make functional statements will not alone ensure change. For change to occur, *action* is essential. You need to test reality and act on your new thoughts and beliefs. For example, assume that you have convinced yourself that your failure to get a certain job does not mean that you are a failure as a person. You can act on this belief by taking the risk of applying for another job that interests you. Rather than avoiding doing new things that you have wanted to do, you might seek out some of these new ventures and take the risk of being less than perfect.

Environmental Sources of Stress for Helpers

In addition to personal, or internal, sources of stress, external factors also can create stress in helpers. **Environmental** sources of stress include the physical aspects of the work setting or the structure of the position itself. A major stressor is the reality of having too much to do in too little time. Other environmental stresses are organizational politics, restrictions imposed by insurance companies, unrealistic demands by the agency, an overwhelming amount of paperwork, critical coworkers, and cutbacks in programs. Since managed care programs have come into existence, helpers experience the stress of addressing critical needs of individual clients and families within a few sessions. Helpers oftentimes feel personally responsible to provide the level of care that is necessary, but they must work within highly restrictive parameters. Attempting to accomplish the impossible in an unrealistically short time can be highly stressful.

Another potential environmental stressor is the quality of your working relationships with colleagues. Dealing with coworkers and supervisors can be a source either of support or of stress. Some of your coworkers may be difficult to get along with because of their negative personality traits or toxic behaviors. Some events can be extremely stressful, such as legal actions, financial pressures, major life transitions, threats of layoffs, and change of job responsibilities. Certain client behaviors, such as suicidal threats or attempts and severe depression, are highly stressful. Other client-induced stresses include anger toward the helper, aggression and hostility, apathy or lack of motivation, a client's premature termination, and lack of client cooperation. Consider the following case as an example of how stress can take its toll on a helper who faces many demands.

Case example: An overburdened counselor. Wendy works in a very busy county social service agency and carries a large caseload. The agency is understaffed, and she is constantly asked to take on more clients than she can adequately attend to. When Wendy is asked to take on extra work, she has a difficult time saying "no." She likes being seen as a hard worker by her colleagues. She skips meals, works overtime to complete paperwork, functions on only a few hours of sleep each night, and worries about how her schedule is affecting her family. At a recent physical examination, Wendy's physician prescribed blood-pressure medication and cautioned that her health is at risk. Although Wendy is aware of her stressful situation, she does not see any way to change it. Her husband is disabled, and she is the sole provider for the family. In addition, her supervisor is also overworked and has no time to deal with Wendy's problems.

Your stance. Consider your own position. If Wendy consulted with you, what would you suggest she do? If you were in Wendy's situation, what would you do? What ethical issues, if any, do you see in this case?

Stress in an Agency Environment

Because you may work for some kind of organization, it is useful to reflect on the major sources of frustration, dissatisfaction, and tension that are likely to be part of this work. Working in an agency setting involves a major commitment on your part, and you need to understand the intricacies of your agency, including its policies and practices. Once you know what the agency is about, it will be easier for you to develop coping strategies for dealing with the demands of being a part of this system (Alle-Corliss & Alle-Corliss, 2006). It helps to look at ways for you to retain your power and vitality within the agency setting. A rehabilitation counselor who works with veterans told us of the stress he experiences as a result of the demands placed on him by his agency to see more clients in a shorter amount of time. He feels pressured to "close a case quickly and efficiently," yet his clients often want more from him than he can give. In fact, he reports that many of his clients see him as uncaring in that he does not give them enough time. What he did not tell his clients was that he would have liked to spend more time with them. Instead, he took on full responsibility for how his clients were reacting, and he typically felt unappreciated by both his staff and his clients. Had he said more to his clients about what he was thinking and feeling, they would have had a basis to perceive him differently.

During the initial years of employment as a professional helper in an organization, it is common to experience a high level of stress and anxiety. Many helpers have reported frustration and disappointment over their job's unexpected stressors and demands. We asked former students who had entered the helping professions to identify some of the main frustrations and stresses they were facing. Most often they identified the slowness of the system, the resistance of administrators and fellow staff members to new ideas, and unrealistic expectations and demands. One woman in her mid-20s made this comment:

> I get frustrated with the slow process of the system. New ideas are often over-looked. My age is a source of frustration when working with other people who will not take me seriously. Because of my age, I sometimes have difficulty gain-ing credibility. My biggest source of dissatisfaction, however, is watching chil-dren that I have worked with and have seen improve go back into the system (or family) and regress to where they started.

A young social worker observed, "My greatest frustration is with the admin-istration and its lack of support, common purpose, or teamwork." And a woman who was managing a volunteer staff of student interns had this to report:

> I am most frustrated when the staff is resistant to new ideas. Dealing with governmental bureaucracy is another major source of stress. They make it very difficult to get things done.

Agencies often make unrealistic demands, especially insisting that prob-lems be solved quickly. For those who work with clients sent by the courts or those on probation, for instance, the helper is under pressure to see that behav-ioral changes take place in a specified time so that more people can be seen, which means more funding.

Organizations tend to make too many demands on workers by restricting their autonomy, by providing little positive feedback for their job performance, and by setting unrealistic policies. Poor management and inadequate supervi-sion are other factors that increase workers' stress.

Retain Power and Vitality

We cannot prescribe a universal method for getting along in the agency where you work. We can, however, present some strategies we have found helpful and ask you to determine how appropriate these strategies are for you. In addition, we ask you to devise your own strategies to cope with the stresses associated with being part of an organization and ways to preserve your indi-viduality.

Your first opportunity to assert your individuality is in the job interview by asking questions about the requirements and expectations of a position. It is important to recognize that accepting a position with an agency entails agreeing to work within a certain philosophical framework. By asking relevant questions, you begin to assume a stance of power: you are exploring how much you want a particular job and what you are willing to sacrifice to get it.

In our experience established organizations tend to resist major attempts at change. Realize that small and subtle changes can be quite significant. When you devote most of your energy to trying to change the people who defend the status quo, your positive programs may become a lesser priority. You will need to decide for yourself how much energy you are willing to expend on dealing with the negative forces you encounter. When you attempt radical, systemwide changes, you may be overwhelmed or paralyzed. If you focus instead on making changes within the scope of your position, you stand a better chance of succeeding.

Study the reasons for the policies of the organization for which you work. Perhaps there are good reasons certain rules have been established, even if they seem more restrictive than necessary. However, if a policy is not in the best interest of your clients, you can begin to question the assumptions on which the policy is based. You can suggest alternative policies, and you can find out whether others on the staff share your view. Forming alliances with colleagues can put you in a better position to bring about change than operating in isolation.

Establish Priorities and Cultivate Support

People often remain powerless because they do not establish priorities and work on them systematically. We have found it helpful to first determine what we *most* want to accomplish in a given position. By reflecting on our priorities, we can decide which compromises we can make without sacrificing our integrity and which positions we are not willing to negotiate. Knowing what we consider to be most important puts us in a much better position to ask for what we want. In addition, good communication with directors and supervisors is essential. Doing this may not be an easy matter, especially when we are expected to juggle a multitude of tasks in an agency setting.

One essential element in learning how to work effectively in any organization is to realize that *you* are a vital part of that system: "The institution" is not something that can be divorced from you. Your relationships with other staff members are a central part of the system, and working with your colleagues will most likely enhance your effectiveness. Colleagues can be nourishing and supportive, and your interactions with them can give you a fresh perspective on some of your activities. Furthermore, genuine relationships with your coworkers can be a way of gaining influence.

Although interactions with others in the institution can be energizing, they can also be debilitating, draining, and a chronic source of stress. Instead of developing support groups within an agency, some people form cliques, harbor unspoken hostility, and generally refuse to confront the conflicts or frictions that keep the staff divided. There are often hidden agendas at staff meetings, resulting in discussion of superficial matters while real issues remain unaddressed. We want to underscore the importance of finding ways to establish working relationships that enrich your professional life instead of draining your energy. If you feel isolated, you can decide to take the initiative and arrange for helpful interactions with others on the staff. There are resources that can nourish you if you reach out for them.

As you answer these questions, think of ways to increase your influence in an organization while remaining true to your principles:

- What experiences have you had in encountering resistance to your ideas?
- What would you do if the organization you worked for instituted some policies to which you were strongly opposed?

- How would you proceed if you believed that some fundamental changes needed to be made in your institution but your colleagues disagreed?
- What would you do if your supervisor continually blocked most of your activities?
- How would you attempt to create collegiality if members of your staff seemed to work largely in isolation from one another?
- If the agency staff seemed to be divided by jealousies, hostilities, or unspoken conflicts, what would you do about the situation?
- Would you leave an agency if you were being asked to do things that are against your basic philosophy? Do you believe it is ethical to continue your association with this agency?

Understanding Stress and Burnout

People in many different careers experience burnout, but those in the helping professions are especially vulnerable because of the nature of their involvement with people in need. If you increase your awareness of the early warning signs of burnout and develop practical strategies for staving it off, you will be better able to respond effectively to the challenges your work presents. When stresses are not coped with effectively, the end result can be burnout. Burnout is the result of severe, prolonged, mismanaged stress.

The Nature of Burnout

Burnout has been described as a state of physical, emotional, and mental exhaustion that results from constant or repeated emotional pressure associated with an intense, long-term involvement with people. It is characterized by feelings of helplessness and hopelessness and by a negative view of self and negative attitudes toward work, life, and other people. Jenaro, Flores, and Arias (2007) describe burnout as "an answer to chronic labor stress that is composed of negative attitudes and feelings toward coworkers and one's job role, as well as feelings of emotional exhaustion" (p. 80). Maslach (2003) identifies burnout as a type of job stress that results in a condition characterized by physical and emotional exhaustion, depersonalization, and a reduction of personal accomplishments. According to Maslach, factors that lead to a path toward burnout are work overload, lack of control, insufficient reward, breakdown of community, unfairness, and significant value conflicts. Burnout results in personal feelings of depression, loss of morale, feelings of isolation, reduced productivity, and a decreased capacity to cope. The problem of burnout is particularly critical for people working in systems or in community agencies and experiencing the stresses associated with this work. With the emphasis in this kind of work on giving to others, there is often not enough focus on self-care.

Skovholt (2001) distinguishes between two kinds of burnout: meaning burnout and caring burnout. If you are experiencing **meaning burnout**, your work in caring for others no longer gives you sufficient meaning and purpose in life. The meaning of your work has been lost, and the existential purpose for your work is not apparent. If you are experiencing **caring burnout**, your professional attachments are draining your energy. Caring burnout is the result of a cumulative depletion of your energy to the extent that you are left without a spark. In addition, helping professionals who observe and work with people who have experienced traumatic events may suffer **compassion fatigue**, a stress-related syndrome that results from the cumulative drain on the helper's capacity to care for others (Figley, 1995). In *Empathy Fatigue: Healing the Mind, Body, and Spirit of Professional Counselors*, Mark Stebnicki (2008) writes about the stress generated by listening to multiple stories of trauma that clients bring to therapy, which may lead to a deterioration of the counselor's resiliency or coping abilities. Stebnicki has coined the term **empathy fatigue**, which shares some similarities with concepts of other fatigue syndromes such as *compassion fatigue, secondary traumatic stress, vicarious traumatization,* and *burnout*. Stebnicki believes that helpers who are psychologically present for their clients often pay the price of being profoundly affected by clients' stories that are saturated with themes of daily stress, grief, loss, anxiety, depression, and traumatic stress. Practitioners who experience *empathy fatigue* may be heading toward professional burnout. To avoid this outcome, Stebnicki states that "developing a clearer understanding of the risk factors and prevention strategies associated with empathy fatigue is pivotal in developing self-care strategies for the professional counselor" (p. 222).

Burnout does not happen suddenly; it is an ongoing process that begins slowly and progresses through several developmental stages. It might be helpful to think of burnout on a continuum rather than in either/or terms. In the beginning of a helping career, you are often motivated by a high sense of idealism. As you experience the inevitable frustrations and stresses of being a professional helper, your idealism tends to wane.

Those who work with people need to see that what they do is worthwhile, yet the nature of their profession is such that they often don't see immediate or concrete results. This lack of reinforcement can have a debilitating effect as counselors begin to wonder whether anything they do makes a difference. The potential for burnout is greater if helpers practice in isolation, have little interchange with fellow professionals, have demanding or disturbed clients, or have few vital interests outside of work. When helpers find it increasingly difficult to be fully present for their clients and catch themselves responding in rehearsed and detached ways, burnout is not far away.

Helpers feel great pressure to do well. Frequently, the lives and welfare of others are intimately connected to the decisions and recommendations they make. All of this work-related stress can result in serious psychological, physical, and behavioral disorders. A growing body of research reveals the negative toll exacted from mental health practitioners in symptoms such as moderate depression, mild anxiety, emotional exhaustion, and disturbed relationships. It is essential to recognize the hazards of the helping endeavor if we hope to develop effective self-care strategies (Norcross, 2000; Norcross & Guy, 2007). A supervisor can play a key role in assisting trainees in developing an ongoing practice of self-assessment and self-care that will reduce their risk of burnout and impairment (Stebnicki, 2008). Those in the helping professions must be vigilant for the signs of burnout and must engage in self-care to ensure that they are not practicing in an impaired state that may harm clients (Tarvydas & Johnston, 2009).

How Crisis Work Can Affect the Helper

Helpers may be called upon to assist people in many different kinds of crisis situations (see Chapter 13 for a discussion of crisis intervention in the community). According to Brown and O'Brien (1998), crisis intervention and other frontline mental health workers experience sources of stress that often lead to burnout. Some of these include lacking full involvement in the decision-making process related to their work; feeling that their abilities are not being fully utilized on the job; being taxed by regulations, procedures, and paperwork; and being exposed to discomfort and dangers in their work setting. The importance of self-care for helpers doing this kind of work cannot be over-emphasized.

One young social worker we know did crisis intervention primarily with the family members of murder victims. Although she showed concern and empathy for her clients, the nature of her work was affecting her negatively to the extent that she was planning to change jobs. Like other crisis workers, she learned that burnout is an occupational hazard.

Joining a group of peers who are also doing crisis intervention is a great way of dealing with the emotions that surface as a result of crisis intervention. If you are carrying around excess psychological pain, the crises of your clients can soon become your crises. It is absolutely essential that you remain sensitive to the ways in which this work is affecting you personally and that you pay attention to what is happening to you. If you forget to take care of yourself or if you delude yourself into thinking that you don't have time for yourself, you can be certain that you will not be able to function very long in the demanding work of helping others through their crises. You will have become stuck in the quagmire of your own crisis.

Some Causes of Burnout

There is no single cause of burnout; rather, it is best understood by considering the individual, interpersonal, and organizational factors that contribute to it. Recognizing the causes of burnout can be the first step toward dealing with it. These situations often lead to burnout:

- Doing the same type of work with little variation
- Giving a great deal personally and not getting back much in the way of appreciation or other positive responses
- Lacking a sense of accomplishment and meaning in your work
- Being under constant and strong pressure to produce, perform, and meet deadlines—many of which may be unrealistic

- Working with a difficult population, such as highly resistant clients, involuntary clients, or those who show very little progress or change
- Continuing conflict and tension among staff; an absence of support from colleagues and an abundance of criticism
- Lacking trusting relationships between supervisors and workers, creating conflict rather than teamwork toward commonly valued goals
- Lacking opportunities for personal expression or for taking initiative in trying new approaches; a situation in which experimentation, change, and innovations not only are not rewarded but are actively discouraged
- Continuing dissatisfaction with agency goals and few opportunities to create new goals
- Providing substandard services to clients
- Having unrealistic demands on your time and energy
- Having personally and professionally taxing work without much opportunity for supervision, continuing education, or other forms of in-service training
- Experiencing unresolved personal conflicts beyond the job situation, such as marital tensions or chronic health or financial problems

Individual Factors Contributing to Burnout

Helpers play a role in creating their own burnout. Certain personality traits and characteristics can increase your risk for burnout. Some individual factors such as a compelling need for approval, feeling unappreciated, and striving for unrealistically high goals can increase your risk for burnout.

Feeling needed. In Chapter 1 we talked about the helper's need to be needed. This need can work for or against you. There is a considerable expenditure of energy in thinking about and taking care of those who need you. As you are starting out and building a practice, you may be flattered that people seek your help. Indeed, it feels affirming to be sought after and needed. Some helpers have a difficult time taking a vacation, especially when they are convinced that their clients cannot function without them. These helpers forget that they, too, have needs, which are probably not being met because their involvement and commitment to others has overwhelmed their life. There are limits to how much you can take on without paying a price in terms of your physical, mental, and emotional health.

Feeling unappreciated. A major theme heard by those who are suffering from burnout is that they do not feel recognized for who they are or what they do, that they receive little positive feedback, and that they do not feel that their dedication is appreciated. You may be sincerely devoted to helping others, yet your efforts may seem meager at times. You will hear more often about what you are failing to do and about your deficiencies than about what you have done well. If appreciation is lacking on the job, it is difficult over a period of time to know whether what you are doing really makes a difference to anyone. This process tends to erode both your ideals and your enthusiasm, which leads to demoralization.

Feeling overwhelmed. At times you may be expected to carry a heavy workload, and the demands to see more clients, to provide an increasing number of services, and to do more in less time can contribute to a sense of disillusionment. Caseloads may be unrealistically high in some agencies, and no matter how efficient you are, it may not be possible to do all that is expected of you. You may feel alone and isolated and believe that nobody understands or cares.

Feeling discouraged. An important factor in burnout is whether your ideals are working for or against you. In our experience, those who set unrealistically high goals for themselves also tend to have high expectations of others. As long as helpers feel satisfied by their efforts, their energy level remains high. Most health professionals were initially attracted to their careers in large part because of their hope of making a significant difference in the lives of others. One sign of burnout is the dulling of these ideals and the loss of involvement and passion. When helpers' efforts are not recognized, they are likely to become discouraged.

The problem of tarnished idealism increases as you come into contact with cynical colleagues who are threatened by your enthusiasm. It is difficult to stay creative and excited when those around you are continually undermining your efforts to make a difference. If you constantly hear that your proposals for change won't work and if you are without real support for your ideas, your belief that you can make a difference may disappear. If you receive an abundance of negative reactions from others, you may become self-critical and wonder whether you are making any difference to those you are supposedly helping. Being critical of and unkind to yourself usually leads to being critical of and unkind to others.

If you work in a toxic environment, you would do well to actively seek some source of support either in your job setting or away from it. It is not likely that the agency will create this support for you. You could ask colleagues to join you in making the time for regular meetings aimed at providing mutual support. Learning to balance idealism with realism is essential for survival as a helping professional.

Interpersonal and Organizational Factors Contributing to Burnout

Maslach and Leiter (1997) focus on the organizational factors, or the social environment, as the primary cause of burnout. The hallmark of the burnout syndrome is a shift in the way professionals view the people they are helping. They change from feeling positive and caring to feeling negative and uncaring. Continuous contact with clients who are unappreciative, upset, and depressed often leads helpers to view all recipients in helping relationships in negative terms. Practitioners may care less, begin to make derogatory comments about their clients, ignore them, and want to move away from them. Dehumanized responses are a core ingredient of burnout.

According to Maslach and Leiter (1997), organizations have the power and the resources to do a great deal to prevent burnout. For example, agencies can provide child care at the job site, create support groups, offer counseling for staff members, and give workers opportunities for physical exercise during breaks. By creating a positive work environment, organizations can enhance worker productivity. Organizations that allow practitioners some degree of job autonomy, self-direction, and independence will decrease and prevent the risk of organizational burnout (Riggar, 2009). When helpers feel that the organization is concerned for their well-being, they tend to have positive feelings about themselves and others in their workplace.

The Impaired Professional

Burnout is a major contributor to the making of an impaired practitioner. Guy (1987) defines **impairment** as the "diminution or deterioration of therapeutic skills and abilities due to factors which have sufficiently impacted the personality of the therapist to result in potential incompetence" (p. 199). Impairment can also be viewed as the presence of an illness or severe psychological depletion that is likely to block a professional from being able to deliver effective services, which results in the helper consistently functioning below acceptable practice standards. A number of other factors can negatively influence a professional's effectiveness, both personally and professionally, including addictions, substance abuse, and physical illness. **Impaired professionals** are unable to effectively cope with stressful events, and they are unable to adequately carry out their professional duties. Those practitioners whose inner conflicts are consistently activated by client material may respond by trying to stabilize themselves rather than facilitating the growth of their clients.

Impaired practitioners clearly contribute to the suffering of their clients rather than alleviating it. For example, sexually exploitive behavior by counselors is often a manifestation of impairment (Emerson & Markos, 1996). Counselors who become sexually involved with clients show personality patterns similar to those of impaired counselors. These shared characteristics include fragile self-esteem, difficulty establishing intimacy in one's personal life, professional isolation, a need to rescue clients, a need for reassurance about one's attractiveness, and substance abuse.

Because a common characteristic of impairment is denial, professional colleagues may need to confront the behavior of an impaired counselor. Herlihy (1996) suggests confronting the impaired counselor with sensitivity, respect, and preparedness. Caring colleagues can be instrumental in helping impaired practitioners break through their denial. We see it as ethically imperative that impaired professionals recognize and deal with their impairment. Ideally, practitioners themselves will realize that they need help and take steps to deal with problems that are keeping them stuck in dysfunctional patterns.

Most ethics codes of the various professions specifically address the ethical dimensions of professional impairment. Here are three examples, drawn from marriage and family therapy, social work, and counseling:

American Association for Marriage and Family Therapy (2001a)

Marriage and family therapists seek appropriate professional assistance for their personal problems or conflicts that may impair work performance or clinical judgment. (3.3.)

National Association of Social Workers (2008)

Social workers whose personal problems, psychosocial distress, legal problems, substance abuse, or mental health difficulties interfere with their professional judgment and performance should immediately seek consultation and take appropriate remedial action by seeking professional help, making adjustments in workload, terminating practice, or taking any other steps necessary to protect clients and others. (4.05.b.)

American Counseling Association (2005)

Counselors are alert to the signs of impairment from their own physical, mental, or emotional problems and refrain from offering or providing professional services when such impairment is likely to harm a client or others. They seek assistance for problems which reach the level of professional impairment and, if necessary, they limit, suspend, or terminate their professional responsibilities until such time it is determined that they may safely resume their work. (C.2.g.)

Monitor Yourself to Prevent Burnout

Professional burnout is an internal phenomenon that becomes obvious to others only in its advanced stages; therefore, you should take special care to recognize your own limits. How you approach your tasks and what you get from doing them are more important than how much you are doing. Ultimately, whether you experience burnout depends on how well you monitor the effects that the stresses of your work have on you and the choices you make to deal with stress both internally and externally.

Many paths are available to combat burnout and prevent impairment. You can do much personally to lessen the chances of becoming impaired or to restore yourself. You do not need to do this alone; reach out to your colleagues as a source of support. In addition, explore the valuable resources your agency may have available to help you maintain your effectiveness. Maslach and Leiter (1997) point out the steep costs of burnout for the organization. When burnout reaches the stage of a full-blown problem, treatment is difficult and an organization is faced with major damage control. From Maslach and Leiter's perspective, preventive measures by an organization are wise and prudent investments in the future of that organization. By making this investment in the present, the costs and losses of burnout are forestalled.

Taking Action to Change

If you hope to prevent stress from controlling you, it is imperative that you take an active stance in recognizing how your stresses lead to personal depletion and how they eventually lead to burnout. If you give of yourself continually and ignore the signs of stress and the toll it is taking, you will eventually find that you have nothing to give. You cannot give and give without replenishing your reserve. But simply recognizing that you cannot be a universal giver is not enough; you need an action plan and the commitment to carry out this plan. Make some decisions about specific ways you can better manage stress in your life. Monitor how you are affected by stress, and follow up by applying some of the stress management strategies we have discussed.

For an excellent discussion of how to deal with and prevent burnout and begin a program of self-care, we recommend *Empathy Fatigue: Healing the Mind, Body, and Spirit of Professional Counselors* (Stebnicki, 2008).

You Have Control Over Yourself

We have suggested that to a large extent you contribute to creating your own stress by the interpretation you give to events. Although you cannot always control these events, you can control how you respond to them and the stance you take toward them. Become attuned to the warning signals that you are being depleted, and take seriously your own need for nurturing and for recognition. What follows are some thoughts on what you can do not only to prevent burnout but to take good care of yourself.

• Examine your behavior to determine if it is working for you. Ask yourself these questions: "Is what I am doing what I really want to be doing? If not, why am I continuing in this direction?" "What are some things I want to be doing professionally that I am not doing? Who or what is stopping me?" Once you have answered some of these questions, decide what action to take.

• Look at your expectations to determine whether they are realistic. It is essential to temper your ideals with reality if you are to avoid continual frustration.

• You may expect that you can be all things to all people, and you must always to be available for anyone who needs you. Regardless of how much you have to offer others, there is a limit to what you can give and what clients will accept. Identify your limits and learn to work within them.

• Find other sources of meaning besides work. These activities and interests can help you at least temporarily escape from job stresses and develop some balance in your life.

• There may be some unpleasant aspects of your job that are difficult to change, but you can approach your work differently. Find some way to rearrange your schedule to reduce your stress.

• It is easy to become overwhelmed by thinking of all the things that you feel powerless to change. Instead, focus on the aspects of your work that you have the power to change.

• Colleagues who face the same realities as you on the job can provide you with new information, insights, and perspectives. The companionship of colleagues can be a great asset. Take the initiative and create a support group so that your colleagues can listen to one another and provide help.

• Recognize the early signs of burnout and take remedial action. It is best to direct your energies toward preventing this condition.

The real challenge is to learn ways to structure your life so that you can prevent burnout. Prevention is much easier than trying to cure a condition of severe physical and psychological depletion. An important prevention measure to lessen the chance of burnout is to seek diversity in your personal life and in your professional work. By engaging in diverse personal and professional activities, you have a good chance of bringing vitality to your work.

A couple, both social workers, remind themselves continually not to become overwhelmed by myriad demands and not to lose sight of why they are in the agency. They accept that they cannot do everything they want to do. They are creative in finding ways to vary their activities. They work with children and adults, co-lead groups, supervise interns and professionals, teach, administer programs, and give in-service presentations. They attempt to develop a tolerant perspective when the agency acts in a petty way, which they do partly by keeping a sense of humor. They both assess their priorities and maintain limits. To be sure, this is not a simple matter; it involves a commitment to self-assessment and an openness to change.

Staying Alive Personally and Professionally

What can you do to promote your wellness from a holistic perspective? To retain your vitality as a person and as a professional, you must first realize that there are limits to your ability to give to others. Skovholt (2001) notes that those in the helping professions are experts at one-way caring. He warns of the drawbacks involved if one-way caring relationships are characteristic of helpers' personal lives, and he encourages helpers to learn to nurture the personal self. Skovholt points out that self-care involves finding ways to replenish the self: "Personal self-care should focus in part on producing feelings of zest, peace, euphoria, excitement, happiness, and pleasure" (p. 147). Norcross and Guy (2007) state that "self-care is not a narcissistic luxury to be fulfilled as time permits; it is a human requisite, a clinical necessity, and an ethical imperative" (p. 14). Self-care is best viewed as an ongoing preventive activity (Barnett, Baker, Elman, & Schoener, 2007), and it should be a priority for all helpers.

In *Caring for Ourselves: A Therapist's Guide to Personal and Professional Well-Being,* Baker (2003) emphasizes the importance of tending to all facets of our being. This involves paying attention to and being respectful of our needs, which is a lifelong task for mental health professionals. Baker makes the point that for us to have enough to share with others in our personal and professional lives, we need to nourish ourselves. It will be difficult to maintain our vitality if we do not find ways to consistently tend to our whole being.

Rather than thinking in terms of avoiding burnout and impairment, think in terms of taking care of yourself and in striving for wellness. In their study of the characteristics of well-functioning mental health professionals, Coster and Schwebel (1997) surveyed experienced professional psychologists who identified factors that contributed to their ability to function well. The dimensions that were most often mentioned included self-awareness and monitoring; support from peers, spouses, friends, mentors, and colleagues; values; and a balanced life that allowed time for family and friends. Well people are committed to creating a lifestyle that contributes to taking care of their physical selves, challenging themselves intellectually, expressing the full range of their emotions, finding rewarding interpersonal relationships, and searching for a meaning that will give direction to their lives. This holistic approach to well-being requires that we pay attention to the specific aspects of our lifestyle, including how we work and play, how we relax, how and what we eat, how we think and feel, how we keep physically fit, our relationships with others, our values and beliefs, and our spiritual needs. To the degree that we ignore or neglect one or more of these areas, we pay a price in terms of optimal functioning.

One model of wellness that can be applied to practitioners in the helping professions is provided by Myers, Sweeney, and Witmer (2000), who define **wellness** as "a way of life oriented toward optimal health and well-being in which body, mind, and spirit are integrated by the individual to live more fully within the human and natural community. Myers and Sweeney (2005b) believe that high-level wellness is the result of deliberate, conscious choices that are made every day to maintain a lifestyle of tending to the body, mind, and spirit. In their model of the wheel of wellness, Myers and Sweeney (2005c) borrow from the Adlerian perspective and identify five life tasks that are a basic part of healthy functioning: spirituality, self-direction, work and leisure, friendship, and love. We briefly describe each of these components and raise some questions for you to apply to yourself.

- *Spirituality* is an awareness of a being or force that goes beyond the material dimension and gives a deep sense of wholeness or connectedness to the universe. What does spirituality mean to you?

- *Self-direction* involves a sense of mindfulness and intentionality in meeting major life tasks. Meyers and colleagues list a sense of worth, healthy sense of control, realistic beliefs, emotional awareness and coping, problem solving and creativity, sense of humor, nutrition, exercise, self-care, gender identity, and cultural identity as components of self-direction. What value do you place on each of these life tasks?

• *Work and leisure* (or unstructured time) provide a sense of accomplishment. If you were to analyze your weekly activities, what kind of balance would you find between work and leisure?

• *Friendship* incorporates all of one's social relationships that involve a connection with others. Do you have the kind of friends that you want? Are your friendships nourishing you?

• *Love* involves long-term, intimate, trusting, compassionate, and mutually committed relationships. Do you have a quality love relationship in your life? To what degree does that relationship nourish you emotionally?

Self-care is vital to optimal and effective functioning. Learning to cope with personal and professional sources of stress generally involves making some fundamental changes in your lifestyle. At this point, take some time to ask yourself what basic changes, if any, you want to make to promote your wellness.

Your Personal Strategy for Self-Care

You need to find your own way of remaining vital as a professional. Use the following suggestions to stimulate you to think of additional methods of preventing or treating burnout. After you think about each suggestion, rate each one using the following code:

3 = This approach would be *very meaningful* to me.
2 = This approach would have *some value* for me.
1 = This approach would have *little value* for me.

____ 1. Pursue paths to self-care such as meditation, deep relaxation, yoga, and therapeutic massage.
____ 2. Become involved in peer group meetings where a support system is available.
____ 3. Find other interests besides my work.
____ 4. Attend to my health, and take care of my body by exercising and eating well.
____ 5. Determine whether what I am doing is meaningful or draining.
____ 6. Do some of the things now that I plan to do when I retire.
____ 7. Take time for myself to do some of the things that I enjoy.
____ 8. Get involved in some type of personal therapy.
____ 9. Read stimulating books, and do some personal writing.
____ 10. Vary the activities in my work environment.
____ 11. Find nourishment with family and friends.
____ 12. Take short focusing and relaxing breaks during the day.
____ 13. Make time for my spiritual development.
____ 14. Rearrange my schedule to reduce stress.

_____ 15. Learn my limits, and learn to set limits with others.
_____ 16. Do things I truly enjoy.
_____ 17. Begin new projects that have meaning to me.

Keep in mind that burnout is a cumulative process. Recognizing that you are on a path toward impairment demands a high level of honesty. You need to be alert to subtle indications and then be willing to take action to remedy a situation that will inevitably result in burnout. Reflect on ways in which you can take care of yourself as well as being a helper to others. We cannot stress enough how important it is that you act on the awareness you have gained from your reflections. We encourage you to spend some time creating an action plan and make a commitment to carry out your plan.

Our Personal Experiences With Self-Care

We would like to share with you our own struggles with burnout and some measures we use to take care of ourselves. First of all, even though we are aware of the dangers of burnout, we are not immune to it. At different times throughout our professional lives we have wondered about the meaning of our work. We have come to realize that the answer does not lie merely in cutting out activities that we don't enjoy. Much of what we do professionally we like very much, and we have to remind ourselves that we cannot accept all the attractive projects that may interest us. The psychological and financial rewards, however high and tempting, do not always compensate for the emotional and physical depletion that results from an overscheduled professional life. For example, we scheduled too many counseling groups in a given year. Although these groups were professionally rewarding, it took a great deal of energy to organize and facilitate them. We eventually began to reduce the number of groups we conducted. In another instance we became aware that too many of our "vacations" were coupled with professional commitments such as giving a workshop or attending a convention. Although we see this mixture as a good balance, we nevertheless realized that we missed real vacations that were separate from any professional commitments.

Another way in which we attempt to prevent burnout and to take care of ourselves is to pay attention to the early signals that we are overextending ourselves, and we involve ourselves in diverse projects. We engage in a variety of professional tasks, all of which are enjoyable and rewarding to us, yet we had to learn that we could not do all of them at the same time. Besides offering our services to others, we recognize our need for input from others in the field, and we attend workshops for our own personal and professional development. Being aware of the demands that our profession puts on us, we are highly conscious of living a healthy lifestyle. Therefore, we pay attention to our nutritional habits, and no matter how busy we are, we make the time that we need for adequate rest and regular exercise. As part of our lifestyle, we made the decision to live in a remote mountain community. But this remoteness and our busy schedules kept us, at times, from seeing our friends and colleagues. We had to realize that we could easily separate ourselves too much from relationships that were much needed and a source of joy and support for us. Thus, we made extra efforts to schedule blocks of time with our friends and to maintain and to nourish these valued relationships.

By Way of Review

- One of the hazards of the helping professions is that helpers are typically not very good at asking for help for themselves.

- Sensitize yourself to both the external and internal factors that contribute to your experience of stress.

- It is next to impossible to eliminate stress from your life; the crucial question is, "Does stress control you, or do you control stress?"

- Self-monitoring is the first step in developing an effective stress management program. If you recognize situations that lead to stress, you can make decisions about how to think, feel, and behave in response to these situations.

- Some of the most useful ways of managing stress are the cognitive approaches. These include changing your distorted self-talk, learning time management skills, and applying them to daily life in a systematic fashion.

- Learning to recognize and cope with the reality of professional burnout is essential for your survival as a helper. Intense involvement with people over a period of time can lead to physical and psychological exhaustion.

- There is no single cause of burnout; rather, a combination of individual, interpersonal, and organizational factors lead to burnout. Understanding these factors can help you learn how to prevent or cope with burnout.

- Burnout can be the result of the many demands placed on you by an agency. It is important to learn specific ways of surviving with dignity in an agency setting.

- Just as there are many sources of burnout, there are multiple ways to prevent and combat it.

- Coping with stress effectively is a way to lessen the chances of becoming an impaired helper.

What Will You Do Now?

1. Make a list of some of the environmental factors that are most stressful in your life. Once you have identified external stressors, write in your journal about how you might deal with them differently. What can you do now to minimize at

least some of these sources of stress? Develop a plan of action, and try it out for at least a week. Consider making a contract with someone so that you will be accountable for acting to reduce stress in your life.

2. Identify a few of the warning signs that you are not taking care of yourself. What are some specific steps that you are willing to consider in taking better care of yourself?

3. Reflect on the patterns of stress you experience in your life. Think about your responses to the sources-of-stress checklist and the other information presented in this chapter. How does stress affect your life? What are you willing to do to cope with these sources of stress? In your journal, keep track of some stressful activities for a few weeks.

4. We encourage you to look at the factors in you that are most likely to cause burnout. A common denominator in many cases of burnout is the question of *responsibility*. In what ways could your assumption of an inordinate degree of responsibility contribute to burnout?

5. If you have trouble doing everything that you want with the time you have available, consider trying the time management strategies described. Keep a written record of what you do in the coming week. At the end of the week, add up the hours you are spending on personal, social, job, and academic activities. Review your activities, and ask yourself if you are spending the time you have in the ways you want.

6. Arrange an interview with a practicing professional, and ask this person these questions: "What are some of the major stresses you face in your work?" "What are some ways you deal with these stresses?" "What are your thoughts on preventing burnout?"

7. Self-care and self-renewal involve a balanced attention to our physical, emotional, mental, social, and spiritual dimensions. Identify some specific ways you can achieve greater balance in your life to continue your self-renewal process. In your journal, write down some ideas about patterns that you may want to change to enhance the balance in your life. Then make an action plan that will assist you in coping with stress by using some of the preventive and combative strategies discussed in this chapter.

8. For the full bibliographic entry for each of the sources listed here, consult the References at the back of the book. One of the best single sources on burnout and self-care strategies is Skovholt's (2001) book, *The Resilient Practitioner*. See Kottler (1993, 2000a) and Guy (1987) for discussions of how stress affects the personal and professional lives of helpers. For a comprehensive presentation on research and practical clinical skills to manage stress and enhance well-being, see Luskin and Pelletier (2005). For two well-written books on self-care, see Baker (2003) and Norcross and Guy (2007). For an

excellent treatment of empathy fatigue and what you can do to prevent it, see Stebnicki (2008). See George (1998) for a practical guidebook for coping with stress. See G. Corey and M. Corey (2010) for ideas on self-renewal and retaining your vitality. See Ellis (2000, 2001a, 2001b) for cognitive techniques for learning how to dispute dysfunctional beliefs that often lead to stress. For ways of applying cognitive behavioral techniques to your own life, see Ellis (2004a, 2004b).

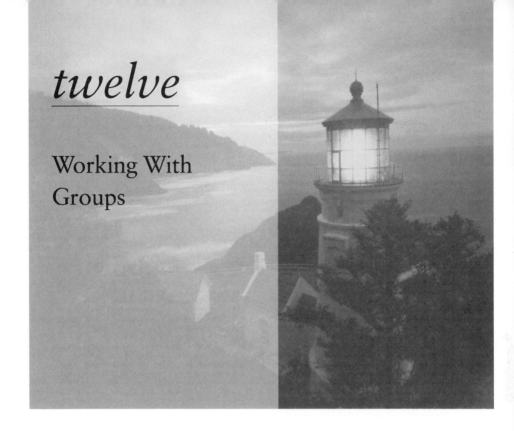

twelve

Working With Groups

Focus Questions

1. Have you participated in a therapeutic group? If so, what was this experience like for you? What did it teach you about groups? about leading groups? about being a member? about yourself?

2. What value do you see in group work for meeting the needs of the various client populations that you hope to serve?

3. What kind of group would you most like to organize? What would be your goals for the group?

4. What specific actions would you take to start your group? What colleagues or other sources would you consult to get this group started?

5. How prepared are you to lead or co-lead a group? What personal qualities do you have that could help or hinder you as a group leader? What knowledge and skills do you possess that will enhance your ability to lead groups? What do you still need to learn?

6. What kind of person would you select to co-lead a group with you? What characteristics would you look for?

7. What ethical issues might you face in setting up or facilitating a group?

8. What are your thoughts about how to work effectively with diversity in a group?

9. What do you think are the most important tasks a group leader needs to accomplish with a group during the early stages of a group's development?

10. What would you see as being a critical task for a group to accomplish prior to termination of the group?

Aim of the Chapter

Group work is recognized as the appropriate modality to be used most frequently by school counselors and in agency settings for a variety of client populations. Your supervisor or the director of your agency may ask you to start a specific kind of group. You may feel unprepared to organize and lead a group, or you may be unclear about the value of groups for special client populations. The main purpose of this chapter is to introduce you to the distinct values of group work. We present a perspective on group process and provide an introduction to how groups can be useful in various settings. We discuss the skills you will need to organize and facilitate groups for the diverse client populations you will serve. This chapter provides an overview of group work, but it is not sufficient to equip you to lead groups on your own without supervision from a person who is skilled in doing group work. This chapter also aims at discussing some of the merits of your becoming involved as a member in a therapeutic group.

Group Work as the Treatment of Choice

In the past two decades, group work has been enjoying a resurgence of interest. In the 1960s and 1970s encounter groups and personal-growth groups were considered one pathway for making human connections and for moving toward greater self-actualization. Today the focus has changed, and structured groups for specific client populations seem to be most in demand. The benefits of therapeutic groups are being increasingly recognized in mental health settings, and they are becoming more widely used for a variety purposes (Piper, 2001). Short-term groups are the treatment of choice for certain types of problems, such as complicated grief, trauma reactions, adjustment problems, and existential concerns (Piper & Ogrodniczuk, 2004). Barlow (2008) reports that group therapy is no longer viewed as a second-choice form of treatment; it is as effective as individual treatment and, in some cases, is more effective.

Group therapy fits well into the managed care scene because groups can be designed to provide brief, cost-effective treatments. In this setting, the group is definitely time limited, and the group will have fairly narrow goals. Many time-limited groups are aimed at symptomatic relief, teaching participants problem-solving strategies and interpersonal skills.

The interpersonal learning that occurs in groups can accelerate personal changes, but groups do not represent the only approach to helping clients to understand and cope with their problems. Practitioners need to assess whether clients are better served in a group or in individual therapy. In some cases, groups may be the most appropriate intervention in a client's life. In other cases, group work may be used as a supplementary form of treatment or as the next step a client takes after completing some individual counseling. From our perspective, groups are the treatment of choice for many client populations. Groups are highly effective, and they offer unique opportunities for new learning. Groups have the power to move people in creative and more life-giving directions. Most client populations can benefit from a properly designed group with a qualified leader or co-leaders, a topic we discuss in more detail later in this chapter.

The Value of Group Work

Many of the problems for which people seek professional assistance are interpersonally rooted. People experience difficulties in forming and maintaining intimate relationships, and they sometimes feel they have few options for changing their predictable patterns. They may be at a loss in how to live well with the ones they love. Groups provide a natural laboratory that demonstrates to people that they are not alone and that skills for interpersonal living can be learned. Groups provide a sense of community, which can be an antidote to the impersonal culture in which many individuals live. Groups are powerful because participants can experience some of their long-term problems being played out in the group sessions. At the same time, a group gives members opportunities to design and try out more effective ways of behaving.

Through the unfolding of the group process, members observe how others interact, and they learn something about themselves by joining in the interaction. The group experience serves as a living laboratory; it becomes a mirror in which members see themselves as they are. For instance, Luigi tends to keep himself isolated in the group, and in many ways he makes it difficult for others to get close to him. Through the feedback of other members and the leader, he has a chance to learn about his part in contributing to his own isolation, not only in the group but also in his everyday life. The safety of the group affords him opportunities to experiment with being different. Instead of ignoring his feelings, he can begin to express them. Rather than being immediately defensive, he can open himself to really hearing others. He can experiment with reaching out to others and asking for what he wants. Others in the group profit from Luigi's work because it enables them to understand the ways they are like him.

Groups offer a forum in which members reveal their confusion, anger, helplessness, guilt, resentment, depression, and anxiety. By expressing and exploring their feelings, members are able to see the similarity of human struggles. Those group members who have difficulty in expressing their feelings are likely to learn by listening to others who are able to express the range of their emotions. For example, Carola has adopted a stoic attitude, thinking that her situation will be more tolerable if she contains her feelings. She may not realize the stress to which she is subjecting herself by doing this. As she begins to express her concerns, she may realize that others experience some of her pain and that she is not alone in the way she feels. Her sharing can help lower the walls that keep her isolated.

Some universal human themes typically become apparent through a group experience. In addition, the differences that do exist within the group can become catalysts for growth among group members. Clients may be separated by differences in age, gender, ability, sexual orientation, social and cultural background, worldview, and life experience. Yet as people risk revealing their deeper concerns and feelings, they begin to recognize similarities with other group members. Although the circumstances leading to pain over disappointment may be different for each person, the emotions associated with certain events have a universal quality.

In groups composed of people with a common concern, such as a support group for women survivors of incest, the shared feelings are often even more intense. Before joining the support group, they probably felt alone in their feelings of hurt, sadness, fright, guilt, resentment, and anger. As each woman reveals her story and her feelings about her situation, others are able to identify and come to understand a pattern that unites them. The bonding that builds within the group creates an atmosphere in which women can see more clearly how they have been affected by incest. It also leads to insights into how their earlier experiences have set the stage for the way they now think, feel, and behave. Members are often at different stages in their healing process, and the group allows members to see what they have achieved and where they can do more work.

Groups offer hope to members that a different kind of life is possible. For example, groups for people who admit that their lives are out of control when they abuse alcohol offer steps leading to recovery. When these clients were abusing substances, they believed that they were powerless to change, and they were without hope. But the modeling of others who are learning to take control of their lives one day at a time is living proof that there is hope for a better life. Having hope that change is possible can lead individuals to significant lifestyle changes; Alcoholics Anonymous is one example of this idea in action.

The acceptance that develops in a group can be a powerful healing force. In a group for children of divorce, compassion and support are given not only by the leader but also by other children. Individuals within this group are able to be vulnerable when they sense that what concerns them has importance for others too.

A distinct advantage of groups is the opportunity for learning from the feedback of many others. If reactions are given with sensitivity and respect, members come to realize the ways in which their behavior affects others. The process of interpersonal feedback shows people how they contribute to both favorable and unfavorable outcomes, and it also gives them new possibilities for relating to others.

The Various Types of Groups

The various kinds of groups differ with respect to goals, techniques used, the role of the leader, training requirements, and the people involved. The range of groups designed to help people cope with specific problems or those aimed at particular client populations is limited only by a practitioner's imagination. We find that such special groups are mushrooming and that they frequently arise from the needs of a particular group or from the interests of the professional who is designing them.

Many groups have both an educational and a therapeutic dimension. These groups are often short term, have some degree of structure, deal with a particular population, and focus on a specific theme. They can serve a number of purposes, such as giving information, sharing common concerns, teaching coping skills, helping people practice better ways of interpersonal communication, teaching problem-solving techniques, and assisting people once they leave the group.

Eventually, as a part of your job as a professional helper, you may be asked to set up and lead one or more groups. Depending on the age and population with which you work, you are likely to find yourself looking for resources to help you design a group. Many creative groups have been designed to meet the special needs of particular populations.

Structured groups, sometimes referred to as **psychoeducational groups,** generally have an educational focus and are designed to deal with an information deficit in a certain area. The aim of such groups is to prevent an array of educational deficits and psychological problems. New information is incorporated through the use of planned skill-building exercises. A few examples of psychoeducational groups are stress management, learning coping skills, managing relationships and ending relationships, and parenting skills groups.

Another type of group is the **counseling group,** which focuses on interpersonal process and problem-solving strategies and attends to conscious thoughts, feelings, and behavior. A counseling group helps participants resolve problems in living or dealing with developmental concerns. This kind of group also uses interactive feedback and support methods in a here-and-now time frame. Members of a counseling group are guided in understanding the interpersonal nature of their problems. With an emphasis on discovering inner personal strengths and constructively dealing with barriers that are preventing optimal development, members develop interpersonal skills that enable them to better cope with both current difficulties and future problems.

The counseling group becomes a microcosm of society, with a membership that is diverse but that shares common problems. The group process provides a sample of reality, with the struggles that people experience in the group resembling their conflicts in daily life. Participants learn to respect differences in cultures and values and discover that, on a deep level, they are more alike than different. Although participants' individual circumstances may differ, their pain and struggles are often similar.

In reality, the kinds of groups you might design are a function of both your interests and the needs of your work setting. For most client populations, a support or structured group can be organized to combine educational and therapeutic aims. Once you determine some areas of need within the community or at the agency where you work, you and your coworkers can launch short-term groups to address these needs.

The Stages of a Group and Tasks of Group Leaders

If you expect to lead groups, understanding the typical patterns during different stages of a group will give you a valuable perspective and help you predict problems and intervene in appropriate and timely ways. Knowledge of the critical turning points in a group can guide you in helping participants mobilize their resources to successfully meet the tasks facing them at each stage. Your tasks as a group worker are different for each of the stages.

The stages of a group include the pregroup, initial, transition, working, and final stages. These stages in the life of a group do not generally flow neatly and predictably in the order described in this section. In actuality there is considerable overlap between the stages. Groups ebb and flow, and both members and leaders need to pay attention to the factors that affect the direction a group takes. We begin with a brief description of each of the stages in the life of a group.

Pregroup Stage

The **pregroup stage** consists of all the factors involved in the formation of a group. Careful thought and planning are necessary to lay a solid foundation for any group. Before a group ever meets as a group, the leader will have designed a proposal for a group, attracted members, and screened and selected members for the group.

Initial Stage

The **initial stage** of a group is a time of orientation and exploration. At the initial sessions members tend to present dimensions of themselves that they consider socially acceptable. This phase is generally characterized by a certain degree of anxiety and insecurity about the structure of the group. Members are tentative because they are discovering and testing limits and are wondering whether they will be accepted. Typically, members bring to the group certain expectations, concerns, and anxieties, and it is vital that they be allowed to express them openly. As members get to know one another and learn how the group functions, they develop the norms that will govern the group, explore fears and expectations pertaining to the group, identify personal goals, clarify personal themes they want to explore, and determine if this group is a safe place.

The manner in which the leader deals with the reactions of members largely determines the degree of trust that develops. Group leaders have the general role of helping the members form a community where they can learn from one another. They carry out this role by teaching members from the beginning of a group to focus on the here and now, by modeling appropriate group behavior, and by assisting members in establishing personal goals.

Group leaders have many tasks during the initial phase of a group, including the following:

- Teach participants how the group works.
- Address matters of informed consent.
- Develop ground rules and set norms.
- Assist members in expressing their fears and expectations and work toward the development of trust.
- Be open with the members and be psychologically present for them.
- Provide a degree of structuring that will neither increase member dependence nor promote excessive floundering.
- Help members establish concrete personal goals.
- Deal openly with members' concerns and questions.
- Teach members basic interpersonal skills such as active listening and responding.

Transition Stage

Before group members can interact at the depths they are capable of, the group generally goes through a **transition stage**. During this stage, members deal with anxiety, reluctance, defensiveness, and conflict, and the leader's task is to help members learn how to begin working on the concerns that brought them to the group. Leaders can help members come to recognize and accept their fear and defensiveness yet, at the same time, challenge them to work through their anxieties and any reluctance they may be experiencing. Members decide whether to take risks and bring out into the open ways they may be holding back, either because of what they might think of themselves or what others could think of them.

Perhaps the central task that leaders face during the transition phase is the need to intervene in the group in a sensitive manner and at the appropriate time. The basic task is to provide both the encouragement and the challenge necessary for the members to face and resolve the conflicts that exist within the group and their own defenses against anxiety and resistance. Some of the major tasks that leaders need to perform during the transition phase include the following:

- Teach group members the importance of recognizing and expressing their anxieties.
- Help participants recognize the ways in which they react defensively and create a climate in which they can deal with this defensiveness openly.
- Provide a model for the members by dealing with them directly, respectfully, and honestly.
- Encourage members to express reactions that pertain to here-and-now happenings in the sessions.

Working Stage

The **working stage** is characterized by productiveness, which builds on the effective work done in the initial and transition stages. Mutuality and self-exploration increase, and the group focuses on making behavioral changes. In actual practice the transition stage and the working stage merge with each other, and there are individual differences among members at all of the stages of a group. During the working stage, the group may return to earlier themes of trust, conflict, and reluctance to participate. Productive work occurs at all stages of a group, not just at the working stage, but the quality and depth of the work takes different forms at various developmental phases of the group.

Some of the central leadership functions at this stage include the following:

- Provide systematic reinforcement of desired group behaviors that foster cohesion and productive work.
- Look for common themes among members.
- Provide opportunities for members to give one another constructive feedback.
- Continue to model appropriate behavior, especially caring confrontation, and disclose ongoing reactions to the group.
- Support the members' willingness to take risks and assist them in carrying this behavior into their daily living.
- Assist members in developing specific homework assignments as practical ways of making changes.
- Focus on the importance of translating insight into action.

Final Stage

The final stage is a time to further identify what was learned and to decide how this new learning can become part of daily living. Group activities include terminating, summarizing, and integrating and interpreting the group experience. As the group is ending, the focus is on conceptualization and bringing closure to the group experience. During the termination process, the group will deal with feelings of separation, address unfinished concerns of members, review the group experience, engage in practicing new behaviors that members may want to take into their daily life, design action plans, identify strategies for coping with relapse, and build a supportive network.

The group leader's central tasks during the ending phase are to provide a structure that allows participants to clarify the meaning of their experiences in the group and to assist members in generalizing their learning from the group to everyday situations.

For an illustration of the stages of an actual group, see the DVD program "Evolution of a Group" in *Groups in Action: Evolution and Challenges—DVD and Workbook* (Corey, Corey, & Haynes, 2006).

Developing Skills as a Group Leader

Many institutions now use groups as their primary approach in helping clients resolve their problems. If you hope to set up and facilitate groups, you must obtain the necessary knowledge and skills to lead groups effectively. Supervised training is an indispensable element in becoming a competent group leader. You are faced with an ethical dilemma if a supervisor asks you to design or lead certain kinds of groups without supervision when you have not had the proper educational preparation. Although you do not need to be an expert when you begin to facilitate groups, you should seek the guidance of experienced group workers.

Effective group leaders are aware of group processes and know how to tap the healing forces within a group. Leading a group is far more complex than working on an individual basis with clients. In addition to the basic skills for individual counseling, group leadership skills include helping members create trust, linking members' work, teaching members how to give and receive feedback, facilitating disclosure and risk taking, intervening to block counterproductive group behavior, identifying common themes, setting up role-playing situations that help members enact and explore their struggles, and preparing members for closure.

Leader Skills in Working With Difficult or Reluctant Group Members

One of the major group leadership skills you need to develop is the ability to intervene effectively when you encounter defensiveness in a group member. It is essential that you not only learn to recognize and deal with members' defenses, but also that you become aware of your own reactions to the defensive behaviors exhibited by members, some of which may include being threatened by what you perceive as a challenge to your leadership role; anger over the members' lack of cooperation and enthusiasm; feelings of inadequacy; and anxiety over the slow pace of the group.

One of the most powerful ways to intervene when you are experiencing intense feelings over what you perceive as defensiveness is to deal with your own feelings and possible defensive reactions to the situation. If you ignore your reactions, you are leaving yourself out of the interactions that occur in the group. Furthermore, by giving the members your reactions, you are modeling a direct style of dealing with conflict and problematic situations rather than bypassing them. Your own thoughts, feelings, and observations can be the most powerful resource you have in dealing with defensive behavior. When you share your reactions pertaining to what is going on in the group—in such a way as not to blame and criticize the members for deficiencies—you are letting the members experience an honest and constructive interaction with you.

Although it is understandable that you will want to learn how to handle "problem members" and the disruption of the group that they can cause, the emphasis should be on actual *behaviors* rather than on labeling members. It is helpful to consider problem behaviors as manifestations of protecting the self that most participants display at one time or another during the history of a group.

As the leader of a group, it is your task to educate members to involve themselves in productive group behaviors that will maximize the benefits of their group experience. In working with problematic behaviors displayed by group members, you need to be mindful of how your interventions can either decrease or escalate these behaviors. Some of the following behaviors can be considered as appropriate interventions when dealing with difficult behaviors of group members. If you keep the following points in mind, you have a good chance of effectively dealing with difficult situations:

- Do not dismiss or put members down.
- Educate the members about how the group works. Strive to be honest with members rather than mystifying the process.
- Encourage members to explore their defensiveness rather than demanding they give up their ways of protecting themselves.
- Challenge group members in a caring and respectful way to do things that may be painful and difficult.
- Do not retreat from conflict in a group.
- Provide a balance between support and challenge.
- Invite group members to state how they are personally affected by problematic behaviors of other members while blocking judgments, evaluations, and criticisms.

In working with difficult group members, you might ask yourself questions such as these:"What am I doing to contribute to the problems?""Does the client remind me of anyone in my personal life?"These questions can help you examine and understand how your personal reactions might be contributing to the client's defensive behaviors. It is good to remind yourself that the very reason people seek a group is to assist them in finding more effective ways of expressing themselves and dealing with others. For examples of how to deal with a variety of difficult group members, see the DVD program "Challenges Facing Group Leaders" in *Groups in Action: Evolution and Challenges—DVD and Workbook* (Corey, Corey, & Haynes, 2006).

The Ethical and Professional Group Leader

The "Best Practice Guidelines" (Association for Specialists in Group Work [ASGW], 2008) provide group workers with suggestions aimed at increasing ethical and professional behavior. What follows is an overview of some of the qualities that we think reflect such standards.

You first spend time thinking about what you most want to accomplish through a group format. If you intend to co-lead your group, make time before you even meet potential members to discuss with your co-leader general group goals and an overall plan for getting your group into motion. You will not be getting a group together unless you believe that your group has real potential for making a difference to those who join.

You then provide information to prospective group candidates. Realizing that some of the people who need your group the most may be reluctant to seek your services, make some provisions for outreach work and getting the word out to a particular target population that could most benefit. You also make some provision for screening prospective group members. In the screening sessions, select members whose needs and goals are compatible with the goals of the group, those who will not impede the group process, and those whose well-being will not be jeopardized by the group experience. You explore with the members the risks of potential life changes, and you help them explore their readiness to face these possibilities. In short, before your group ever meets, you will have spent time laying a foundation and preparing members for a successful learning experience.

Once the group begins to meet, you assess the degree to which its purposes are being met. If you are co-leading the group, arrange to meet with your colleague regularly so that your efforts are coordinated. Ideally, these meetings take place both before and after each group session.

Because you are aware that confidentiality is the cornerstone of any group, you make sure that the participants know what it implies, and you encourage them to bring up any concerns they might have about maintaining confidences. You make some effort to teach members how to become active participants so that they can get the most from the group sessions and also how to apply their newly acquired interpersonal skills in everyday living.

If you have an open group, one characterized by changing membership, you help members who are ready to leave the group integrate their learning, and you allow those who are staying to talk about their feelings about losing a member. As new members join, you attend to them so that they will be able to make use of the group resources. Although members ultimately have the right to leave a group, you discuss with them the possible risks of leaving prematurely, and you encourage them to discuss their reasons for wanting to quit. If your group is made up of involuntary members, you take steps to enlist their cooperation and their continuation on a voluntary basis.

Just as you take care not to impose your values on those clients you see individually, you are also sensitive to the ways in which your own values and needs have an impact on the group process. You exert care not to coerce participants to change in ways they have not chosen. Although you avoid imposing your values on members, you are willing to express your beliefs and values if doing so is likely to benefit the members. Although you are able to meet your needs through your work, you do not do so at the members' expense. You also protect members' rights against coercion and undue pressure from other participants. You teach the members that the purpose of the group is to help them find their own answers rather than yielding to pressure from others.

For the duration of the group, you monitor your own behavior and become aware of what you are modeling to the members. You recognize the importance of teaching members how to evaluate their progress in meeting their goals, and you also design follow-up procedures.

You recognize and respect diversity within the group and encourage members to be sensitive to how differences in culture, race, religion, age, sexual orientation, disability, and gender might be influencing group process. You are able to recognize the limits of your multicultural competency and expertise when working with a diverse range of group members. It is not necessary to know everything about the cultural background of members in your groups. There is a good deal to be said for inviting members to identify what they deem to be significant aspects of their culture with you and other members.

Many individuals live in more than one culture. Oftentimes they have allegiance to their own home culture but find certain aspects of their new culture appealing. These members may experience conflicts in their attempt to integrate the values from the two cultures in which they live. These core struggles can be productively explored in an accepting group if you and other members respect this cultural conflict. If you are a diversity-sensitive group practitioner, the techniques that you employ are appropriate to the cultural background and needs of the members in your group.

Depending on the type of intervention, you are aware of the limits of your competence. You avoid using potentially powerful techniques unless you are trained in their use under supervision. You are willing to seek consultation or supervision when encountering ethical concerns that could interfere with the functioning of the group.

Just as you prepare members for entering a group, you also prepare them for termination from the group in the most efficient period of time. You help members pull together what they have learned from their group experience and assist them in developing an action plan for the period after they leave the group. You are knowledgeable about the resources within your community that can assist members in their special needs, and you help members seek any professional assistance they need. As the group comes to an end, you encourage members to find resources that will enable them to continue the growth they have begun through the group.

Working With Co-Leaders

In our practice of group work, in teaching and supervising group practitioners, and in conducting group-process workshops for students and professionals, we favor working as a team. Although our preference is for the co-leadership model, this is not the only acceptable model of group leadership. Many people facilitate a group alone quite effectively. Realistically speaking, however, there are many institutional barriers to the practice of co-leadership of groups. Budgetary concerns are an ever-increasing barrier to co-facilitated groups. An agency administrator is likely to ask the question, "Why should we pay two staff members to facilitate a group that could be led by one person?"

There are a number of advantages to co-leading groups for all concerned: the group members can gain from the perspectives of two leaders; depending on their styles, the co-leaders can each bring a unique focus to the session and can complement each other's facilitation; and the co-leaders can process what is occurring in the group and plan for future sessions. One of the advantages of co-leading is that it can help you identify and work with countertransference that emerges within the group. As you recall from Chapter 4, countertransference can distort your objectivity to the extent that it interferes with effective counseling. For example, your co-leader may typically react with great impatience to men who are reluctant to express their feelings. You may be better able to make contact with such a man. You can also help your co-leader identify his or her reactions and attachments to a certain member in your private meetings with your co-leader outside of the group.

Along with the advantages of co-leadership, there are also some disadvantages. Co-leader relationships can complicate the group process, which raises a multitude of potential ethical issues. Luke and Hackney (2007) reviewed the literature and identified the following potential disadvantages to the co-leadership model: relationship difficulties between the leaders, competition between the leaders, ineffective communication, and overdependence on the co-leader. Group leaders must attend to their own individual development, their development as a co-leading team, and the development of the group they are facilitating (Luke & Hackney, 2007). It is somewhat demanding for group leaders to divide their time between these multiple areas of development, yet doing so is essential for a successful group. Getting regular supervision is extremely useful as a basic part of learning how to facilitate groups.

The choice of a co-leader is crucial, and it involves far more than attraction and liking. Their functioning as a dyad affects the dynamics of the group, either positively or negatively. If the co-leaders are not working effectively together, the group will likely suffer. Unresolved conflicts between the leaders often result in splitting within the group. If the leaders' energies are directed at competing with each other or at some other power struggle or hidden agenda, there is little chance that the group will be effective. Each of the leaders should be secure enough that the group won't have to suffer as one or both of them try to impress each other. We surely don't think it is essential that co-leaders always agree or share the same perceptions or interpretations; in fact, a group can be given vitality if co-leaders feel trusting enough to express their differences of opinion. Mutual respect and the ability to establish a relationship based on trust, cooperation, and support are most important.

In their study of competency concerns in co-leader relationships, Okech and Kline (2006) found that effective co-leader relationships require commitment to establishing and maintaining these relationships. Co-leaders who are not communicating effectively tend to spend an inordinate amount of time within the group on their relationship issues. Okech and Kline's study underscores the importance of co-leaders being committed to recognizing and working through issues that interfere with them working effectively in the group. They state: "By openly attending to these dynamics outside of group, co-leaders may be less likely to use their groups to play out and ineffectively attend to their relationship issues" (p. 177).

We emphasize the value of co-leaders spending some time together immediately following a group session to assess what has happened. Similarly, they should meet at least briefly before each session to talk about anything that might affect their functioning in the group. Although we like a co-leading model, we think it is important that the two leaders have some say in deciding to work as a team.

Consider a Group Experience for Yourself

Most of this chapter has been addressing ways that you could employ group approaches in your professional work. At this point we ask you to consider the value of experiencing a group as a participant. One of the best ways to learn how to facilitate a group is to actively participate in a group as a member. Take a few moments to reflect on your openness to being a group member. How willing are you to define goals that will enable you to participate actively and fully in learning about yourself and others? Would you be willing to recognize your own vulnerabilities and to reveal them in the context of the group?

If you participate in experiential groups as a part of your training, you can use your experience for personal change and also for working on concerns you have as a helper. Other members can help you take an honest look at yourself and help you to better understand how you come across to others. Your own honesty about who you are is the most significant factor in your ability to change. It is up to you to make any group you enter personally meaningful.

In Chapter 4 we discussed dealing with the transference reactions your clients may have, as well as ways of recognizing any countertransference reactions you may have to them. An experiential group is an ideal place to explore your feelings toward clients and the effects that they have on you. The group can be useful in bringing about an awareness of your blind spots that make it difficult for you to be objective. A group experience that is connected to your training program may not be an appropriate place to work through unfinished business from your past, but it can serve you by sensitizing you to how your vulnerabilities could interfere with your work as a helper. For instance, assume that you become aware of being uncomfortable and seeking approval when you are in the company of older persons, much like you did with your parents. You will probably need to work outside the group in your own therapy to understand your vulnerability and to heal in this area, but the group can draw your attention to this way of responding. In a group you can learn about your defensiveness when you feel vulnerable, and this awareness of your own defenses can be extremely useful in teaching you how to work with clients that you perceive as being difficult.

One of our colleagues (Kristin) tells us that she felt extremely anxious the first time she co-led an incest survivors' group. Kristin remembers saying to herself, "What if they ask me if I was molested? Will they believe I can help them if I tell them I wasn't?" "How will I be able to handle the painful things I'm going to hear?" She worked on these concerns both in her supervision and with her co-leader, who also shared many of these concerns. As the group progressed, it didn't take long for Kristin to realize that there were many ways for her to relate and be helpful to the members. Her initial fears did not paralyze her because she was able to express them and work through them outside of the group.

You don't have to be seriously psychologically impaired to profit from a group experience designed for personal growth. Your willingness to seek input from others and to accept feedback can start a pattern that will encourage you to continue seeking out others when the demands on you in your helping role are great. Being in a group as a part of your program provides an avenue for talking about the feelings, fears, and uncertainties that characterize the developing helper you are becoming. Your capacity to receive constructive feedback from others can better equip you to give quality service to clients. When you are a reluctant group participant yourself, you will probably have trouble inspiring others, especially clients who seem reluctant. If you are able to become an active group member yourself, you can use this experience later in teaching members in your groups how to make the most of their group experience.

Teaching Group Members How to Get the Most From a Group Experience

We are convinced that those who participate in groups will get more from the experience if they are given some instructions of how to become involved participants. We offer some recommendations for group members here that you can use to teach members in a group you are facilitating how to best participate. For a more detailed discussion, we refer you to *Groups: Process and Practice* (M. Corey, Corey, & Corey, 2010).

1. Recognize that trust is not something that just happens in a group; you have a role in creating this climate of trust. If you are aware of anything getting in the way of a sense of safety, share your hesitations with the group.

2. Commit yourself to getting something from your group by focusing on your personal goals. Before each meeting, think about how you can get involved, what personal concerns you want to explore, and other ways to use the time in group meaningfully.

3. Although it is useful to have a tentative agenda of what you want to discuss, do not stick strictly to your agenda if you are affected by what others are exploring and if this suggests moving in a different direction.

4. If the work other members are doing is affecting you, it is important to let them know in what ways you are being affected. If you are able to identify with the struggles or pains of others, it generally helps both you and them to share your feelings and thoughts.

5. Express persistent feelings that you are having that pertain to what is emerging in the group in the here and now. For example, if you have difficulty sharing yourself personally in your group, let others know what makes it hard for you to self-disclose.

6. Decide for yourself what, how much, and when you will disclose personal facets of yourself. Others will not have a basis for knowing you unless you tell them about yourself.

7. Avoid getting lost and overwhelming others with detailed information about you or your history. Disclose struggles that are significant to you at this time in your life, especially as these concerns pertain to what others in the group are exploring.

8. Practice your attending and listening skills. If you can give others your attention and understanding, you are contributing a great deal to the group process.

9. Try to challenge yourself if you judge that you are "taking too much group time for yourself." If you become overly concerned about measuring how much you are taking and receiving, you will inhibit your spontaneity and you will hold yourself back.

10. Use your group as a place to experiment with new behaviors. Allow yourself to try out different ways of being to determine ways that you may want to change. Think of ways to carry these new ways of thinking, feeling, and acting into your outside life by giving yourself your own homework assignments.

11. Understand that making changes will not be instantaneous. You can also expect some setbacks in the progress you make. Keep track of the progress you are making, and remember to give yourself credit for your efforts and the subtle changes that you are making.

12. Be aware of using questions as your main style of interacting. If you are inclined to ask a question, let others know what is behind your question.

13. Avoid giving advice. If you become aware of wanting to tell others what to do, reveal to them what your investment is in giving this advice. Learn to speak *for* yourself and *about* yourself.

14. Concentrate on making personal and direct statements to others in your group. Direct communication with a member is more effective than "talking about" that person through the leader.

15. In giving feedback to others, avoid categorizing or labeling them. Instead of telling others who or what they are, tell them what you are observing and how this is affecting you.

16. Pay attention to any consistent feedback you might receive. For example, if you hear that others perceive you as being somewhat judgmental and critical, do not be too quick to try to convince others that you are open and accepting. Instead, take in what you are hearing and consider their input to determine how what they are saying fits for you, especially in your life away from group.

17. Respect your defenses and understand that they have served a purpose for you. However, when you become aware of feeling or acting defensively in your group, challenge your defenses by seeing what will occur if you become less guarded.

18. Provide support for others by expressing your care for them, but do not quickly intervene by trying to comfort others when they are experiencing feelings, such as expressing pain over an event. Let them know how their pain is affecting you.

19. Take responsibility for what you are accomplishing in your group. Spend some time thinking about what is taking place in these meetings and evaluating the degree to which you are attaining your goals. If you are not satisfied with your group experience, look at what you can do to make the group a more meaningful experience.

20. Be aware of respecting and maintaining the confidentiality of what goes on inside your group. The way that you handle confidentiality says a great deal about your character. If you have any concerns that what you are disclosing is not staying within the group, be willing to bring this matter up in a session.

21. Keep a personal journal in which you record impressions of your own explorations and learning in your group. A journal will be invaluable in keeping track of your progress and noting changes in your ways of thinking, feeling, and acting.

By Way of Review

• For many target populations and certain purposes, groups are the treatment of choice, not a second-rate approach to helping people change.

• Inherent values in the group process lead to self-acceptance, deeper understanding of oneself, and change. Some of these values are learning that one is not alone, receiving feedback from many sources, gaining opportunities for experimenting with new behavior, and using the group as an interpersonal laboratory.

• Become familiar with the stages of development of groups so that interventions are effective and meet the needs of the group. Group development includes the pregroup and initial, transition, working, and final stages.

• Helpers are expected to follow ethical guidelines in forming and conducting group sessions. It is important to know the limits of your competency if you are asked to work with groups.

• Skills in working with groups can be acquired and refined. These skills can be applied to working with a wide array of special populations in a variety of settings.

• As a student in a training program, you have a great deal to gain from groups in your personal and professional development. If you expect to make group work a part of your practice, training and supervision are essential.

What Will You Do Now?

1. Investigate the services that are offered in a local community agency or facility. Ask about how the groups are organized, what services are available to special client groups, and what outcomes these groups have had. If you are doing fieldwork in an agency now, inquire about group work.

2. If a group experience is not part of your training program, join a group in your college or university, in the community, or through private practice. Even if you decide not to join a group, this exercise can be useful in learning about community resources.

3. If you are working in an agency or if you have a fieldwork placement, see whether you can observe a group. Of course, both the group members and the leader would have to agree before you could visit a session. The purpose of this visit is to acquaint you with the potential of groups for meeting the needs of various client populations.

4. If you are currently involved in a group, or have been in a group in the past, in your journal describe the kind of group member that you are (or were). What might this teach you about your ability to lead or co-lead groups? You might also write about your concerns or fears in doing group work. Let yourself brainstorm as you write about the possible advantages of working with people in groups. Think about your interests, and see if you can identify some general ideas for ways to employ small groups as a vehicle for branching out from your interests.

5. For the full bibliographic entry for each of the sources listed here, consult the References at the back of the book. For a practical handbook on the evolution of a group and key group process issues at each stage, see M. Corey, Corey, and Corey (2010). For a practical book on ways of creating, implementing, and evaluating techniques for therapeutic groups, see Corey, Corey, Callanan, and Russell (2004). For a useful treatment of group skills and strategies, see Jacobs, Masson, and Harvill (2009). For a comprehensive overview of a wide variety of topics in the field of group counseling, see DeLucia-Waack, Gerrity, Kalodner, and Riva (2004). For a treatment of the practice of multicultural

group work, see DeLucia-Waack and Donigian (2004). Consult Yalom and Leszcz (2005) for an in-depth treatment of theoretical and practical issues dealing with interpersonal therapy groups. For an overview of 11 major theories of group counseling, with practical applications to various groups, see Corey (2008). For educational video programs showing the Coreys co-leading two different groups, see *Groups in Action: Evolution and Challenges—DVD and Workbook* (Corey, Corey, & Haynes, 2006).

thirteen

Working in the Community

Focus Questions

1. What role do you see yourself playing in your community? To what degree do you focus on the needs of the community as well as on those of individuals?

2. Many helpers direct their efforts to helping clients understand factors within themselves that contribute to their problems. Others focus on the environmental factors that may be influencing an individual's problems. Still others focus on a combination of individual empowerment and environmental change. What are the advantages or disadvantages of combining both individual and environmental factors?

3. Community workers devote some time to educating the community about pressing social problems and about making use of the human services within the community. What interests might lead to your involvement in the local community?

4. Outreach work is a basic community intervention. If you were working in a community agency, what group would you target? What possible advantages do you see of going into the community to provide services for a client population that might not otherwise seek your services?

5. What challenges do you expect to face as a community worker with respect to delivering your services to diverse clients? What kinds of helping roles might you have to assume as a worker in the community?

6. What do you understand by the term *social activism?* Could you make a difference in a community if you assumed a social activist role as a helper?

7. Crisis intervention is a short-term helping strategy that has particular relevance for dealing with many of the problems individuals in a community face. Do you think these methods for bringing about change in a community are efficient and effective?

8. If you had a field placement in a community agency, how prepared would you be in dealing with clients in various crisis situations?

Aim of the Chapter

For professional helpers to foster real and lasting changes, many argue that they must have an impact on the total milieu of people's lives. Working with people who come for individual counseling is one way professionals can use their helping skills, but helpers can foster change in both individuals and the community if they use a systems approach. The aspirations and difficulties of individual clients are intertwined with those of many other people in a community system. By focusing on the capabilities and strengths within a community, community workers can help to empower people in the community.

But what is a community, and how will you find members of it? In *Promoting Community Change,* Mark Homan (2008) captures the spirit of **community** in this definition:

> A community is a number of people who share a distinct location, belief, interest, activity, or other characteristic that clearly identifies their commonality and differentiates them from those not sharing it. This common distinction is sufficiently evident that members of the community are able to recognize it, even though they may not currently have this recognition. Effectively acting on their recognition may lead members to more complete personal and mutual development. (p. 98)

When we use the term **community agency,** we include any institution—public or private, nonprofit or for-profit—designed to provide a wide range of social and psychological services to the community. Likewise, when we speak of **community workers,** we refer to a diverse pool of human service workers and community health workers whose primary duties revolve around serving individuals within their community and serving the community as a whole.

In this chapter we focus on the special responsibilities associated with working in a community. The aim of this chapter is to help you recognize how the external environment is affecting your clients. We cannot treat individuals in isolation from the context of their lives because the community has an impact on how individuals think, feel, and act. As helpers, we have a responsibility to address the conditions that create problems for the individuals who come to see us.

Community **change agents** play an active role in creating community programs and agencies from the bottom up. They base their efforts on the needs of the members of the community in which they work. By listening to your clients, you will become aware of environmental factors that limit the changes many of your clients want to make in their lives. You will hear your clients' aspirations and begin to recognize some of the roadblocks to their success. You may not specialize in community interventions, but you can still play a significant role in helping to bring changes to the community you serve.

The first step is to become aware of the communities that touch your clients' lives. Ask yourself how you would answer the following questions:

- How are the human services needs in your community met?
- What are the special needs of low-income people?
- Where can people go for the social and psychological services they need?

- If people ask you what resources are available to assist them, can you direct them?
- What forces within your community do you see as contributing to the problems individuals and groups are experiencing?
- What assets are available to empower people in the community?
- What institutional barriers exist that serve to deter individuals from gaining equitable access and participation in society?
- What are some of the prevailing attitudes of people in your community toward the range of services provided?
- If these attitudes are positive, how would you build on them? How can you change these attitudes if they are negative?

Traditional psychotherapy focuses on resolution of internal conflicts as a pathway to individual change; the community approach focuses on social change rather than merely helping people adapt to their circumstances. A **community orientation** encourages designing interventions that go beyond the office. Helpers trained in individual helping models who work in the community will need to develop a more expansive notion of who the client is. The community itself is the most appropriate focus of attention because resources, strengths, and abilities for solutions lie within the community. When addressing unmet community needs, helpers must work closely with community members to identify and develop community resources and employ measures that ultimately strengthen the community itself.

The Scope of the Community Approach

The helping process does not take place in a vacuum. Human services specialists develop intervention strategies that deal with the societal factors that adversely affect the lives of many diverse members of the community. This is in keeping with the traditional social work perspective of working with the "person in the environment." A process that considers both individual and environmental factors is consistent with the **community mental health movement,** which began in the 1950s and was based on the premise that human problems result primarily from failures in the social system. This movement called for community control of human services and focused on prevention, early detection, and providing services to people who had traditionally been underserved (Trull, 2005).

Many of the problems people face are the result of being disenfranchised as individuals or as members of a group from systems that hold valued resources for them. The goal of community workers is to work toward greater degrees of enfranchisement. Culturally skilled community workers particularly understand how the sociopolitical influences impinge on the experiences of persons from diverse cultural groups. These workers strive to ameliorate social injustices that adversely affect the mental health of persons in oppressed and marginalized groups in contemporary society (Crethar, Torres Rivera, & Nash, 2008).

Helpers must demonstrate a willingness to deal with clients' economic survival needs from the outset. Too often practitioners ignore the fact that before people can be motivated toward growth and actualization their basic needs must be met. Mental health services should no longer be tailor-made for the upper-middle class. Many community workers believe that all people are equally entitled to high-quality treatment programs. Consequently, community workers advocate for services for people of all ages and backgrounds and with all types and degrees of problems.

The traditional approach tends to treat dysfunctions as belonging to the individual, and the helper teaches the individual to adjust to the "realities" of living in a society. In contrast, the community approach assesses these dysfunctions in the context of a larger system; individuals are taught ways of empowering themselves so that they can be less affected by some of the inequities in society (Lewis, Lewis, Daniels, & D'Andrea, 2003). The traditional approach to understanding and treating human problems focuses on resolution of internal conflicts as a pathway to individual change, whereas the community approach focuses on ways of changing the environmental factors that are causing individuals' problems. Practitioners who operate from this broader community perspective "are able to liberate themselves from a myopic view of counseling that has historically overemphasized an individual, intrapsychic approach and move to more comprehensive, culturally respectful helping methods that include strategies to foster a greater level of social justice in their clients' lives" (Crethar et al., 2008, p. 270). The community mental health perspective is relevant to all communities, but it is particularly relevant to historically marginalized, oppressed, and underserved communities. Community work involves practitioners learning a range of skills, some of which include connecting people, developing leadership, inspiring confidence, and promoting a culture of learning. Members of the community are encouraged to take control of and master their own problems so that traditional individual intervention becomes less necessary (Trull, 2005).

Homan (2008) stresses that we need to change the conditions that affect people rather than trying to change the people who are affected by the conditions. He believes that all human services workers are called upon to work for change when there are injustices in the system. If we are interested in changing societal conditions, Hogan (2007) believes that we must first work on better understanding ourselves as cultural beings. We need to recognize that our personal cultural framework is the starting point for how we engage the world and for the methods we use in our professional work.

Multiple Roles of Community Workers

By creating opportunities for community members to develop skills and abilities that contribute to the vitality of their community, community workers help to develop the community, not merely attend to some of its problems. This elevates the quality of life in the community and expands the members' capacity to confront current and future challenges.

Working with the community usually means working with a specific group or in a situation in which competing or collaborating groups are dealing with an issue or set of issues in a community. These groups usually have a strong identity or a potential for one and can be readily organized. In fact, the work of community change is really the work of small groups. That is, within the community groups with whom you are working you will find a smaller group of people who take an active part in change efforts. Most of the work of this group will be done in a small group context. In Chapter 12 we describe how important it is for human services workers to capitalize on the value of group approaches. In functioning as a change agent within the community, small group skills are essential and powerful.

Various Perspectives on the Roles of Helper

Atkinson, Thompson, and Grant (1993) believe the conventional role of psychotherapist is appropriate "only for a client who is highly acculturated and now wants relief from an existing problem that has an internal etiology" (p. 269). There are criticisms of the conventional approaches to therapy because they place undue responsibility on the client for his or her plight. At the extreme, some interventions place the major responsibility of client problems entirely on the individual without regard for environmental factors that may be contributing to the problem.

The helping professions must recognize that many problems—such as prejudice, oppression, and discrimination—reside outside, not within, the person. Community-oriented work emphasizes the necessity of recognizing and dealing with environmental conditions that often create problems for ethnically diverse client groups. Helpers are encouraged to embrace the roles of environmental change agents and sociopolitical activists to reform social systems and ameliorate unnecessary suffering. To do this, helpers need to acquire new professional roles in delivering a broad range of services aimed at promoting the mental health of people from diverse groups and backgrounds (Crethar et al., 2008). Atkinson (2004) suggests that it is appropriate for community workers to assume some or all of the following alternative roles to traditional helping models as needed to benefit clients: (1) advocate, (2) change agent, (3) consultant, (4) adviser, (5) facilitator of indigenous support systems, and (6) facilitator of indigenous healing methods. In selecting a role and strategies to use with racial or ethnic minority clients, it is useful to take into account the client's level of acculturation, the etiology of the problem, and the goal of counseling. All of these alternative roles embody fundamental principles of social justice and activism that are aimed at client empowerment (Constantine, Hage, Kindaichi, & Bryant, 2007). Let's briefly examine these alternative helper roles.

1. **Advocate.** Because ethnic minority clients are often oppressed by the dominant society, helpers can speak on their behalf. Helpers especially need to function as advocates for clients who are low in acculturation, people who need remediation of a problem resulting from discrimination and oppression, and for

disenfranchised individuals whose backgrounds make it difficult for them to utilize professional services. Crethar and colleagues (2008) define **advocacy** as "proactive efforts carried out by counseling professionals in response to institutional, systemic, and cultural impediments to their clients' well-being" (p. 274). Helpers function in an advocacy role when they use their skills in helping clients to effectively deal with institutional barriers that impede their personal, social, academic, or career goals. Practitioners are called upon to act *with* and *on behalf of* their clients and others in the community.

Client advocacy should be carried out by practitioners who have multicultural competence. Helpers can get involved in social and political activism to help client groups learn how to overcome barriers and empower themselves (Lee, 2006a). Lee and Ramsey (2006) state that helper-advocates must have the awareness, knowledge, and skills to effectively address the range of issues that clients may present.

> Counselors who work with culturally diverse client groups, therefore, have been called on to become agents of systemic change by channeling energy and skill into helping clients from diverse backgrounds break down institutional and social barriers to optimal development. When necessary, mental health professionals must be willing to act on behalf of disenfranchised clients in an advocacy role, actively challenging long-standing traditions and preconceived notions that may stand in the way of optimal mental health and development. (p. 7)

2. **Change agent.** Functioning in this role, community workers do what they can to confront and bring about change within the system that contributes to, if not creates, the problems clients face. Lee (2006a) contends that the cause of problems is not so much within individuals as it is in intolerant or restrictive environments. Thus, the best way to address problems is to eradicate the impediments in the system. In the role of change agents, helpers assist clients in recognizing oppressive forces in the community as a source of their problem and also teach clients strategies for dealing with these problems.

The main purpose of community change is to foster healthy communities. A change agent recognizes that healthy communities produce healthy people. As systemic change agents, community workers assist clients in developing power, particularly political power, to bring about change in the clients' social and physical environment. When operating in the role of a change agent, community workers must sometimes educate organizations to change their culture to meet the needs of the community (Homan, 2008).

3. **Consultant.** Operating as consultants, helpers can encourage individuals from diverse cultures to learn useful skills to interact successfully with various forces within their community. In this role, the client and the helper cooperate in addressing unhealthy forces within the system. As consultants, helpers can work with clients from diverse racial, ethnic, sexual/affectional, ability, gender, and cultural backgrounds to design preventive programs to reduce the negative impact of racism and oppression.

4. **Adviser.** This role is similar to that of consultant. It differs in that the community worker as adviser initiates the discussion with clients about ways to deal with environmental problems that contribute to their personal problems. For example, recent immigrants may need advice on immigration paperwork, coping with problems they will face in the job market, problems that their children may encounter at school, and resources for the acquisition of language skills. Helpers need to acquire knowledge about these topics and know when and where to refer clients for further assistance.

5. **Facilitator of indigenous support systems.** Many ethnically diverse clients, people in rural environments, and older people would not consider seeking professional counseling or therapy. They may not feel comfortable or safe with mental health professionals who are not members of their indigenous framework of helping (Constantine et al., 2007). However, they may turn to help from family members, close friends, or social support systems within their own communities. Community workers can play an important role by encouraging clients to make full use of resources within their own communities, including community centers, churches, extended families, neighborhood social networks, friendship networks, and ethnic advocacy groups. Community workers can work with church leaders in influencing social policy and community change.

6. **Facilitator of indigenous healing systems.** In many cultures human service professionals have little hope of reaching individuals with problems due to their mistrust of traditional mental health approaches and professionals. If helpers are aware of the kinds of healing resources that exist within a client's culture (indigenous resources), they can refer a client to a folk or spiritual healer from his or her culture. At times it may be difficult for helpers to adopt the worldview of their clients. In such instances it could be helpful to work collaboratively with an indigenous healer (such as religious leaders and institutions, energy healers, and respected community leaders). Becoming a culturally competent helper requires being open to indigenous health and healing practices (Stebnicki, 2008). Helpers who develop an understanding of indigenous healing systems are likely to find that this profoundly affects their practice in working with others. Stebnicki also notes that many indigenous healing practices may benefit the helper's self-care program.

In their article on indigenous mental health practices, Constantine, Myers, Kindaichi, and Moore (2004) present a comprehensive literature review and discuss the cultural relevance of indigenous healing practices in promoting psychological, physical, and spiritual well-being for people of color. They encourage counselors to be open to learning about indigenous healing resources. However, Constantine and her colleagues caution practitioners to exercise due care in making referrals to indigenous helping resources so as not to jeopardize clients' physical and mental health. By assuming an open stance, "counselors may be able to recognize potential similarities and differences between indigenous and Western approaches to helping and may begin to bridge gaps between traditional helping institutions and the cultures of the individuals they serve" (p. 120).

Community Intervention

A comprehensive community perspective involves four levels of intervention: (1) direct client services, (2) indirect client services, (3) direct community services, and (4) indirect community services.

Direct client services focus on *outreach activities* to a population that might be at risk for developing mental health problems. Community workers provide help to clients either facing crises or dealing with ongoing stressors that impair their coping ability. Target populations for such programs are school dropouts, alcohol and drug abusers of all ages, people who are homeless, victims and perpetrators of child and elder abuse, suicidal individuals, victims of violent crimes, older people, persons with AIDS, and adolescent mothers. By reaching out to those schools and communities, helpers can offer a variety of personal, career, and family counseling services to at-risk groups (Lewis et al., 2003).

Indirect client services consist of *client advocacy*, which involves active intervention for and with an individual or a group. The community agency works to empower disenfranchised groups that have become split off from the mainstream community. These include, but are not limited to, the unemployed, the homeless, older people, persons with disabilities, and persons living with AIDS. Helpers need to become advocates, speaking up on their clients' behalf and actively intervening in their clients' situation (Lewis et al., 2003). The advocacy process is best conceived of as a way to assist groups who typically do not have power to move in the direction of acquiring tools to find and use resources, both within the community and within themselves.

Direct community services in the form of *preventive education* are geared to the population at large. Examples of these programs include life planning workshops, AIDS prevention workshops, the creative use of leisure, and training in interpersonal skills. Because the emphasis is on prevention, these programs help people develop a wider range of competencies.

Indirect community services are attempts to *change the social environment* to meet the needs of the population as a whole and are carried out by influencing public policy. Community intervention deals with the victims of poverty, sexism, and racism, which typically leave people feeling powerless. The focus is on promoting systemic change by working closely with those in the community who develop public policy.

Community intervention calls for helpers who (a) are familiar with resources within the community they can refer clients to, when necessary, (b) have a basic knowledge of the cultural background of their clients, (c) possess skills that can be used as needed by clients, (d) have the ability to balance various roles as professionals, (e) are able to identify nonprofessionals in the community who have the ability to be change agents for their community, (f) have the willingness to be advocates for policy changes in the community, and (g) have the ability to connect with the community and to connect community members with each other.

Outreach

As mental health professionals have become more aware of the need to provide services to a wider population, effective outreach strategies have received increased attention. These strategies are particularly useful for reaching ethnic minorities because of the traditional mistrust of primarily White mental health professionals who have often been seen as mislabeling people from diverse groups and excluding them from services.

As you saw in Chapter 7, if practitioners hope to reach and effectively deal with a cultural group different from their own, they must acquire a broad understanding of culturally diverse client populations. It is essential that culturally competent helpers use intervention techniques that are consistent with the life experiences and cultural values of diverse groups in the community if they hope to succeed in their outreach efforts (Lee & Ramsey, 2006).

The community psychology model, with its emphasis on creating responsive social systems, is perhaps best suited for people of color. White and Parham (1990) write that this kind of outreach model differs from the traditional model used in the helping professions in the sense that the community worker does not wait for people to come in for help. Instead, the worker reaches out to the community with a coordinated package of preventive mental health services aimed at improving the psychological health of people throughout the life cycle.

The outreach approach includes developmental and educational efforts, such as skills training, stress management training, education of the community about mental health and the benefits of counseling, and consultation in a variety of settings. These efforts must be made in a way that makes sense to the community, not just the practitioner. If people in the community do not utilize services, it is appropriate to question the value of the services or the appropriateness of the way these services are delivered. Community workers need to be willing to learn *from* and *with* the community when organizing services.

You do not have to be all things to potential clients in the community. If you work in a community agency, you will most likely be part of a team working with individual clients. The case management approach involves a number of helping professionals, each with a different specialty. Managed care systems also utilize a team approach, so you need to learn how to build collaborative relationships with the members of a professional team at your agency. Once a need is identified within a community, a group of workers has more power to reach client groups than does a single worker functioning in isolation.

Explore the kinds of outreach work you might be inclined to do in your own community. If you have a field placement or a job in a community agency, what ideas do you have for outreach projects? Can you seek out mental health professionals in your community, or faculty members at your college, who have the expertise to provide you with direction in meeting critical needs of certain client groups? How might you and fellow students combine your talents and efforts to develop a program for reaching a neglected segment of your community? What agencies and resources within your community could you use in developing such an outreach project? Your program does not have to involve a grand design; even a small change can help individuals who might never ask for assistance.

Educating the Community

Educating the community includes educating the professionals regarding the existence and dimensions of problems as well as some steps for dealing with them. This effort also entails educating the broader community about the same things and, in addition, about the costs to the community of maintaining the problem. Professionals need to educate potential consumers about the availability of services as well as their right to demand that they be delivered with quality.

There are many reasons people do not make use of available resources: they may not be aware of them, they may not be able to afford these services, they may have misconceptions about the nature and purpose of counseling, they may be reluctant to recognize their problems, they may harbor the attitude that they should be able to take charge of their lives on their own, they may believe professional helpers are attempting to control their lives, they may perceive that these services are not intended for them because they view such services as culturally insensitive, or they may believe they are not worthy to receive services. There are also practical limiting factors that make it difficult to use community services. For example, if clients are required to travel to the agency to receive services, community members without access to transportation may be unable to make use of the programs.

One goal of the community approach is to educate the public and attempt to change the attitudes of the community toward mental health programs. Perhaps the most important task in this area is to demystify the notion of mental illness. Many people still cling to misconceptions and archaic notions of mental illness. Professionals face a real challenge in combating these faulty notions. Helpers also need to be able to present the array of services they offer to the community in terms that the target groups can understand. Many people still consider seeking any form of professional psychological treatment as something only for those who are seriously mentally ill. Others think professional helpers have answers to every problem a client brings to the agency. Others hold the belief that professional help is only for the weak or for those who simply cannot solve their own problems. Unless professionals actively work on presenting helping services in a way that is understandable, acceptable, and culturally appropriate to the community at large, many people who could benefit from professional help may not seek it. Educating the community can awaken people to the resources that are available to assist and empower them.

One small grassroots nonprofit agency in Orange County, California, has applied outreach strategies to educate the community and meet its critical needs (Hogan-Garcia & Scheinberg, 2000). The Coalition for Children, Adolescents and Parents (CCAP) is a community agency aimed at the prevention of adolescent pregnancy. For the past 20 years, CCAP has provided after-school recreational services, tutoring, academic enrichment programs, physical examinations, parenting education, conflict resolution, cultural diversity training, school-based group counseling, a homeless shelter, drug abuse prevention, and child care training—to mention a few services. All members of the agency staff have demonstrated a commitment to clarifying and understanding personal values, beliefs, and behaviors. Because the individuals on the staff believe in the value of understanding cultural diversity, they have been able to serve as a bridge between mainstream and other segments of their community.

One of the early projects designed by CCAP involved outreach and education in the Latino community to prevent the spread of HIV. A Latina staff member conducted interviews with 30 mothers in the community regarding their understanding of HIV, human sexuality, and teen pregnancy. From this contact with these mothers, a group of leaders (comadres) was formed, and they took steps to educate the community. The women who served as leaders met for monthly meetings, which were held at a neighborhood center. Eventually, the women invited their husbands into the classes.

This is an example of an effective collaborative effort by an agency that is committed to ensuring that the members of the community have a full voice in determining the nature of the services. The projects that are a part of CCAP are based on a set of culturally competent practice principles in a culturally diverse community.

Hogan (2007, chap. 5) identifies the following tasks that practitioners might be involved in when educating the community:

- Support the needs of minority groups in the community.
- Assist client groups to become true partners with professionals in the development and delivery of services with shared decision-making authority.
- Promote community organization and development activities as fundamental agency responsibilities and see that this is reflected in agency budgets.
- Actively reach out to people with special needs and initiate programs aimed at preventing problems rather than merely treating them.
- Draw on and improve the skills of community workers and laypeople to help meet the many different needs of clients and discover and use the many abilities of clients.
- Develop strategies to deal effectively with poverty, drug and alcohol abuse, child sexual/physical abuse, child neglect, and domestic violence.
- Develop strategies that will empower the disenfranchised in the community.
- Consult with a variety of social agencies about programs in gerontology, welfare, child care, and chemical dependence and rehabilitation and help community workers apply psychological knowledge in their work.
- Evaluate human-service programs to assess agency intervention efforts.
- Work with members of a particular community to develop and build on community assets to promote communities and instill self-reliance.

Influencing Policymakers

The need for community-based programs is compounded by such problems of our contemporary society as poverty, homelessness, crime, drive-by shootings, gang activities, AIDS, absent parents, divorce, domestic violence, child abuse, unemployment, tension and stress, alienation, addictions to drugs and alcohol, delinquency, and neglect of older persons. These are just a few of the major challenges that communities need to address in preventing and treating human problems. Community helpers can shape social policy by working within the sociopolitical arena to instigate change. For instance, research into the prevention of AIDS has come about largely through lobbying efforts and political pressure.

If you have not already done so, you will inevitably come in contact with people who have tested positive for HIV, people who have AIDS, people who have had sexual contact with someone who is HIV-positive, and people who are close to individuals with HIV or AIDS. You simply cannot afford to be unaware of the many issues that have emerged from the AIDS epidemic. You might be expected to offer direct services to clients with the disease or to provide indirect services in the community geared to education and prevention. You will not be able to educate those with whom you come in contact unless you are educated about the problem yourself. Keep up to date on recent findings as they affect clinical practice. Although it is not realistic to expect that you will have in-depth knowledge of the range of problems confronting a community, you can have a general knowledge of these problems and familiarize yourself with resources valuable to people with specific needs. In working in a community you will probably be part of a team of human services professionals. Each member of the team will have different areas of expertise, and through interprofessional collaboration the combined strengths of practitioners can bring a diverse range of resources to a problem such as preventing HIV/AIDS. Professional training programs have a responsibility to prepare helpers to become competent advocates for at-risk individuals and groups and teach students the skills they will need to influence policymaking.

Community workers can easily feel overwhelmed, and community agencies are often underfunded and understaffed. Without adequate funding, creative programs remain on the drawing board, and agencies resort to crisis work, treating rather than preventing problems. Because helpers are frequently overworked and have many conflicting demands on their time, it may be difficult for them to do much work in the areas of education, influencing policymakers, outreach, and advocacy. However, helpers must find a way to legitimize the use of time for these activities. One way community workers can initiate change is by organizing within an agency and developing a collective voice.

Mobilizing Community Resources

In *Promoting Community Change: Making It Happen in the Real World,* Homan (2008) suggests that if you want to assume an active role in mobilizing the resources within a community it is useful to have certain knowledge and skills. To maximize your efforts in a community, hone your skills in these areas:

- Achieve credibility and standing within the community.
- Promote meaningful involvement of members of the community being served in community change efforts.

- Develop and build on the strengths or capabilities of members of the community.
- Know your target, your issue, your troops, and your resources.
- Identify the stakeholders, those who are potential allies and opponents.
- Establish and maintain a personal network, especially involving people who may be in a position to assist client groups.
- Understand the transferability of skills used in working with individual clients to working with the community.
- Understand planning and its relationship to action.
- Acknowledge that power is used to maintain or change conditions within the community.
- Learn that power *with* is at least as important as power *over*.
- Assist the community to declare its needs in a way that enables people to act on them.
- Keep people who are involved in the change effort connected to one another.
- Make sure that your strategies and tactics fit the situation.
- Understand that people must *feel* something before they will *do* something.
- Use the "cycle of empowerment": involvement, communication, decisions, action.
- Listen as assertively as you speak.
- Assume responsibility for instigating change.
- Avoid setting arbitrary limits on yourself. Believe in your own capabilities.
- Commit yourself to learning—about yourself, your community, your issue, your strategies and tactics.
- Focus on the commonalities among community members rather than on their differences.
- Remember that it's not only "they" who need to change but "we" who must change what we are doing.
- Accept the reality of certain problems or conditions without letting these barriers stop productive efforts.
- Address ethical issues in the delivery of services.
- Believe in the rights of members of the community to lead full and satisfying lives.

The most successful programs include community members in determining the direction their communities need to take. As a community worker you will assume an active role, but remember that it is the community members themselves who are the "experts" on their own needs. Viewing community members as the experts is a way of fostering a sense of empowerment. Rather than deciding for a community what is needed, your role might be more to facilitate connections within a community and to help individuals learn to use available resources to effect changes in their community.

Some uncertainty is natural when you are trying to decide how you can make a difference in your community. Remind yourself of the skills you have to help you analyze situations and build relationships. It is also important to recognize that idealism can be a valuable asset. Like any other asset, it is strengthened when put into practice.

Working With Special Populations in the Community

We encourage you to think about diverse special groups, especially neglected or unpopular client groups, within your community and see how you could mobilize community resources in meeting their needs. Keep in mind the importance of being willing to pay attention to similar feelings you are experiencing with your clients who may differ from you in a number of significant respects, even if you have not experienced their same problems.

Learn to work *with* the community as well as *for* the community. Any program that you design must incorporate ways of reaching out to the target population as well as ways for potential clients to gain access to your services. How might you develop educational programs in your community to provide services to these client groups? Realize that education is only a first step and that educational efforts must be directed toward action programs that will bring about community improvement. How might you mobilize the community to take action that will improve the plight of certain at-risk groups?

Regardless of the client population, these questions illustrate principles that you can apply in understanding and working with any target group in the community:

- What specific populations in your community are most in need of help? What kind of help do they need?
- To what degree do you understand the special needs of these target groups? What resources and capabilities of the community can be brought to bear on resolving the plight of a target group?
- What are your assumptions and attitudes toward this target group? What possible prejudices, biases, and stereotypes might you harbor toward this group?
- Identify some of your fears or concerns in working with a client group. How will you deal with your own fears?
- How might you deal with the strong reactions of those within the community who may be shocked that you are working with such unpopular client populations?
- In what ways might society stigmatize at-risk groups such as people who are homeless? people who abuse substances? veterans? children from alcoholic families? those who are unemployed?
- In what ways might individuals within certain groups continue to stigmatize themselves?
- As a helper, how can you remove stigmas that block effective programs?

Take a moment to reflect on what you have already read about the community approach. Think of your educational background, level of professional training, and work experiences. If you plan to go into the human services field, you are likely to spend some time working in a community agency setting, and you will be working with many different groups within the community. If you are working in such a setting at this time, how prepared are you, both personally and academically, to assume a broader view of helping that encompasses being an agent for change within the community? How can you learn what you will need to know to assume such a role? What specific skills do you need to acquire? What fears would you need to challenge to work effectively in the community? How might you translate your idealism into a practical set of strategies to bring about constructive change within the community?

Social Activism and Making a Difference

In his article "Making a Difference," Rob Waters (2004) profiles the work of five community-oriented therapists who became social activists. These five "citizen-therapists" exemplify people who are deeply engaged in their own communities and who are actively working to promote change. Each of these therapists has taken a different path to change the community, yet each of them has been motivated by the question, "How can I make a difference?"

Ramon Rojano (cited in Waters, 2004) is convinced that the direction the helping profession needs to take is for therapists to become active agents of social change. As a psychiatrist who worked primarily with rich Anglo Americans, Rojano shifted his focus to working in a child guidance clinic with Latinos and African Americans. He quickly realized that relying on traditional psychotherapy approaches to deal with a family's psychological needs was pointless unless he addressed poverty, violence, and the social and economic crises that were part of the lives of these family members. Referring to his approach as "community family therapy," Rojano has shifted from the traditional role for which he was trained as a psychiatrist to an alternative role for bettering the mental health system for the poor.

Diane Sollee (cited in Waters, 2004) is a leader in the marriage education movement. Part of her work has involved seminars aimed at training people to become marriage educators, who have the task of teaching basic communication skills to couples. To avoid becoming identified with any political faction, Sollee has refused to accept funding from anyone. The core of her work is to get couples the information and skills they need to succeed in their marriage and family life.

Kenneth Hardy (cited in Waters, 2004) is a family therapist who over the years has developed projects in schools, churches, corporations, and the United States military to help groups deal with diversity issues. Hardy's goal is to help people acknowledge the reality of social injustice and the inequalities of race, gender, and social class in ways that help develop a true understanding of diversity. In his professional work, Hardy has focused increasingly on those who are disenfranchised and disempowered.

Jack Saul (cited in Waters, 2004) is the director of New York University's International Trauma Studies Program, and he is committed to helping people survive disaster. In reflecting on the aftermath of 9/11, Saul contends that "collective suffering requires a collective response" (p. 40). In disaster situations, Saul believes that therapists need to think in broader terms and develop models for mobilizing a community's own resources for healing. He met with officials to set up Project Liberty, which was the commission established to distribute $100 million in mental health funds that Congress provided for recovery from the 9/11 disaster. Currently, Saul is devoting his energies to developing community resources for healing the 6,000 Liberian refugees living on Staten Island. He operates largely behind the scenes to help organize drop-in centers, job-placement programs, and family support programs that bring together various community leaders. Saul says, "The key thing in doing this kind of work is to bring your therapeutic skills to the community in a way that promotes the community's own capacities, without becoming too central" (p. 41).

Barbara Lee (cited in Waters, 2004), a graduate of the School of Social Welfare at the University of California at Berkeley, is now a member of Congress on Capitol Hill. Lee has learned that she is able to have the widest possible impact by exercising political power. Lee brings a clinician's perspective to bear on the running of her congressional office. She and her staff advocate for low-income people. Lee cosponsored a bill that authorized AIDS relief to Africa, which was signed into law by President Bush in 2003. This achievement is but one example of what Lee means when she says, "I didn't go into politics to be part of the system, but to change the system, to shake it up and make things better" (p. 43).

These five social activists have demonstrated that systems can be changed and that communities have a built-in capacity for healing. Helpers who adopt a social activist and social justice perspective do not restrict themselves to thinking in terms of remediation of problems in individual clients' lives. They are concerned with implementing preventive strategies aimed at fostering systemic changes in their clients' environmental contexts (Crethar et al., 2008).

Crisis Intervention in the Community

Crisis intervention is one of the main models utilized in community agency work. You will learn methods of dealing with a variety of crisis situations in your supervised field placements, and chances are that you will have many opportunities to practice these skills. In writing about the development of the crisis intervention model, Kanel (2007) shows how this model is linked to community-based mental health programs. The community mental health movement emphasized prevention programs, and much of crisis intervention theory is based on interventions aimed at minimizing psychological impairment and promoting psychological health.

Although the Community Mental Health Centers Act of 1963 was originally intended to serve chronically mentally ill patients, community workers soon began seeing clients who were experiencing psychological problems that were typically dealt with in the private practices of therapists. Later, the Lanterman Petris Short bill of 1968 established more specific requirements for providing mental health services in the community, emphasizing short-term crisis intervention for people who were not chronically mentally ill. The short-term crisis intervention model is considered more cost effective than traditional forms of psychotherapy, which made crisis intervention a preferred approach for most health maintenance organizations (Kanel, 2007).

The Context of Crisis

After reviewing many different definitions of **crisis**, James (2008) summarized these definitions thusly: "Crisis is a perception or experiencing of an event or situation as an intolerable difficulty that exceeds the person's current resources and coping mechanisms" (p. 3). Several authors present models of crisis intervention (see James, 2008; Kanel, 2007). The crisis model can be applied to working with the community as the "client" as well as working with individuals who are in crisis.

Crisis intervention is a short-term approach to helping that is the treatment of choice in cases where clients are experiencing a state of acute psychological disequilibrium. Individuals in crisis, or a community that is faced with a crisis, are temporarily disrupted cognitively, emotionally, and behaviorally, and they are in need of immediate and skilled help. This helping process should last as long as it typically takes people to bounce back to their previous level of functioning, which is generally up to 6 weeks.

Most clients who come to a community agency will be experiencing either a developmental or a situational crisis. A **developmental crisis** pertains to some expected difficulty at a particular stage of life. As you saw in Chapter 3, Erikson's developmental stages present opportunities for transformation and also represent a potential crisis. Developmental crises include the trauma of early childhood, getting married or divorced, the stresses of parenthood, coping with children leaving home, finding meaning in life after retirement, and adjusting to the death of friends and family members. Events such as these do not necessarily lead to crises; the person's interpretations and responses to these life transitions are the determining factors.

In crisis theory, the term *crisis* is not considered negative; rather, it is an essential ingredient in human growth and development. Crisis is a time in one's life for making choices. Situations do not merely happen to us. The stance we take toward life situations is what determines our quality of life. The word *crisis* is derived from the Greek word *krinein*, which means "to decide." Crisis situations can represent both a danger and an opportunity. For example, being confronted by a serious illness can result in a reevaluation of one's priorities and a major change in the way one is living. How people respond to these critical turning points is what makes the difference. A utopian existence is not one without any crises, for crisis is an essential element in human development. The crises that we face at various phases of life are frequently catalysts that awaken us to the richer possibilities awaiting us if we have the courage to go through a transformation.

In addition to the expected developmental crises associated with the various stages of life, we also must endure unexpected events that can have the impact of paralyzing our will to act or can result in new directions for living once the crisis situation is over. Such **situational crises** can include sexual assault, discovery of a serious illness in oneself or a loved one, the breakup of an intimate relationship, a serious financial setback, or a natural disaster such as an earthquake or a hurricane. As a helper employed in a community agency, you may be called on to counsel suicidal clients, deal with clients with posttraumatic stress disorders, help those with severe physical limitations, or offer strategies for those who abuse drugs and alcohol.

In some communities, crisis teams meet regularly to update information and work out procedures for responding to crisis situations. It is clear that those in the helping professions need to have the knowledge, skills, and training to provide immediate assessment, intervention, referral, and follow-up.

The Process of Crisis Intervention

There are two levels of crisis intervention. **First-order intervention** can be thought of as psychological first aid. This level of intervention is carried out by mental health professionals and a network of others such as ministers, judges, police and fire personnel, nurses, paramedics, physicians, school counselors, parole officers, teachers, and a wide range of human services workers. **Second-order intervention,** or crisis therapy, requires considerably more specialized training and expertise.

First-order intervention involves immediate assistance and may take only one session. The major goal of this level of intervention is to reestablish an individual's immediate coping capacity. To accomplish this goal, helpers offer support, do what they can to reduce the chances of death, and link people in crisis to other helping resources. There are many settings where the staff must be equipped to handle a wide range of crises, such as the hospital emergency room or the crisis intervention hot line. Staff members and nonlicensed workers can be given training to respond quickly and effectively when they initially encounter people in crisis.

The task of helpers who offer psychological first aid is to help individuals tap any resources available to them to restore a sense of equilibrium, which will eventually enable them to work through their reactions so that they can meet future challenges. Helpers create support through their attitudes and behaviors. Perhaps what helpers most have to offer is their gift of presence. This is the capacity "to be fully there" for individuals in crisis as they tell their story and seek human connection to guide them to some sense of stability amid the temporary chaos they are experiencing.

In your initial encounter with a client in crisis, you can give the gift of presence partially by what you say but even more by a manner that reflects genuine caring and a deep sense of compassion. You may often feel helpless to change a tragic situation, and you could burden yourself with thoughts that what you are *doing* is not enough. Yet presence is powerful and often transcends what you can actually do to change the situation. Your willingness to fully connect with others as they strive to put their lives back together can be most healing and necessary.

It is important that your clients feel invited to tell their stories and also that you avoid assuming that you know exactly what they need or what is best for them. As they tell their stories, listen with as much understanding as possible. The real task is for you to encourage them to talk and for you to understand what they are going through from their perspective. Try to get a sense of where your clients want to go and what options for action they would consider. As clients express themselves, it is important that you also make an assessment of the immediate situation, especially of their coping resources.

Your primary task in crisis intervention is to ensure your clients' safety. Some clients may feel so distraught and so unable to cope with the crisis that they see suicide as their only way out. Suicidal urges may last for only a short time in the face of despair, and it is your job to intervene to prevent any deadly actions. People in crisis frequently provide clues to the depth of their despair. In making an assessment of the client's potential for taking lethal action, you must know the appropriate questions to ask as well as be aware of danger signs. Develop contracts with clients who pose a danger to themselves, and plan specific methods of follow-up after a session. Arranging for referrals is a very important part of this work. Ask yourself if you have enough knowledge and skill to assist your clients in crisis. Know your limits and the resources within the community that can serve as a lifeline for people who are experiencing a crisis.

The first-order level of crisis intervention often entails a short-range plan of what to do next. People in crisis can overwhelm themselves with the feeling that everything has to be attended to at once. You can help clients focus on what must be done now and what can wait until later. Clients often feel immobilized to the degree that they cannot see any options. You can calm them and help them identify a network of resources available to them, such as family, friends, and community. Through the process of receiving psychological first aid, people often get the understanding, support, and guidance they need so as not to harm themselves or others. At this level, one of your tasks is to help clients identify and examine possible routes they can later use to work through the crisis.

According to Kristi Kanel (personal communication, November 3, 2008), for some individuals a crisis can be resolved through this first level of intervention, especially when the crisis worker can connect the client to community resources that can be utilized throughout the client's life. These community agencies, schools, churches, health clubs, and many other natural support systems existing in the community are a more natural way for people to cope with the many and never-ending stressors (possible precipitating events that often lead to crisis states). First-level crisis intervention creates the opportunity for clients to learn what the community has to offer them in the future when life becomes too difficult for them to manage on their own. These community services create a sense of social connectedness, which is vital for successful management of life's struggles.

Although mental health counseling centers are considered community services, not all people need a professional person to be there for them in times of crisis. Having a strong infrastructure of community programs in place may be preferable for populations who might not feel comfortable seeking the services of a professional therapist. Just having community agencies available may serve not only to intervene with crises but to prevent people from entering into impaired states of functioning in the first place. For example, communities with easily accessible teen centers designed from the bottom up offer teens opportunities to become involved there rather than pursuing risky behaviors that often lead to crises, such as teen pregnancy, sexually transmitted infections, gangs, runaways, and suicide.

Sometimes, this initial level of intervention does not resolve their crisis. The effects of the crisis can linger, and vestiges must be worked through. This is where second-order intervention, also known as **crisis therapy**, becomes necessary. This is a short-term therapeutic process that goes beyond immediate coping and aims at crisis resolution and change. The main goals of this level of intervention are to help people in crisis better face their future and to minimize their chances of becoming a psychological casualty. It is critical that clients learn from the crisis and that they be given opportunities to work through unfinished business. Ideally, they will be given the assistance that will result in their remaining open to life and to new choices rather than closing themselves off to the vast range of future possibilities.

In crisis counseling, clients are encouraged to express and deal with feelings, some of which may have been repressed. It can be very freeing for clients to let go of these feelings and convert them into positive emotional energy to be used constructively. Typically, it is feelings that are denied expression (such as guilt or anger) that cause people the most difficulties. Venting pent-up feelings in itself often facilitates psychological healing.

Another task of second-order crisis intervention consists of helping clients attain a realistic perspective on the crisis event. There is a need to develop an understanding of how the event has affected them, including the meaning of the crisis in their lives. Clients typically must rebuild cognitions that have been damaged by the crisis. Part of the process of crisis therapy involves clients' learning how their thought patterns have resulted in certain behaviors. Clients are helped to cognitively reframe events, which allows for a new range of behavioral possibilities. As can be seen, this advanced phase of crisis work demands a great deal of expertise and is provided by helping professionals who have specialized knowledge and skills.

By Way of Review

• The community perspective emphasizes social change rather than merely helping people adapt to their circumstances.

• It is not useful to focus on individual client treatment and neglect the institutional or social conditions that contribute to an individual's problems. A process that considers both the internal conflicts of the individual and the social factors within the community will provide a balanced perspective for helpers.

• It is essential that training programs prepare students to assume a proactive stance toward community intervention, especially with reference to early prevention approaches for at-risk groups in the community.

• A comprehensive community counseling program has four aspects. Direct client services focus on outreach activities for at-risk groups in the community. Direct community services in the form of preventive education are geared to the population at large. Indirect client services consist of intervening actively for an individual or a group. Indirect community services focus on influencing policymakers and bringing about positive changes within the community.

• Helpers need to assume an advocacy role for disenfranchised clients whose background makes it difficult for them to utilize professional assistance.

• Helpers who work in the community will be expected to develop skills in the areas of engaging in outreach, providing education to community members, assuming an advocacy role, and influencing policymakers.

• You do not have to be all things to potential clients in the community. If you work in a community agency, you will most likely be part of a team working with individual clients.

• Social activism is a powerful way to make a significant difference in the community.

• Crisis intervention is one of the main modalities in community agencies. Many at-risk groups are in need of immediate short-term help in working through both situational and developmental crises.

What Will You Do Now?

1. Select an at-risk population in your community. As a class project, you and several classmates can explore strategies for dealing with a particular client population by using a community approach. What can be done to awaken people in your community to the needs of the at-risk group you have identified?

2. Spend some time thinking about how you might get involved in your community by doing some kind of volunteer work or selecting a field placement that will get you directly involved in community projects. Brainstorm possible ways of making even small changes in some facet of your community. How can you involve yourself in projects that are already under way or with fellow students who are doing some form of work in the community? Write ideas in your journal of how you can use your interests and talents in the service of others in your community.

3. Investigate the services available in your community for people in crisis. Look into what is offered in your own college or university. Ask about the crisis services provided by one of your community agencies. Inquire about what is being done by way of training volunteers for crisis intervention, such as working on a telephone hot line. You might consider doing volunteer work in your community as part of a crisis team. Ask about training programs and the possibility of serving as an "on-call" worker in times of special need.

4. For the full bibliographic entry for each of the sources listed here, consult the References at the back of the book. Homan (2008) views the community as the client and offers the basic knowledge and skills needed to face the challenge of community change. See Lewis, Lewis, Daniels, and D'Andrea (2003) for a

comprehensive description of the community counseling perspective. For a variety of topics pertaining to community agency counseling, see MacCluskie and Ingersoll (2001). For an excellent resource outlining the theory and practice of crisis intervention, see James (2008); for a practical guide to crisis intervention techniques, see Kanel (2007).

Concluding Comments

If this book has been instrumental in giving you some ideas about the kind of helper you want to become, we have met our objectives. We encourage you to dream and to allow yourself to envision the helper you want to become. Set clear priorities, and remember that the challenges we have presented throughout these chapters do not have to be addressed immediately or all at once. Refrain from being overly ambitious; remember that the "ideal helper" we described in Chapter 1 is just that—an ideal to strive toward. You can begin now to reach your visions by becoming an active and questioning student and by putting yourself fully into your fieldwork activities. We hope you will become excited by your journey of self-exploration as you learn about the helping professions.

The process of becoming a helper is intrinsically related to the process of becoming a person. We have emphasized the importance of looking at your life and of understanding your motivations. Although it is not essential for you to be problem-free, we have stressed the importance of being a model for your clients. Reflect on whether what you do in your own life is what you encourage your clients to do. If you urge your clients to take the risks that growth entails, it is essential that you do this in your own life.

This is a good time to reflect on the personal meaning this book has for you. Ask yourself these questions: Do you still think the helping professions are for you? What do you think you can bring to your work? How might your work affect your personal life? What are the greatest challenges you expect to face? Do you now have a different perspective on the concerns that were addressed in this book? At this point, what do you see as your major strengths and some of your limitations? What steps could you take to address your limitations? How can you build on your strengths?

Now that you have completed the book, we have a few specific suggestions for consolidating your learning. If you are not inclined to do all of these things, choose the exercises that seem most useful to you. Return to Chapter 1 and once again complete the *Self-Assessment: An Inventory of Your Attitudes and Beliefs About Professional Helping*. You took this inventory as a pretest at the beginning of the course. Now, as the course is ending, you can use this self-inventory to determine the degree to which your attitudes and beliefs about helping may have changed.

Take time to read the *Focus Questions* at the beginning of each chapter again. Can you answer all of these questions now? Have your answers to some of these questions changed as you have acquired new knowledge from the book and in your course? We recommend that you review the key points at the end of each chapter in the *By Way of Review* section to help you consolidate your key learning. Finally, choose one activity from the *What Will You Do Now?* section at the end of each chapter and pursue it on your own. Challenge yourself to extend your learning experience by taking the initiative to complete these projects. If you have been keeping a journal, continue to write about the experiences you are having in your training program as a way to extend the self-reflection process.

We dedicate this book to you, our readers, as you prepare for a career in one of the helping professions. We hope that you see more clearly now how the kind of person you are is so vitally linked to the kind of helping professional you will become. We wish our best to you in your continuing journey!

References*

*This list contains both references cited and suggestions for further reading. An asterisk (*) before an entry indicates a source that we highly recommend as supplementary reading.

*Acuff, C., Bennett, B. E., Bricklin, P. M., Canter, M. B., Knapp, S. J., Moldawsky, S., & Phelps, R. (1999). Considerations for ethical practice of managed care. Professional Psychology: Research and Practice, 30(6), 563–575.

*Ainslie, R. (2007). Psychoanalytic psychotherapy. In A. B. Rochlen (Ed.), Applying counseling theories: An online case-based approach (pp. 5–20). Upper Saddle River, NJ: Pearson Prentice-Hall.

*Alle-Corliss, L., & Alle-Corliss, R. (2006). Human service agencies: An orientation to fieldwork (2nd ed.). Belmont, CA: Brooks/Cole, Cengage Learning.

*American Association for Marriage and Family Therapy. (2001). AAMFT code of ethics. Alexandria, VA: Author.

American Counseling Association. (2005). ACA code of ethics. Alexandria, VA: Author.

American Psychiatric Association. (2000). Diagnostic and statistical manual of mental disorders: Text revision (4th ed.). Washington, DC: Author.

American Psychological Association. (2002). Ethical principles of psychologists and code of conduct. American Psychologist, 57(12), 1060–1073.

American Psychological Association. (2003). Guidelines on multicultural education, training, research, practice, and organizational change for psychologists. American Psychologist, 58(5), 377–402.

American Psychological Association, Division 44. (2000). Guidelines for psychotherapy with lesbian, gay, and bisexual clients. American Psychologist, 55(12), 1440–1451.

American School Counseling Association. (2004). Ethical standards for school counselors. Alexandria, VA: Author.

Anderson, M. J., & Ellis, R. (1988). On the reservation. In N. A. Vacc, J. Wittmer, & S. B. DeVaney (Eds.), Experiencing and counseling multicultural and diverse populations (2nd ed., pp. 107–126). Muncie, IN: Accelerated Development.

Anderson, S. K., & Kitchener, K. S. (1996). Nonromantic, nonsexual posttherapy relationships between psychologists and former clients: An exploratory study of critical incidents. Professional Psychology: Research and Practice, 27(1), 59–66.

*Armstrong, T. (2007). The human odyssey: Navigating the twelve stages of life. New York: Sterling.

Arredondo, P., Toporek, R., Brown, S., Jones, J., Locke, D., Sanchez, J., & Stadler, H. (1996). Operationalization of multicultural counseling competencies. *Journal of Multicultural Counseling and Development, 24*(1), 42–78.

Association for Counselor Education and Supervision. (1993, Summer). Ethical guidelines for counseling supervisors. *Spectrum, 53*(4), 3–8.

Association for Counselor Education and Supervision. (1995). Ethical guidelines for counseling supervisors. *Counselor Education and Supervision, 34*(3), 270–276.

Association for Lesbian, Gay, Bisexual and Transgender Issues in Counseling. (2008). *Competencies for counseling gay, lesbian, bisexual and transgendered (GLBT) clients.* Retrieved January 1, 2008, from www.algbtic .org/resources/competencies.html

Association for Specialists in Group Work. (2008). Best practice guidelines. *Journal for Specialists in Group Work, 33*(2), 111–117.

Atkinson, D. R. (2004). *Counseling American minorities* (6th ed.). Boston, MA: McGraw-Hill.

Atkinson, D. R., Thompson, C. E., & Grant, S. K. (1993). A three-dimensional model for counseling racial/ethnic minorities. *The Counseling Psychologist, 21*(2), 257–277.

*Baker, E. K. (2003). *Caring for ourselves: A therapist's guide to personal and professional well-being.* Washington, DC: American Psychological Association.

Barlow, S. H. (2008). Group psychotherapy specialty practice. *Professional Psychology: Research and Practice, 39*(2), 240–244.

Barnett, J. E. (2007). Psychological wellness: A guide for mental health practitioners. *Ethical Issues in Professional Counseling, 10*(2), 9–18.

*Barnett, J. E. (2008). Impaired professionals: Distress, professional impairment, self-care, and psychological wellness. In M. Hersen & A. M. Gross (Eds.), *Handbook of clinical psychology* (pp. 857–884). New York: Wiley.

Barnett, J. E., Baker, E. K., Elman, N. S., & Schoener, G. R. (2007). In pursuit of wellness: The self-care imperative. *Professional Psychology: Research and Practice, 38*(6), 603–612.

Barnett, J. E., Behnke, S. H., Rosenthal, S. L., & Koocher, G. P. (2007). In case of ethical dilemma, break glass: Commentary on ethical decision making in practice. *Professional Psychology: Research and Practice, 38*(1), 7–12.

Barnett, J. E., Cornish, J. A. E., Goodyear, R. K., & Lichtenberg, J. W. (2007). Commentaries on the ethical and effective practice of clinical supervision. *Professional Psychology: Research and Practice, 38*(3), 268–275.

Barnett, J. E., Doll, B., Younggren, J. N., & Rubin, N. J. (2007). Clinical competence for practicing psychologists: Clearly a work in progress. *Professional Psychology: Research and Practice, 38*(5), 510–517.

*Barnett, J. E., & Johnson, W. B. (2008). *Ethics desk reference for psychologists.* Washington, DC: American Psychological Association.

*Barnett, J. E., & Johnson, W. B. (2010). *Ethics desk reference for counselors.* Alexandria, VA: American Counseling Association.

Barnett, J. E., Lazarus, A. A., Vasquez, M. J. T., Moorehead-Slaughter, O., & Johnson, W. B. (2007). Boundary issues and multiple relationships: Fantasy and reality. *Professional Psychology: Research and Practice, 38*(4), 401–410.

Barnett, J. E., Wise, E. H., Johnson-Greene, D., & Bucky, S. F. (2007). Informed consent: Too much of a good thing or not enough? *Professional Psychology: Research and Practice, 38*(2), 179–186.

Beck, A. T. (1976). *Cognitive therapy and the emotional disorders.* New York: New American Library.

Beck, A. T. (1987). Cognitive therapy. In J. K. Zeig (Ed.), *The evolution of psychotherapy* (pp. 149–178). New York: Brunner/Mazel.

Beck, A. T., & Weishaar, M. E. (2008). Cognitive therapy. In R. J. Corsini & D. Wedding (Eds.), *Current psychotherapies* (8th ed., pp. 263–294). Belmont, CA: Brooks/Cole, Cengage Learning.

Bemak, F., & Chung, R. C-Y. (2007). Training social justice counselors. In C. Lee (Ed.), *Counseling for social justice* (pp. 239–258). Alexandria, VA: American Counseling Association.

Bennett, A. G., & Werth, J. L., Jr. (2006). Working with clients who may harm themselves. In B. Herlihy & G. Corey, (Eds.), *ACA ethical standards casebook* (6th ed., pp. 223–228). Alexandria, VA: American Counseling Association.

*Bennett, B. E., Bricklin, P. M., Harris, E., Knapp, S., VandeCreek, L., & Younggren, J. N. (2006). *Assessing and managing risk in psychological practice: An individualized approach.* Rockville, MD: The Trust.

*Bernard, J. M., & Goodyear, R. K. (2009). *Fundamentals of clinical supervision* (4th ed.). Upper Saddle River, NJ: Pearson.

*Bersoff, D. N. (2003). *Ethical conflicts in psychology* (3rd ed.). Washington, DC: American Psychological Association.

Bitter, J. R. (1987). Communication and meaning: Satir in Adlerian context. In R. Sherman & D. Dinkmeyer (Eds.), *Systems of family therapy: An Adlerian integration* (pp. 109–142). New York: Brunner/Mazel.

Bitter, J. R. (1988). Family mapping and family constellation: Satir in Adlerian context. *Individual Psychology: The Journal of Adlerian Theory, Research, and Practice, 44*(1), 106–111.

*Bitter, J. R. (2009). *Theory and practice of family therapy and counseling.* Belmont, CA: Brooks/Cole, Cengage Learning.

Bobbitt, B. L. (2006). The importance of professional psychology: A view from managed care. *Professional Psychology: Research and Practice, 37*(6), 590–597.

Bowen, M. (1978). *Family therapy in clinical practice.* New York: Jason Aronson.

*Brammer, L. M., & MacDonald, G. (2003). *The helping relationship: Process and skills* (8th ed.). Boston: Allyn & Bacon.

*Brems, C. (2001). *Basic skills in psychotherapy and counseling.* Belmont, CA: Brooks/Cole, Cengage Learning.

Brislin, D. C., & Herbert, J. T. (2009). Clinical supervision for developing counselors. In I. Marini & M. A. Stebnicki (Eds.), *The professional counselor's desk reference* (pp. 39–47). New York: Springer.

Brockett, D. R., & Gleckman, A. D. (1991). Countertransference with the older adult: The importance of mental health counselor awareness and strategies for effective management. *Journal of Mental Health Counseling, 13*(3), 343–355.

Brown, C., & O'Brien, K. M. (1998). Understanding stress and burnout in shelter workers. *Professional Psychology: Research and Practice, 29*(4), 383–385.

Brown, C., & Trangsrud, H. B. (2008). Factors associated with acceptance and decline of client gift giving. *Professional Psychology: Research and Practice, 39*(5), 505–511.

Burke, M. T., & Miranti, J. G. (Eds.). (1995). *Counseling: The spiritual dimension.* Alexandria, VA: American Counseling Association.

Calhoun, K. S., Moras, K., Pilkonis, P. A., & Rehm, L. P. (1998). Empirically supported treatments: Implications for training. *Journal of Consulting and Clinical Psychology, 66,* 151–162.

Campbell, C. D., & Gordon, M. C. (2003). Acknowledging the inevitable: Understanding multiple relationships in rural practice. *Professional Psychology: Research and Practice, 34*(4), 430–434.

Canadian Counselling Association. (2007). *CCA code of ethics.* Toronto, Canada: Author.

*Cashwell, C. S., & Young, J. S. (2005). *Integrating spirituality and religion into counseling: A guide to competent practice.* Alexandria, VA: American Counseling Association.

*Cochran, J. L., & Cochran, N. H. (2006). *The heart of counseling: A guide to developing therapeutic relationships.* Belmont, CA: Wadsworth, Cengage Learning.

Codes of ethics for the helping professions (4th ed.). (2011). Belmont, CA: Brooks/Cole, Cengage Learning.

Commission on Rehabilitation Counselor Certification. (2003). *Scope of practice for rehabilitation counseling.* Schaumburg, IL: Author. Retrieved October 14, 2008, from http://www.crccertification.com/pages/31research.html

Commission on Rehabilitation Counselor Certification. (2009). *About CRCC.* Retrieved April 28, 2009, from http://www.crccertification.com

Commission on Rehabilitation Counselor Certification. (2010). *Code of professional ethics for rehabilitation counselors.* Schaumburg, IL: Author.

Constantine, M. G., Hage, S. M., Kindaichi, M., & Bryant, R. M. (2007). Social justice and multicultural issues: Implications for the practice and training of counselors and counseling psychologists. *Journal of Counseling and Development, 85*(1), 24–29.

Constantine, M. G., Myers, L. J., Kindaichi, M., & Moore, J. L. (2004). Exploring indigenous mental health practices: The role of healers and helpers in promoting well-being in people of color. *Counseling and Values, 48*(2), 110–125.

*Conyne, R. K., & Bemak, F. (Eds.). (2005). *Journeys to professional excellence: Lessons from leading counselor educators and practitioners.* Alexandria, VA: American Counseling Association.

Cooper, C. C., & Gottlieb, M. C. (2000). Ethical issues with managed care: Challenges facing counseling psychology. *The Counseling Psychologist, 28*(2), 179–236.

*Corey, G. (2008). *Theory and practice of group counseling* (7th ed.) and *Manual.* Belmont, CA: Brooks/Cole, Cengage Learning.

*Corey, G. (2009a). *The art of integrative counseling* (2nd ed.). Belmont, CA: Brooks/Cole, Cengage Learning.

*Corey, G. (2009b). *Case approach to counseling and psychotherapy* (7th ed.). Belmont, CA: Brooks/Cole, Cengage Learning.

*Corey, G. (2009c). *Theory and practice of counseling and psychotherapy* (8th ed.) and *Manual.* Belmont, CA: Brooks/Cole, Cengage Learning.

*Corey, G., & Corey, M. (2010). *I never knew I had a choice* (9th ed.). Belmont, CA: Brooks/Cole, Cengage Learning.

*Corey, G., Corey, M., & Callanan, P. (2011). *Issues and ethics in the helping professions* (8th ed.). Belmont, CA: Brooks/Cole, Cengage Learning.

*Corey, G., Corey, M., Callanan, P., & Russell, J. M. (2004). *Group techniques* (3rd ed.). Belmont, CA: Brooks/Cole, Cengage Learning.

*Corey, G., Corey, M., & Haynes, R. (2003). *Ethics in action CD-ROM.* Belmont, CA: Brooks/Cole, Cengage Learning.

*Corey, G., Corey, M., & Haynes, R. (2006). *Groups in action: Evolution and challenges—DVD and Workbook.* Belmont, CA: Brooks/Cole, Cengage Learning.

*Corey, G., Haynes, R., Moulton, P., & Muratori, M. (2010). *Clinical supervision in the helping professions: A practical guide* (2nd ed.). Alexandria, VA: American Counseling Association.

Corey, G., & Herlihy, B. (2006a). Client rights and informed consent. In B. Herlihy & G. Corey, *ACA ethical standards casebook* (6th ed., pp. 151–153). Alexandria, VA: American Counseling Association.

Corey, G., & Herlihy, B. (2006b). Competence. In B. Herlihy & G. Corey, *ACA ethical standards casebook* (6th ed., pp. 179–182). Alexandria, VA: American Counseling Association.

Corey, G., Herlihy, B., & Henderson, K. (2008). Perspectives on ethical counseling practice. *Ethical Issues in Professional Counseling, 11*(1), 1–11. [Published by the Hatherleigh Company, Long Island City, New York.]

*Corey, M., Corey, G., & Corey, C. (2010). *Groups: Process and practice* (8th ed.). Belmont, CA: Brooks/Cole, Cengage Learning.

*Cormier, S., & Hackney, H. (2005). *Counseling strategies and interventions* (6th ed.). Boston: Allyn & Bacon.

Cornish, J. A. E., Gorgens, K. A., Monson, S. P., Olkin, R., Palombi, B. J., & Abels, A. V. (2008). Perspectives on ethical practice with people who have disabilities. *Professional Psychology: Research and Practice, 39*(5), 488–497.

*Corsini, R., & Wedding, D. (Eds.). (2008). *Current psychotherapies* (8th ed.). Belmont, CA: Brooks/Cole, Cengage Learning.

Coster, J. S., & Schwebel, M. (1997). Well-functioning in professional psychologists. *Professional Psychology: Research and Practice, 28*(1), 5–13.

Cottone, R. R. (2001). A social constructivism model of ethical decision making in counseling. *Journal of Counseling and Development, 79*(1), 39–45.

*Cottone, R. R., & Tarvydas, V. M. (2007). *Counseling ethics and decision making* (3rd ed.). Upper Saddle River, NJ: Merrill/Prentice-Hall.

Council on Rehabilitation Education. (2009). *CORE history.* Retrieved April 28, 2009, from http://www.core-rehab.org

Crespi, T. D., Fischetti, B. A., & Butler, S. K. (2001, January). Clinical supervision in the schools. *Counseling Today, 7, 28, 34.*

Crethar, H. C., & Ratts, M. J. (2008, June). Why social justice is a counseling concern. *Counseling Today, 50*(12), 24–25.

Crethar, H. C., Torres Rivera, E., & Nash, S. (2008). In search of common threads: Linking multicultural, feminist, and social justice counseling paradigms. *Journal of Counseling and Development, 86*(3), 269–278.

Cummings, N. A. (1995). Impact of managed care on employment and training: A primer for survival. *Professional Psychology: Research and Practice, 26*(1), 10–15.

Dattilio, F. M., & Norcross, J. C. (2006). Psychotherapy integration and the emergence of instinctual territoriality. *Archives of Psychiatry and Psychotherapy, 8*(1), 5–16.

*Davis, S. R., & Meier, S. T. (2001). *The elements of managed care: A guide for helping professionals.* Belmont, CA: Brooks/Cole, Cengage Learning.

Dearing, R. L., Maddux, J. E., & Tangney, J. P. (2005). Predictors of psychological help seeking in clinical and counseling psychology graduate students. *Professional Psychology: Research and Practice, 36*(3), 323–329.

*DeJong, P., & Berg, I. (2008). *Interviewing for solutions* (3rd ed.). Belmont, CA: Brooks/Cole, Cengage Learning.

DeLucia-Waack, J. L., & Donigian, J. (2004). *The practice of multicultural group work: Visions and perspectives from the field.* Belmont, CA: Brooks/Cole, Cengage Learning.

*DeLucia-Waack, J. L., Gerrity, D., Kalodner, C. R., & Riva, M. T. (Eds). (2004). *Handbook of group counseling and psychotherapy.* Thousand Oaks, CA: Sage.

DePoy, E., & Gilson, S. F. (2004). *Rethinking disability: Principles for professional and social change.* Belmont, CA: Brooks/Cole, Cengage Learning.

Dew, D. W., & Peters, S. (2002). Survey of master's level rehabilitation counselor programs: Relationship to public vocational rehabilitation recruitment and retention of state vocational rehabilitation counselors. *Rehabilitation Education, 16,* 61–65.

*Diller, J. V. (2007). *Cultural diversity: A primer for the human services* (3rd ed.). Belmont, CA: Brooks/Cole, Cengage Learning.

*Dolgoff, R., Loewenberg, F. M., & Harrington, D. (2009). *Ethical decisions for social work practice* (8th ed.). Belmont, CA: Brooks/Cole, Cengage Learning.

Duran, E., Firehammer, J., & Gonzalez, J. (2008). Liberation psychology as a path toward healing cultural soul wounds. *Journal of Counseling and Development, 86*(3), 288–295.

Egan, G. (2006). *Skilled helping around the world: Addressing diversity and multiculturalism.* Belmont, CA: Brooks/Cole, Cengage Learning.

*Egan, G. (2010). *The skilled helper* (9th ed.). Belmont, CA: Brooks/Cole, Cengage Learning.

*Ellis, A. (1999). *How to make yourself happy and remarkably less disturbable.* San Luis Obispo, CA: Impact.

*Ellis, A. (2000). *How to control your anxiety before it controls you.* New York: Citadel.

*Ellis, A. (2001a). *Feeling better, getting better, and staying better.* Atascadero, CA: Impact.

*Ellis, A. (2001b). *Overcoming destructive thoughts, feelings, and behaviors.* Amherst, NY: Prometheus Books.

*Ellis, A. (2002). *Overcoming resistance: A rational emotive behavior therapy integrated approach* (2nd ed.). New York: Springer.

*Ellis, A. (2004a). *Rational emotive behavior therapy: It works for me—It can work for you.* Amherst, NY: Prometheus Books.

*Ellis, A. (2004b). *The road to tolerance: The philosophy of rational emotive behavior therapy.* Amherst, NY: Prometheus Books.

*Ellis, A. (2008). Rational emotive behavior therapy. In R. Corsini & D. Wedding (Eds.), *Current psychotherapies* (8th ed., pp. 187–222). Belmont, CA: Brooks/Cole, Cengage Learning.

Ellis, A., & Dryden, W. (1997). *The practice of rational-emotive therapy* (Rev. ed.). New York: Springer.

*Ellis, A., & Harper, R. A. (1997). *A new guide to rational living* (3rd ed.). North Hollywood, CA: Wilshire Books.

*Ellis, A., & MacLaren, C. (2005). *Rational emotive behavior therapy: A therapist's guide* (2nd ed). Atascadero, CA: Impact.

Emerson, S., & Markos, P. A. (1996). Signs and symptoms of the impaired counselor. *Journal of Humanistic Education and Development, 34,* 108–117.

Erikson, E. (1963). *Childhood and society* (2nd ed.). New York: Norton.

Erikson, E. (1982). *The life cycle completed.* New York: Norton.

*Faiver, C. M., Eisengart, S., & Colonna, R. (2004). *The counselor intern's handbook* (3rd ed.). Belmont, CA: Brooks/Cole, Cengage Learning.

Faiver, C. M., Ingersoll, R. E., O'Brien, E., & McNally, C. (2001). *Explorations in counseling and spirituality: Philosophical, practical, and personal reflections.* Belmont, CA: Brooks/Cole, Cengage Learning.

Faiver, C. M., & O'Brien, E. M. (1993). Assessment of religious beliefs form. *Counseling and Values, 37*(3), 176–178.

Ferguson, A. (2009). Cultural issues in counseling lesbians, gays, and bisexuals. In I. Marini & M. A. Stebnicki (Eds.), *The professional counselor's desk reference* (pp. 255–262). New York: Springer.

Figley, C. R. (1995). Compassion fatigue: Toward a new understanding of the costs of caring. In B. H. Stamm (Ed.), *Secondary traumatic stress.* Lutherville, MD: Sidran Press.

Ford, M. P., & Hendrick, S. S. (2003). Therapists' sexual values for self and clients: Implications for practice and training. *Professional Psychology: Research and Practice, 34*(1), 80–87.

Foster, D., & Black, T. G. (2007). An integral approach to counseling ethics. *Counseling and Values, 51*(3), 221–234.

*Frame, M. W. (2003). *Integrating religion and spirituality into counseling: A comprehensive approach.* Belmont, CA: Brooks/Cole, Cengage Learning.

Frame, M. W., & Williams, C. B. (2005). A model of ethical decision making from a multicultural perspective. *Counseling and Values, 49*(3), 165–179.

Francis, P. C. (2009). Religion and spirituality in counseling. In I. Marini & M. A. Stebnicki (Eds.), *The professional counselor's desk reference* (pp. 839–849). New York: Springer.

Gabbard, G. (1995, April). What are boundaries in psychotherapy? *The Menninger Letter, 3*(4), 1–2.

Garcia, J. G., Cartwright, B., Winston, S. M., & Borzuchowska, B. (2003). A transcultural integrative model for ethical decision making in counseling. *Journal of Counseling and Development, 81*(3), 268–277.

George, M. (1998). *Learn to relax: A practical guide to easing tension and conquering stress.* San Francisco: Chronicle Books.

Getz, J. G., & Protinsky, H. O. (1994). Training marriage and family counselors: A family-of-origin approach. *Counselor Education and Supervision, 33*(3), 183–200.

Gill-Wigal, J., & Heaton, J. A. (1996). Managing sexual attraction in the therapeutic relationship. *Directions in Mental Health Counseling, 6*(8), 4–15.

*Gladding, S. T. (2009). *Becoming a counselor: The light, the bright, and the serious* (2nd ed.). Alexandria, VA: American Counseling Association.

Glosoff, H. L., Corey, G., & Herlihy, B. (2006). Avoiding detrimental multiple relationships. In B. Herlihy & G. Corey, *ACA ethical standards casebook* (6th ed., pp. 209–215). Alexandria, VA: American Counseling Association.

*Goldenberg, H., & Goldenberg, I. (2008). *Family therapy: An overview* (7th ed.). Belmont, CA: Brooks/Cole, Cengage Learning.

Goldenberg, I., & Goldenberg, H. (2004). *Family exploration: Personal viewpoints from multiple perspectives, a workbook for family therapy: An overview* (6th ed.). Belmont, CA: Brooks/Cole, Cengage Learning.

*Goleman, D. (1995). *Emotional intelligence*. New York: Bantam Books.

Goodman, R. W., & Carpenter-White, A. (1996). The family autobiography assignment: Some ethical considerations. *Counselor Education and Supervision, 35*(3), 230–238.

Goodwin, L. R., Jr. (2006). Rehabilitation counselor specialty areas offered by rehabilitation counselor education programs. *Rehabilitation Education, 20,* 133–143.

Griffin, M. (2007). On writing progress notes. *The Therapist, 19*(2), 24–28.

Gutheil, T. G., & Gabbard, G. O. (1993). The concept of boundaries in clinical practice: Theoretical and risk-management dimensions. *American Journal of Psychiatry, 150*(2), 188–196.

*Guy, J. D. (1987). *The personal life of the psychotherapist.* New York: Wiley.

*Hackney, H., & Cormier, S. (2005). *The professional counselor: A process guide to helping* (5th ed.). Boston: Allyn & Bacon (Pearson).

Hage, S. M. (2006). A closer look at the role of spirituality in psychology training programs. *Professional Psychology: Research and Practice, 37*(3), 303–310.

Haley, W. E., Larson, D. G., Kasl-Godley, J., Neimeyer, R. A., & Kwilosz, D. M. (2003). Roles for psychologists in end-of-life care: Emerging models of practice. *Professional Psychology: Research and Practice, 34*(6), 626–633.

Hall, C. R., Dixon, W. A., & Mauzey, E. D. (2004). Spirituality and religion: Implications for counselors. *Journal of Counseling and Development, 82*(4), 504–507.

Hamilton, J. C., & Spruill, J. (1999). Identifying and reducing risk factors related to trainee–client sexual misconduct. *Professional Psychology: Research and Practice, 30*(3), 318–327.

*Hanna, F. J. (2002). *Therapy with difficult clients: Using the precursors model to awaken change.* Washington, DC: American Psychological Association.

*Hanna, S. M. (2007). *The practice of family therapy: Key elements across models* (4th ed.). Belmont, CA: Brooks/Cole, Cengage Learning.

Hansen, N. D., Pepitone-Arreola-Rockwell, E., & Greene A. F. (2000). Multicultural competence: Criteria and case example. *Professional Psychology: Research and Practice, 31*(6), 652–660.

Harper, M. C., & Gill, C. S. (2005). Assessing the client's spiritual domain. In C. S. Cashwell & J. S. Young (Eds.), *Integrating spirituality and religion into counseling: A guide to competent practice* (pp. 31–62). Alexandria, VA: American Counseling Association.

Hathaway, W. L., Scott, S. Y., & Garver, S. A. (2004). Assessing religious/spiritual functioning: A neglected domain in clinical practice? *Professional Psychology: Research and Practice, 35*(1), 97–104.

*Hazler, R. J., & Kottler, J. A. (2005). *The emerging professional counselor: Student dreams to professional realities* (2nd ed.). Alexandria, VA: American Counseling Association.

Herlihy, B. (1996). When a colleague is impaired: The individual counselor's response. *Journal of Humanistic Education and Development, 34,* 118–127.

*Herlihy, B., & Corey, G. (2006a). *ACA ethical standards casebook* (6th ed.). Alexandria, VA: American Counseling Association.

*Herlihy, B., & Corey, G. (2006b). *Boundary issues in counseling: Multiple roles and responsibilities* (2nd ed.). Alexandria, VA: American Counseling Association.

Herlihy, B., & Corey, G. (2006c). Confidentiality. In B. Herlihy & G. Corey, *ACA ethical standards casebook* (6th ed., pp. 159–163). Alexandria, VA: American Counseling Association.

*Herlihy, B., & Corey, G. (2008). Boundaries in counseling: Ethical and clinical issues. *Ethical Issues in Professional Counseling, 11*(2), 13–24. [Published by the Hatherleigh Company, Long Island City, New York.]

*Herlihy, B. R., & Watson, Z. E. P. (2004). Assisted suicide: Ethical issues. In D. Capuzzi (Ed.), *Suicide across the life span: Implications for counselors* (pp. 163–184). Alexandria, VA: American Counseling Association.

*Herlihy, B. R., & Watson, Z. E. P. (2007). Social justice and counseling ethics. In C. C. Lee (Ed.), *Counseling for social justice* (pp. 181–199). Alexandria, VA: American Counseling Association.

*Herlihy, B. R., Watson, Z. E. P., & Patureau-Hatchett, M. P. (2008). Ethical concerns in diagnosing culturally diverse clients. *Ethical Issues in Professional Counseling, 11*(3), 25–34. [Published by the Hatherleigh Company, Long Island City, New York.]

*Hermann, M. A. (2006a). Legal perspectives on dual relationships. In B. Herlihy & G. Corey, *Boundary issues in counseling: Multiple roles and responsibilities* (2nd ed.). Alexandria, VA: American Counseling Association.

*Hermann, M. A. (2006b). The relationship between law and ethics. In B. Herlihy & G. Corey, *ACA ethical standards casebook* (6th ed., pp. 247–249). Alexandria, VA: American Counseling Association.

Ho, D. Y. F. (1985). Cultural values and professional issues in clinical psychology: Implications from the Hong Kong experience. *American Psychologist, 40*(11), 1212–1218.

*Hogan, M. (2007). *The four skills of cultural diversity competence: A process for understanding and practice* (3rd ed.). Belmont, CA: Brooks/Cole, Cengage Learning.

Hogan-Garcia, M., & Scheinberg, C. (2000). Culturally competent practice principles for planned intervention in organizations and communities. *Practicing Anthropology, 22*(2), 27–29.

*Homan, M. (2008). *Promoting community change: Making it happen in the real world* (4th ed.). Belmont, CA: Brooks/Cole, Cengage Learning.

*Ivey, A. E., D'Andrea, M., Ivey, M. B., & Simek-Morgan, L. (2007). *Theories of counseling and psychotherapy: A multicultural perspective* (6th ed.). Boston: Allyn & Bacon.

Ivey, A. E., & Ivey, M. B. (1998). Reframing DSM IV: Positive strategies from developmental counseling and therapy. *Journal of Counseling and Development, 76*(3), 334–350.

*Ivey, A. E., Ivey, M. B., & Zalaquett, C. P. (2010). *Intentional interviewing and counseling: Facilitating client development in a multicultural society* (7th ed.). Belmont, CA: Brooks/Cole, Cengage Learning.

*Jacobs, E. F., Masson, R. L., & Harvill, R. L. (2009). *Group counseling: Strategies and skills* (6th ed.). Belmont, CA: Brooks/Cole, Cengage Learning.

Jaffe, D. T. (1986). The inner strains of healing work: Therapy and self-renewal for health professionals. In C. D. Scott & J. Hawk (Eds.), *Heal thyself: The health of health care professionals.* New York: Brunner/Mazel.

*James, R. K. (2008). *Crisis intervention strategies* (6th ed.). Belmont, CA: Brooks/Cole, Cengage Learning.

*Jenaro, C., Flores, N., & Arias, B. (2007). Burnout and coping in human service practitioners. *Professional Psychology: Research and Practice, 38*(1), 80–87.

Jensen, J. P., & Bergin, A. E. (1988). Mental health values of professional therapists: A national interdisciplinary survey. *Professional Psychology: Research and Practice, 19*(3), 290–297.

*Kanel, K. (2007). *A guide to crisis intervention* (3rd ed.). Belmont, CA: Brooks/Cole, Cengage Learning.

Kaplan, D. (2009). New concepts in counseling ethics. In I. Marini & M. A. Stebnicki (Eds.), *The professional counselor's desk reference* (pp. 59–67). New York: Springer.

Kelly, E. W. (1995a). Counselor values: A national survey. *Journal of Counseling and Development, 73*(6), 648–653.

Kelly, E. W. (1995b). *Spirituality and religion in counseling and psychotherapy.* Alexandria, VA: American Counseling Association.

Kirland, K., Kirkland, K. L., & Reaves, R. P. (2004). On the professional use of disciplinary data. *Professional Psychology: Research and Practice, 35*(2), 179–184.

*Kiser, P. M. (2008). *The human services internship: Getting the most from your experience* (2nd ed.). Belmont, CA: Brooks/Cole, Cengage Learning.

*Kleespies, P. M. (2004). *Life and death decisions: Psychological and ethical considerations in end-of-life care.* Washington, DC: American Psychological Association.

Kleist, D., & Bitter, J. R. (2009). Virtue, ethics, and legality in family practice. In J. R. Bitter, *Theory and practice of family therapy and counseling* (pp. 43–65). Belmont, CA: Brooks/Cole, Cengage Learning.

Knapp, S., Gottlieb, M., Berman, J., & Handelsman, M. M. (2007). When law and ethics collide: What should psychologists do? *Professional Psychology: Research and Practice, 38*(1), 54–59.

*Knapp, S., & VandeCreek, L. (2003). *A guide to the 2002 revision of the American Psychological Association's ethics code.* Sarasota, FL: Professional Resource Press.

*Koocher, G. P., & Keith-Spiegel, P. (2008). *Ethics in psychology and the mental health professions: Standards and cases* (3rd ed.). New York: Oxford University Press.

*Kottler, J. A. (1992). *Compassionate therapy: Working with difficult clients.* San Francisco, CA: Jossey-Bass.

*Kottler, J. A. (1993). *On being a therapist* (Rev. ed.). San Francisco, CA: Jossey-Bass.

*Kottler, J. A. (Ed.). (1997). *Finding your way as a counselor.* Alexandria, VA: American Counseling Association.

*Kottler, J. A. (2000a). *Doing good: Passion and commitment for helping others.* Philadelphia, PA: Brunner-Routledge (Taylor & Francis).

*Kottler, J. A. (2000b). *Nuts and bolts of helping.* Boston: Allyn & Bacon.

*Kottler, J. A., & Jones, W. P. (Eds.). (2003). *Doing better: Improving clinical skills and professional competence.* New York: Brunner-Routledge.

*Kottler, J. A., & Shepard, D. S. (2008). *Introduction to counseling: Voices from the field* (6th ed.). Belmont, CA: Brooks/Cole, Cengage Learning.

Lamb, D. H., Catanzaro, S. J., & Moorman, A. S. (2003). A preliminary look at how psychologists identify, evaluate, and proceed when faced with possible multiple relationship dilemmas. *Professional Psychology: Research and Practice, 35*(3), 248–254.

Lasser, J. S., & Gottlieb, M. C. (2004). Treating patients distressed regarding their sexual orientation: Clinical and ethical alternatives. *Professional Psychology: Research and Practice, 35*(2), 194–200.

Lawson, D. M., & Gaushell, H. (1988). Family autobiography: A useful method for enhancing counselors' personal development. *Counselor Education and Supervision, 28*(2), 162–167.

Lawson, D. M., & Gaushell, H. (1991). Intergenerational family characteristics of counselor trainees. *Counselor Education and Supervision, 30*(4), 309–321.

Lazarus, A. A. (2001). Not all "dual relationships" are taboo: Some tend to enhance treatment outcomes. *The National Psychologist, 10*(1), 16.

Lazarus, A. A. (2006). Transcending boundaries in psychotherapy. In B. Herlihy & G. Corey, *Boundary issues in counseling: Multiple roles and responsibilities* (2nd ed., pp. 16–19). Alexandria, VA: American Counseling Association.

*Lazarus, A. A., & Zur, O. (Eds.). (2002). *Dual relationships and psychotherapy.* New York: Springer.

*Lee, C. C. (2006a). Entering the cross-cultural zone: Meeting the challenges of culturally responsive counseling. In C. C. Lee (Ed.), *Multicultural issues in counseling: New approaches to diversity* (3rd ed., pp. 13–22). Alexandria, VA: American Counseling Association.

*Lee, C. C. (2006b). Ethical issues in multicultural counseling. In B. Herlihy & G. Corey, *ACA ethical standards casebook* (6th ed., pp. 159–164). Alexandria, VA: American Counseling Association.

*Lee, C. C. (2006c). *Multicultural issues in counseling: New approaches to diversity* (3rd ed.). Alexandria, VA: American Counseling Association.

*Lee, C. C. (2007). *Counseling for social justice* (2nd ed.). Alexandria, VA: American Counseling Association.

Lee, C. C., & Hipolito-Delgado, C. P. (2007). Introduction: Counselors as agents of social justice. In C. C. Lee (Ed.), *Counseling for social justice* (pp. xiii–xxviii). Alexandria, VA: American Counseling Association.

Lee, C. C., & Ramsey, C. J. (2006). Multicultural counseling: A new paradigm for a new century. In C. C. Lee (Ed.), *Multicultural issues in counseling: New approaches to diversity* (3rd ed., pp. 3–11). Alexandria, VA: American Counseling Association.

*Lewis, J. A., Lewis, M. D., Daniels, J. A., & D'Andrea, M. J. (2003). *Community counseling: Empowerment strategies for a diverse society* (3rd ed.). Belmont, CA: Brooks/Cole, Cengage Learning.

Luborsky, E. B., O'Reilly-Landry, M., & Arlow, J. A. (2008). Psychoanalysis. In R. J. Corsini & D. Wedding (Eds.), *Current psychotherapies* (8th ed., pp. 15–62). Belmont, CA: Brooks/Cole, Cengage Learning.

Luke, M., & Hackney, H. (2007). Group coleadership: A critical review. *Counselor Education and Supervision, 46*(4), 280–293.

*Lum, D. (2004). *Social work practice and people of color: A process-stage approach* (5th ed.). Belmont, CA: Brooks/Cole, Cengage Learning.

*Lum, D. (2007). *Culturally competent practice: A framework for understanding diverse groups and justice issue* (3rd ed.). Belmont, CA: Brooks/Cole, Cengage Learning.

Luskin, F., & Pelletier, K. R. (2005). *Stress free for good.* New York: Harper Collins.

MacCluskie, K. C., & Ingersoll, R. E. (2001). *Becoming a 21st century agency counselor: Personal and professional explorations.* Belmont, CA: Brooks/Cole, Cengage Learning.

*Mackelprang, R. W., & Salsgiver, R. O. (1999). *Disability: A diversity model approach in human service practice.* Belmont, CA: Brooks/Cole, Cengage Learning.

Margolin, G. (1982). Ethical and legal considerations in marital and family therapy. *American Psychologist, 37*(3), 788–801.

Marini, I. (2007). Cross-cultural counseling issues of males who sustain a disability. In A. E. Dell Orto & P. W. Power (Eds.), *The psychological and social impact of illness and disability* (5th ed., pp. 194–213). New York: Springer.

*Maslach, C. (2003). *Burnout: The cost of caring.* Cambridge: Malor Books.

*Maslach, C., & Leiter, M. P. (1997). *The truth about burnout.* San Francisco: Jossey-Bass.

McCarthy, P., Sugden, S., Koker, M., Lamendola, F., Maurer, S., & Renninger, S. (1995). A practical guide to informed consent in clinical supervision. *Counselor Education and Supervision, 35*(2), 130–138.

*McClam, T., & Woodside, M. R. (2010). *Elements of interviewing.* Belmont, CA: Brooks/Cole, Cengage Learning.

*McGoldrick, M., & Carter, B. (2005). Self in context: The individual life cycle in systemic perspective. In B. Carter & M. McGoldrick (Eds.), *The expanded family life cycle: Individual, family, and social perspectives* (3rd ed., pp. 27–46). Boston: Allyn & Bacon.

McGoldrick, M., Gerson, R., & Petry, S. (2008). *Genograms: Assessment and intervention* (3rd ed.). New York: Norton.

*Meier, S. T., & Davis, S. R. (2008). *The elements of counseling* (6th ed.). Belmont, CA: Brooks/Cole, Cengage Learning.

Melnick, J., & Fall, M. (2008). A Gestalt approach to group supervision. *Counselor Education and Supervision, 48*(1), 48–60.

Miller, E., & Marini, I. (2009). Brief psychotherapy. In I. Marini & M. A. Stebnicki (Eds.), *The professional counselor's desk reference* (pp. 379–387). New York: Springer.

Miller, W. R. (Ed.). (1999). *Integrating spirituality into treatment: Resources for practitioners.* Washington, DC: American Psychological Association.

Miller, W. R., & Thoresen, C. E. (1999). Spirituality and health. In W. R. Miller (Ed.), *Integrating spirituality into treatment: Resources for practitioners* (pp. 3–18). Washington, DC: American Psychological Association.

Millner, V. S., & Hanks, R. B. (2002). Induced abortion: An ethical conundrum for counselors. *Journal of Counseling and Development, 80*(1), 57–63.

*Moleski, S. M., & Kiselica, M. S. (2005). Dual relationships: A continuum ranging from the destructive to the therapeutic. *Journal of Counseling and Development, 83*(1), 3–11.

Mosak, H., & Shulman, B. (1988). *Life style inventory*. Muncie, IN: Accelerated Development.

*Moursund, J. P., & Erskine, R. G. (2004). *Integrative psychotherapy: The art and science of relationship*. Belmont, CA: Brooks/Cole, Cengage Learning.

*Murphy, B. C., & Dillon, C. (2008). *Interviewing in action in a multicultural world* (3rd ed.). Belmont, CA: Brooks/Cole, Cengage Learning.

Myers, J. E., & Sweeney, T. J. (Eds.). (2005a). *Counseling for wellness: Theory, research, and practice*. Alexandria, VA: American Counseling Association.

Myers, J. E., & Sweeney, T. J. (2005b). Introduction to wellness theory. In J. E. Myers & T. J. Sweeney (Eds.), *Counseling for wellness: Theory, research, and practice* (pp. 7–14). Alexandria, VA: American Counseling Association.

Myers, J. E., & Sweeney, T. J. (2005c). The wheel of wellness. In J. E. Myers & T. J. Sweeney (Eds.), *Counseling for wellness: Theory, research, and practice* (pp. 15–28). Alexandria, VA: American Counseling Association.

Myers, J. E., Sweeney, T. J., & Witmer, J. M. (2000). The wheel of wellness counseling for wellness: A holistic model. *Journal of Counseling and Development, 78*(3), 251–266.

National Association of Alcohol and Drug Abuse Counselors. (2004). *NAADAC code of ethics*. Alexandria, VA: Author.

National Association of Social Workers. (2008). *Code of ethics*. Washington, DC: Author.

National Organization for Human Services. (2000). Ethical standards of human service professionals. *Human Service Education, 20*(1), 61–68.

Neimeyer, R. A. (2000). Suicide and hastened death: Toward a training agenda for counseling psychology. *The Counseling Psychologist, 28*(4), 551–560.

*Neukrug, E. (2007). *The world of the counselor: An introduction to the counseling profession* (3rd ed.). Belmont, CA: Brooks/Cole, Cengage Learning.

*Neukrug, E. (2008). *Theory, practice, and trends in human services: An introduction* (4th ed.). Belmont, CA: Brooks/Cole, Cengage Learning.

*Newman, B. M., & Newman, P. R. (2009). *Development through life: A psychosocial approach* (10th ed.). Belmont, CA: Wadsworth, Cengage Learning.

*Nichols, M. P. (with Schwartz, R. C.). (2008). *Family therapy: Concepts and methods* (8th ed.). Boston: Allyn & Bacon.

Norcross, J. C. (2000). Psychotherapist self-care: Practitioner-tested, research-informed strategies. *Professional Psychology: Research and Practice, 31*(6), 710–713.

*Norcross, J. C. (2005). The psychotherapist's own psychotherapy: Educating and developing psychologists. *American Psychologist, 60*(8), 840–850.

*Norcross, J. C., & Guy, J. D. (2007). *Leaving it at the office: A guide to psychotherapist self-care*. New York: Guilford Press.

*Nystul, M. S. (2006). *Introduction to counseling: An art and science perspective* (3rd ed.). Boston: Allyn & Bacon.

Oakes, K., & Raphel, M. M. (2008). Spiritual assessment in counseling: Methods and practice. *Counseling and Values, 52*(3), 240–252.

Okech, J. E. A., & Kline, W. B. (2006). Competency concerns in group co-leader relationships. *Journal for Specialists in Group Work, 31*(2), 165–180.

*Okun, B. F., & Kantrowitz, R. E. (2008). *Effective helping: Interviewing and counseling techniques* (7th ed.). Belmont, CA: Brooks/Cole, Cengage Learning.

Olkin, R. (2009). Disability-affirmative therapy. In I. Marini & M. A. Stebnicki (Eds.), *The professional counselor's desk reference* (pp. 355–369). New York: Springer.

Pack-Brown, S. P., Thomas, T. L., & Seymour, J. M. (2008). Infusing professional ethics into counselor education programs: A multicultural/ social justice perspective. *Journal of Counseling and Development, 86*(3), 296–302.

*Parham, T. A., & Caldwell, L. D. (2006). Dual relationships revisited: An African centered imperative. In B. Herlihy & G. Corey, *Boundary issues in counseling: Multiple roles and responsibilities* (2nd ed., pp. 131–136). Alexandria, VA: American Counseling Association.

*Pedersen, P. (2000). *A handbook for developing multicultural awareness* (3rd ed.). Alexandria, VA: American Counseling Association.

Pedersen, P. (2003). Culturally biased assumptions in counseling psychology. *The Counseling Psychologist, 31*(4), 396–403.

Pedersen, P. (2008). Ethics, competence, and professional issues in cross-cultural counseling. In P. B. Pedersen, J. G. Draguns, W. J. Lonner, & J. E. Trimble (Eds.), *Counseling across cultures* (6th ed., pp. 5–20). Thousand Oaks, CA: Sage.

*Pedersen, P., Crethar, H., & Carlson, J. (2008). *Inclusive cultural empathy: Making relationships central in counseling and psychotherapy.* Washington, DC: APA Press.

Piper, W. E. (2001). Commentary on my editorship (1993–2001). *International Journal of Group Psychotherapy, 51,* 165–168.

Piper, W. E., & Ogrodniczuk, J. S. (2004). Brief group therapy. In J. L. DeLucia-Waack, D. Gerrity, C. R. Kalodner, & M. T. Riva (Eds.), *Handbook of group counseling and psychotherapy* (pp. 641–650). Thousand Oaks, CA: Sage.

Polster, E. (1995). *A population of selves: A therapeutic exploration of personal diversity.* San Francisco, CA: Jossey-Bass.

Ponterotto, J. G., Casas, J. M., Suzuki, L. A., & Alexander, C. M. (1995). *Handbook of multicultural counseling.* Thousand Oaks, CA: Sage.

Pope, K. S., Sonne, J. L., & Holroyd, J. (1993). *Sexual feelings in psychotherapy: Explorations for therapists and therapists-in-training.* Washington, DC: American Psychological Association.

*Pope, K. S., & Vasquez, M. J. T. (2007). *Ethics in psychotherapy and counseling: A practical guide for psychologists* (3rd ed.). San Francisco, CA: Jossey-Bass.

Powers, R. L., & Griffith, J. (1986). *The individual psychology client workbook.* Chicago: The Americas Institute of Adlerian Studies.

Powers, R. L., & Griffith, J. (1987). *Understanding life-style: The psycho-clarity process.* Chicago: The Americas Institute of Adlerian Studies.

*Prochaska, J. O., & Norcross, J. C. (2010). *Systems of psychotherapy: A transtheoretical analysis* (7th ed.). Belmont, CA: Brooks/Cole, Cengage Learning.

Radeke, J. T., & Mahoney, M. J. (2000). Comparing the personal lives of psychotherapists and research psychologists. *Professional Psychology: Research and Practice, 31*(1), 82–84.

Ray, D., & Altekruse, M. (2000). Effectiveness of group supervision versus combined group and individual supervision. *Counselor Education and Supervision, 40*(1), 19–30.

*Remley, T. P., & Herlihy, B. (2010). *Ethical, legal, and professional issues in counseling* (3rd ed.). Upper Saddle River, NJ: Merrill/Prentice-Hall.

Remley, T. P., & Sparkman, L. B. (1993). Student suicides: The counselor's limited legal liability. *The School Counselor, 40,* 164–169.

Richards, P. S., & Bergin, A. E. (2005). *A spiritual strategy for counseling and psychotherapy* (2nd ed.). Washington, DC: American Psychological Association.

Richards, P. S., Rector, J. M., & Tjeltveit, A. C. (1999). Values, spirituality, and psychotherapy. In W. R. Miller (Ed.), *Integrating spirituality into treatment: Resources for practitioners* (pp. 133–160). Washington, DC: American Psychological Association.

*Ridley, C. R. (2005). *Overcoming unintentional racism in counseling and therapy: A practitioner's guide to intentional intervention* (2nd ed.). Thousand Oaks, CA: Sage.

Riggar, T. F. (2009). Counselor burnout. In I. Marini & M. A. Stebnicki (Eds.), *The professional counselor's desk reference* (pp. 831–837). New York: Springer.

Rivas-Vasquez, R. A., Blais, M. A., Rey, G. J., & Rivas-Vazquez, A. A. (2001). A brief reminder about documenting the psychological consultation. *Professional Psychology: Research and Practice, 32*(2), 194–199.

Robles, B. (2009). A synopsis of the Health Insurance Portability and Accountability Act. In I. Marini & M. A. Stebnicki (Eds.), *The professional counselor's desk reference* (pp. 801–812). New York: Springer.

Roessler, R. & Rubin, S. E. (1998). *Case management and rehabilitation counseling.* Austin, TX: PRO-ED.

Roysircar, G., Arredondo, P., Fuertes, J. N., Ponterotto, J. G., & Toporek, R. L. (2003). *Multicultural counseling competencies 2003: Association for multicultural counseling and development.* Alexandria, VA: American Counseling Association.

*Russell-Chapin, L. A., & Ivey, A. E. (2004). *Your supervised practicum and internship.* Belmont, CA: Brooks/Cole, Cengage Learning.

Salisbury, W. A., & Kinnier, R. T. (1996). Posttermination friendship between counselors and clients. *Journal of Counseling and Development, 74*(5), 495–500.

Sampson, E. E. (2000). Reinterpreting individualism and collectivism: Their religious roots and monologic versus dialogic person other relationships. *American Psychologist, 55*(12), 1425–1432.

*Satir, V. (1983). *Conjoint family therapy* (3rd ed.). Palo Alto, CA: Science and Behavior Books.

*Satir, V. (1989). *The new peoplemaking.* Palo Alto, CA: Science and Behavior Books.

Satir, V., & Baldwin, M. (1983). *Satir: Step by step.* Palo Alto, CA: Science and Behavior Books.

Satir, V., Banmen, J., Gerber, J., & Gomori, M. (1991). *The Satir model.* Palo Alto, CA: Science and Behavior Books.

Satir, V., Bitter, J. R., & Krestensen, K. K. (1988). Family reconstruction: The family within—a group experience. *Journal for Specialists in Group Work, 13*(4), 200–208.

Schank, J. A., & Skovholt, T. M. (1997). Dual-relationship dilemmas of rural and small community psychologists. *Professional Psychology: Research and Practice, 28*(1), 44–49.

Schreier, B., Davis, D., & Rodolfa, E. (2005). Diversity-based psychology with lesbian, gay and bisexual patients: Clinical and training issues—practical actions. *California Department of Consumer Affairs (Board of Psychology), 12*, 1–13.

Shafranske, E. P., & Sperry, L. (2005). Future directions: Opportunities and challenges. In L. Sperry & E. P. Shafranske (Eds.), *Spiritually oriented psychotherapy* (pp. 351–354). Washington, DC: American Psychological Association.

*Sharf, R. S. (2008). *Theories of psychotherapy and counseling: Concepts and cases* (4th ed.). Belmont, CA: Brooks/Cole, Cengage Learning.

Shulman, B., & Mosak, H. (1988). *Manual for life style assessment.* Muncie, IN: Accelerated Development.

*Shulman, L. (2009). *The skills of helping individuals, families, groups, and communities* (6th ed.). Belmont, CA: Brooks/Cole, Cengage Learning.

*Skovholt, T. M. (2001). *The resilient practitioner: Burnout prevention and self-care strategies for counselors, therapists, teachers, and health professionals.* Boston: Allyn & Bacon.

*Skovholt, T. M., & Jennings, L. (2004). *Master therapists: Exploring expertise in therapy and counseling.* Boston: Pearson Education.

Sleek, S. (1994, December). Ethical dilemmas plague rural practice. *APA Monitor, 25*(12), 26–27.

Smart, J. (2009). Counseling individuals with disabilities. In I. Marini & M. A. Stebnicki (Eds.), *The professional counselor's desk reference* (pp. 637–644). New York: Springer.

Smith, A. J., Thorngren, J., & Christopher, J. C. (2009). Rural mental health counseling. In I. Marini & M. A. Stebnicki (Eds.), *The professional counselor's desk reference* (pp. 263–273). New York: Springer.

Smith, D., & Fitzpatrick, M. (1995). Patient-therapist boundary issues: An integrative review of theory and research. *Professional Psychology: Research and Practice, 26*(5), 499–506.

Sonne, J. L., & Pope, K. S. (1991). Treating victims of therapist-patient sexual involvement. *Psychotherapy, 28*, 174–187.

*Sperry, L., & Shafranske, E. P. (2005). (Eds.). *Spiritually oriented psychotherapy.* Washington, DC: American Psychological Association.

*Stebnicki, M. A. (2008). *Empathy fatigue: Healing the mind, body, and spirit of professional counselors.* New York: Springer.

Stebnicki, M. A. (2009a). A call for integral approaches in the professional identity of rehabilitation counseling: Three specialty areas, one profession. *Rehabilitation Counselor Bulletin, 99*(4), 64–68.

Stebnicki, M. A. (2009b). Empathy fatigue in the counseling profession. In I. Marini & M. A. Stebnicki (Eds.), *The professional counselor's desk reference* (pp. 801–812). New York: Springer.

Stebnicki, M. A. (2009c). Empathy fatigue: Assessing risk factors and cultivating self-care. In I. Marini & M. A. Stebnicki (Eds.), *The professional counselor's desk reference* (pp. 813–830). New York: Springer.

Strauch, B. (2003). *The primal teen: What the new discoveries about the teenage brain tell us about our kids.* New York: Doubleday.

Stone, C. (2002). Negligence in academic advising and abortion counseling: Courts rulings and implications. *Professional School Counseling, 6,* 28–35.

Sue, D. (1997). Counseling strategies for Chinese Americans. In C. C. Lee (Ed.), *Multicultural issues in counseling: New approaches to diversity* (2nd ed., pp. 173–187). Alexandria, VA: American Association for Counseling and Development.

Sue, D. W. (2005). Racism and the conspiracy of silence: Presidential address. *The Counseling Psychologist, 33*(1), 100–114.

Sue, D. W. (2006). Multicultural perspectives on multiple relationships. In B. Herlihy & G. Corey, *Boundary issues in counseling: Multiple roles and responsibilities* (2nd ed.). Alexandria, VA: American Counseling Association.

Sue, D. W., Arredondo, P., & McDavis, R. J. (1992). Multicultural counseling competencies and standards: A call to the profession. *Journal of Counseling and Development, 70*(4), 477–486.

Sue, D. W., Bernier, Y., Durran, A., Feinberg, L., Pedersen, P. B., Smith, E. J., & Vasquez- Nuttal, E. (1982). Position paper: Cross-cultural counseling competencies. *The Counseling Psychologist, 10*(2), 45–52.

Sue, D. W., Carter, R. T., et al. (1998). *Multicultural counseling competencies: Individual and organizational development.* Thousand Oaks, CA: Sage.

*Sue, D. W., Ivey, A., & Pedersen, P. (1996). *A theory of multicultural counseling and therapy.* Belmont, CA: Brooks/Cole, Cengage Learning.

*Sue, D. W., & Sue, D. (2008). *Counseling the culturally diverse: Theory and practice* (5th ed.). New York: Wiley.

Sumerel, M. B., & Borders, L. D. (1996). Addressing personal issues in supervision: Impact of counselors' experience level on various aspects of the supervisory relationship. *Counselor Education and Supervision, 35*(4), 268–286.

Sutter, E., McPherson, R. H., & Geeseman, R. (2002). Contracting for supervision. *Professional Psychology: Research and Practice, 33*(5), 495–498.

*Sweitzer, H. F., & King, M. A. (2009). *The successful internship: Personal, professional, and civic development* (3rd ed.). Belmont, CA: Brooks/Cole, Cengage Learning.

Szasz, T. (1986). The case against suicide prevention. *American Psychologist, 41*(7), 806–812.

Szymanski, E. M., & Parker, R. M. (2003). *Work and disability: Issues and strategies in career development and job placement* (2nd ed.). Austin, TX: PRO-ED.

Tan, S. Y. (1997). The role of the psychologist in paraprofessional helping. *Professional Psychology: Research and Practice, 28*(4), 368–372.

Tarvydas, V. M., & Johnston, S. P. (2009). Managing risk in ethical and legal situations. In I. Marini & M. A. Stebnicki (Eds.), *The professional counselor's desk reference* (pp. 99–111). New York: Springer.

*Teyber, E. (2006). *Interpersonal process in psychotherapy: An integrative model* (5th ed.). Belmont, CA: Brooks/Cole, Cengage Learning.

Thomas, J. L. (2002). Bartering. In A. A. Lazarus & O. Zur (Eds.), *Dual relationships and psychotherapy* (pp. 394–408). New York: Springer.

Thomas, J. T. (2007). Informed consent through contracting for supervision: Minimizing risks, enhancing benefits. *Professional Psychology: Research and Practice, 38*(3), 221–231.

Thomlison, B. (2002). *The family assessment workbook: A beginner's practice guide to family assessment and intervention.* Belmont, CA: Brooks/Cole, Cengage Learning.

Thorne, B. (2002). *The mystical power of person-centred therapy: Hope beyond despair.* Hoboken, NJ: Wiley.

Trull, T. J. (2005). *Clinical psychology* (7th ed.). Belmont, CA: Wadsworth, Cengage Learning.

Waters, R. (2004). Making a difference: Five therapists who've taken on the wider world. *Psychotherapy Networker, 28*(6), 356–359.

Watson, Z. E. P., Herlihy, B. R., & Pierce, L. A. (2006). Forging the link between multicultural competence and ethical counseling practice: A historical perspective. *Counseling and Values, 50*(2), 99–107.

Watts, R. E., Trusty, J., Canada, R., & Harvill, R. L. (1995). Perceived early childhood family influence and counselor effectiveness: An exploratory study. *Counselor Education and Supervision, 35,* 104–110.

Weihenmayer, E. (2001). *Touch the top of the world.* New York: Dutton.

*Welfel, E. R. (2010). *Ethics in counseling and psychotherapy: Standards, research, and emerging issues* (4th ed.). Belmont, CA: Brooks/Cole, Cengage Learning.

Welfel, E. R., & Patterson, L. E. (2005). *The counseling process: A multitheoretical integrative approach* (6th ed.). Belmont, CA: Brooks/Cole, Cengage Learning.

Werth, J. L., & Holdwick, D. J. (2000). A primer on rational suicide and other forms of hastened death. *The Counseling Psychologist, 28*(4), 511–539.

Werth, J. L., Jr., & Rogers, J. R. (2005). Assessing for impaired judgment as a means of meeting the "duty to protect" when a client is a potential harm-to-self: Implications for clients making end-of-life decisions. *Mortality, 10,* 7–21.

*Werth, J. L., Jr., Welfel, E. R., & Benjamin, G. A. H. (Eds.). (2009). *The duty to protect: Ethical, legal, and professional considerations for mental health professionals.* Washington, DC: American Psychological Association.

*Wheeler, N., & Bertram, B. (2008). *The counselor and the law: A guide to legal and ethical practice* (5th ed.). Alexandria, VA: American Counseling Association.

White, J. L., & Parham, T. A. (1990). *The psychology of blacks: An African-American perspective* (2nd ed.). Englewood Cliffs, NJ: Prentice-Hall.

Wiederman, M. W., & Sansone, R. A. (1999). Sexuality training for professional psychologists: A national survey of training directors of doctoral programs and predoctoral internships. *Professional Psychology: Research and Practice, 30*(3), 312–317.

Wilcoxon, S. A., Walker, M. R., & Hovestadt, A. J. (1989). Counselor effectiveness and family-of-origin experiences: A significant relationship? *Counseling and Values, 33*(3), 225–229.

*Woodside, M., & McClam, T. (2009). *An introduction to human services* (6th ed.). Belmont, CA: Brooks/Cole, Cengage Learning.

Woody, R. H. (1998). Bartering for psychological services. *Professional Psychology: Research and Practice, 29*(2), 174–178.

Wrenn, C. G. (1962). The culturally encapsulated counselor. *Harvard Educational Review, 32,* 444–449.

Wrenn, C. G. (1985). Afterword: The culturally encapsulated counselor revisited. In P. Pedersen (Ed.), *Handbook of cross-cultural counseling and therapy* (pp. 323–329). Westport, CT: Greenwood Press.

Wubbolding, R. E. (1988). *Using reality therapy.* New York: Harper & Row (Perennial Library).

*Wubbolding, R. E. (2000). *Reality therapy for the 21st century.* Philadelphia, PA: Brunner-Routledge (Taylor & Francis).

Wubbolding, R. E. (2006). Case study: A suicidal teenager. In B. Herlihy & G. Corey, *ACA ethical standards casebook* (6th ed., pp. 231–234). Alexandria, VA: American Counseling Association.

*Yalom, I. D. (1997). *Lying on the couch: A novel.* New York: Perennial.

*Yalom, I. D. (2003). *The gift of therapy.* New York: Perennial.

*Yalom, I. D. (with Leszcz, M.). (2005). *The theory and practice of group psychotherapy* (5th ed.). New York: Basic Books.

Yarhouse, M. A., & VanOrman, B. T. (1999). When psychologists work with religious clients: Applications of the general principles of ethical conduct. *Professional Psychology: Research and Practice, 30*(6), 557–562.

Younggren, J. N., & Gottlieb, M. C. (2008). Termination and abandonment: History, risk, and risk management. *Professional Psychology: Research and Practice, 39*(5), 498–504.

Zalaquett, C. P., Fuerth, K. M., Stein, C., Ivey, A. E., & Ivey, M. B. (2008). Reframing the DSM-IV-TR from a multicultural/social justice perspective. *Journal of Counseling and Development, 86*(3), 364–371.

Zinnbauer, B. J., & Pargament, K. I. (2000). Working with the sacred: Four approaches to religious and spiritual issues in counseling. *Journal of Counseling and Development, 78*(2), 162–171.

*Zur, O. (2007). *Boundaries in psychotherapy: Ethical and clinical explorations.* Washington, DC: American Psychological Association.

Name Index

Subject Index